D0712796

# HANDBOOK OF HEALTH PSYCHOLOGY AND AGING

# HANDBOOK OF HEALTH PSYCHOLOGY AND AGING

Edited by
CAROLYN M. ALDWIN
CRYSTAL L. PARK
AVRON SPIRO III

Foreword by
Ronald P. Abeles

THE GUILFORD PRESS
New York     London

© 2007 The Guilford Press
A Division of Guilford Publications, Inc.
72 Spring Street, New York, NY 10012
www.guilford.com

Printed in the United States of America

This book is printed on acid-free paper.

Last digit is print number:   9   8   7   6   5   4   3   2   1

Handbook of health psychology and aging / edited by Carolyn M.
    Aldwin, Crystal L. Park, and Avron Spiro III.
        p. ; cm.
    Includes bibliographical references and index.
    ISBN-13: 978-1-59385-057-9 (alk. paper)
    ISBN-10: 1-59385-057-3 (alk. paper)
    1. Older people—Health and hygiene—Psychological aspects—
Handbooks, manuals, etc.  2. Clinical health psychology—Handbooks,
manuals, etc.  I. Aldwin, Carolyn M.  II. Park, Crystal L.  III. Spiro,
Avron.
    [DNLM: 1. Behavioral Medicine. 2. Aged. 3. Aging—psychology.
4. Attitude to Health. 5. Health Behavior. 6. Health Promotion.
WB 103 H2364 2007]
RA564.8.H36 2007
616.001'9—dc22

                                                    2006030429

# About the Editors

**Carolyn M. Aldwin, PhD,** is Professor and Chair of the Department of Human Development and Family Sciences at Oregon State University. She received her doctorate from the University of California, San Francisco, in 1982 and was a National Institute of Mental Health postdoctoral scholar in Human Development, Environmental Demands, and Health at the University of California, Irvine. Dr. Aldwin received a FIRST award from the National Institute on Aging for her study of psychosocial factors affecting health in aging early in her career, and has published over 60 articles and chapters in this area. She is a fellow of both Divisions 20 (Adult Development and Aging) and 38 (Health Psychology) of the American Psychological Association, as well as the Gerontological Society of America. The second edition of her book *Stress, Coping, and Development: An Integrative Perspective* will be published by The Guilford Press in the Spring of 2007.

**Crystal L. Park, PhD,** is Associate Professor of Psychology at the University of Connecticut. She received her doctorate in clinical psychology from the University of Delaware in 1993 and completed a 2-year National Institute of Mental Health postdoctoral fellowship in health psychology at the University of California, San Francisco, in 1995. Dr. Park's research focuses on stress, coping, and adaptation, particularly on how people's beliefs, goals, and values affect their ways of perceiving and dealing with stressful events. She has developed a comprehensive model of meaning and meaning making, and has been applying this model to a variety of health-related problems, particularly cancer and heart failure. Dr. Park has published articles on the roles of religious beliefs and coping in response to stressful life events, the phenomenon of stress-related growth, and people's attempts to find meaning in or to create meaning out of negative life events. She is on the editorial boards of the *Journal of Clinical and Consulting Psychology* and *Psychology and Health,* and coeditor of *Handbook of the Psychology of Religion and Spirituality* (published by The Guilford Press in 2005) and *Positive Life Changes in the Context of Medical Illness* (to be published by the American Psychological Association in 2007).

**Avron Spiro III, PhD,** is a Senior Research Scientist at the Normative Aging Study, part of the Massachusetts Veterans Epidemiology Research and Information Center (MAVERIC), at the Department of Veterans Affairs Boston Healthcare System. He is also Associate Professor of Epidemiology at the Boston University School of Public Health as well as Associate Professor of Health Policy and Health Services Research at the Boston University Goldman School of Dental Medicine.

# Contributors

**Glenn Affleck, PhD,** is Professor of Community Medicine and Healthcare at the University of Connecticut Health Center.

**Carolyn M. Aldwin, PhD,** is Professor and Chair of the Department of Human Development and Family Sciences at Oregon State University.

**Charles C. Benight, PhD,** is Associate Professor of Psychology and Director of CU Trauma Studies and Resource Center at the University of Colorado at Colorado Springs.

**Cynthia A. Berg, PhD,** is Professor of Psychology at the University of Utah.

**Daria K. Boeninger, BA,** is a doctoral student in the Department of Human and Community Development at the University of California, Davis.

**Heather M. Burke, PhD,** is a postdoctoral scholar in the Health Psychology Program at the University of California, San Francisco.

**David A. Chiriboga, PhD,** is Professor in the Department of Aging and Mental Health at the Florida Mental Health Institute, University of South Florida.

**Denise C. Cooper, MA,** is a clinical psychology/behavioral medicine doctoral candidate in the Department of Psychology at the University of Maryland, Baltimore County.

**Mary C. Davis, PhD,** is Associate Professor of Psychology at Arizona State University.

**Elissa S. Epel, PhD,** is Assistant Professor in the Department of Psychiatry at the University of California, San Francisco, Health Psychology Program.

**Richard H. Fortinsky, PhD,** is Professor of Medicine and Physicians Health Services Chair in Geriatrics and Gerontology at the University of Connecticut Health Center.

**Rachel Forster, BA,** is a doctoral student and Excellence Fellow at the Institute for Health and Department of Psychology, Rutgers, The State University of New Jersey.

**Natalie Frank, PhD,** is Assistant Professor of Psychology at the University of Hartford.

**Howard S. Friedman, PhD,** is Distinguished Professor of Psychology at the University of California, Riverside.

**Sarit A. Golub, PhD, MPH,** is Assistant Professor in the Psychology Department at Queens College, City University of New York.

**Tara L. Gruenewald, PhD, MPH,** is Assistant Professor in the Department of Medicine, Division of Geriatrics, at the University of California, Los Angeles.

**Nancy J. M. Henry, MA,** is a doctoral candidate in the Department of Psychology at the University of Utah.

**Lisa M. Johnson, MA,** is a doctoral student in clinical psychology at Arizona State University.

**Robert M. Kaplan, PhD,** is Professor and Chair in the Department of Health Services at the University of California, Los Angeles, School of Public Health.

**Leslie I. Katzel, PhD,** is Associate Professor of Medicine in the Division of Gerontology, Department of Medicine, at the University of Maryland School of Medicine and Baltimore VA Medical Center.

**Margaret E. Kemeny, PhD,** is Professor in the Department of Psychiatry and Director of the Health Psychology Program at the University of California, San Francisco.

**Ellen J. Langer, PhD,** is Professor of Psychology at Harvard University.

**Elaine Leventhal, MD, PhD,** is Professor of Medicine and Director of the Geriatric Assessment Center, Robert Wood Johnson Medical School, at the University of Medicine and Dentistry of New Jersey.

**Howard Leventhal, PhD,** is Board of Governors Professor of Health Psychology at the Institute for Health, Health Care Policy and Aging Research, Rutgers, The State University of New Jersey.

**Leslie R. Martin, PhD,** is Chair of the Psychology Department at La Sierra University.

**Shahrzad Mavandadi, PhD,** is a Research Scientist in the Department of Psychiatry at the University of Pennsylvania.

**Kate E. Murray, BA,** is a doctoral student in clinical psychology at Arizona State University.

**Heather A. Okvat, MA,** is a doctoral student in clinical psychology at Arizona State University.

**Crystal L. Park, PhD,** is Associate Professor of Psychology at the University of Connecticut at Storrs.

**Gale E. Pearce, PhD,** is a postdoctoral fellow in the Department of Psychology at the University of Utah.

**Sara Honn Qualls, PhD,** is Kraemer Family Professor of Aging Studies; Director of Clinical Training, Psychology Department; and Director of the Gerontology Center at the University of Colorado at Colorado Springs.

**Karen S. Rook, PhD,** is Professor in the Department of Psychology and Social Behavior at the University of California, Irvine.

**Marilyn McKean Skaff, PhD,** is Assistant Professor in the Department of Family and Community Medicine at the University of California, San Francisco.

**Timothy W. Smith, PhD,** is Professor of Psychology at the University of Utah.

**Dara H. Sorkin, PhD,** is Assistant Adjunct Professor in the College of Medicine at the University of California, Irvine.

**Avron Spiro III, PhD,** is a Senior Research Scientist at the Normative Aging Study, Massachusetts Veterans Epidemiology Research and Information Center (MAVERIC), Department of Veterans Affairs Boston Healthcare System, Boston, Massachusetts

**Howard Tennen, PhD,** is Board of Trustees Distinguished Professor at the University of Connecticut Health Center.

**Peter Vitaliano, PhD,** is Professor of Psychiatry and Behavioral Sciences, Psychology, and Health Services in the Department of Psychiatry and Behavioral Sciences at the University of Washington.

**Shari R. Waldstein, PhD,** is Associate Professor of Psychology at the University of Maryland, Baltimore County, and Adjunct Associate Professor of Medicine in the Division of Gerontology, University of Maryland School of Medicine and Baltimore VA Medical Center.

**Owen M. Wolkowitz, MD,** is Professor in the Department of Psychiatry at the University of California, San Francisco.

**Loriena A. Yancura, PhD,** is Assistant Professor in the Department of Family and Consumer Sciences at the University of Hawaii at Manoa.

**Barbara W. K. Yee, PhD,** is Professor and Chair, Department of Family and Consumer Sciences, at the University of Hawaii at Manoa.

**Heather Young, PhD, GNP, FAAN,** is the Grace Phelps Distinguished Professor and Director of the John A. Hartford Center for Geriatric Nursing Excellence at the School of Nursing, Oregon Health Sciences University.

**Alex J. Zautra, PhD,** is Foundation Professor of Clinical Psychology at Arizona State University.

**Laura A. Zettel, PhD,** is Assistant Professor in the Department of Psychology at California State University, Fullerton.

# Foreword

Almost three decades ago Julius Richmond, then the U.S. Surgeon General, published the report *Healthy People: The Surgeon General's Report on Health Promotion and Disease Prevention* (U.S. Department of Health, Education and Welfare, 1979), which highlighted the significance of lifestyles in the etiology and prevention of morbidity and mortality. The report noted that among "the 10 leading causes of death in 1976 . . . perhaps as much as half of U.S. mortality . . . was due to unhealthy behavior or life style; 20 percent to environmental factors; 20 percent to human biological factors; and only 10 percent to inadequacies in health care" (p. 9).[1] Based on this information, the Surgeon General established health goals for the nation, organized by periods of the life course, including "healthy adults" and "healthy older adults."

In response to *Healthy People*, and to their credit, the National Institutes of Health (NIH) and the Alcohol, Drug Abuse, and Mental Health Administration (ADAMHA) commissioned the Institute of Medicine (IOM) to recommend a research agenda to be used in guiding NIH and ADAMHA extramural research funding. Again, "aging and health" received prime attention as the focus of one of the major workshops and chapters in the resulting report, *Health and Behavior: Frontiers of Research in the Biobehavioral Sciences* (Hamburg, Elliott, & Parron, 1982).

During this period, Matilda White Riley (1911–2004)[2] became the founding Associate Director of the Social and Behavioral Research Program (SBR) at the National Institute on Aging (NIA).[3] With her biopsychosocial and life-course perspectives as guiding principles (Riley, 1992), she moved quickly to establish initiatives to foster research on aging, health, and behavior at the NIA, and to bring aging to the forefront of thought among behavioral medicine researchers. Her initial efforts are reflected in the NIA program announcement "Health and Effective Functioning in Middle and Later Years of Life" (National Institutes of Health, 1983) and in the Academy of Behavioral Medicine Research publication on aging (Riley, Matarazzo, & Baum, 1987).

One of Riley's early accomplishments was the appointment of Marcia G. Ory as the chief of the newly constituted branch on "Psychosocial Geriatrics Research" within the NIA. Ory proceeded to develop this branch into one of the major supporters of health and behavior research at the NIH. The program encouraged and supported research addressing the origins, correlates, and malleability of health-related attitudes and behaviors of older people and their caregivers. It was particularly concerned with beliefs about the nature of the aging process and how older people perceive, interpret, or act upon symptoms of illness (Ory, Abeles, & Lipman, 1992). It sought to understand how particular behaviors and attitudes influence the health of people as they age; how health attitudes and behaviors interact with physiological and psychosocial aging processes to influence health and functioning; and how social conditions affect the development, maintenance, and potential modification of these attitudes and behaviors. Over time, the program supported research that provided evidence for three main conclusions:

1. Lifestyle risk factors continue even at older ages to be predictive of subsequent health and functioning.
2. Even at older ages, reductions in lifestyle risk factors are associated with subsequent improvements in health and functioning.
3. It is possible to design and implement interventions that successfully change the lifestyle behaviors of older people (i.e., you *can* "teach an old dog new tricks").

In summary, the relevance of psychosocial factors to the health of older people was among the initial foci of research and public health policy from a health-and-behavior perspective. Perhaps the swing in balance from acute to chronic conditions as primary population health concerns, which accompanied the aging of the population, facilitated the recognition of social and behavioral influences on health. This transition has also resulted in a shift away from the search for a single infectious germ and its corresponding "magic bullet" cure toward an emphasis on complex interactions among social, behavioral, and biological causes and interventions. Moreover, an emphasis on chronic conditions leads to questions about life-course processes and the potential for disease prevention and for health promotion in the later years of life.

As ably demonstrated by the chapters in this handbook, we have made considerable progress in the scientific study of health and behavior, and are now facing the challenges of translating our understanding into practical interventions. We need to continue to develop and employ rigorous methodologies for the testing of psychosocial interventions and to report these in a fashion that permits the evaluation of this accumulating evidence base through systematic reviews. (See the CONSORT statement [Begg et al., 1996] and the publication policy of the American Psychological Association [Dittman, 2004].) That is, health psychology of aging needs to be part of the evidence-based medicine movement to gain acceptance and to be integrated into standard medical practice. Of course, "standard medical practice" needs to be changed to facilitate the inclusion of effective behavioral treatments. Clearly, the "5-minute" encounter between a patient and a doctor is not conducive to effective lifestyle interventions! Perhaps the aging of the baby boomers will increase pressure on biomedical practice and policies to include behavioral medicine; that is, the baby boomer cohorts have come to maturity and majority during a historical shift in values and attitudes toward the patient being an active participant in his or her health and health care, and toward a greater recognition of behavioral and social factors in health over the life course. Maybe increased consumer demand will lead to a better product in health care. We can only hope.

RONALD P. ABELES, PHD
*Office of Behavioral and Social Sciences Research*
*National Institutes of Health*

## ACKNOWLEDGMENTS

The opinions expressed in this foreword are those of the author and do not necessarily reflect the position or policies of the NIH. The author prepared these comments as part of his official duties; consequently, the foreword is in the public domain.

## NOTES

1. More recent analyses by McGinnes and others have continued to document the oft-cited fact that "50% of U.S. mortality is attributable to behavioral and social factors" (McGinnes & Foege, 1993; Mokdad, Marks, Stroop, & Gerberding, 2004).
2. For a description of Matilda Riley's remarkable life and accomplishments, see Abeles (2005).
3. The NIA changed the program's name first to Behavioral Sciences Research and ultimately to Behavioral and Social Research in response to the anti-social-science atmosphere at the White House during the early 1980s.

# REFERENCES

Abeles, R. P. (2005). Soaring: Celebrating Matilda White Riley. *American Sociological Association Footnotes, 33*(1), 1–2.

Begg, C. B., Cho, M. K., Eastwood, S., Horton, R., Moher, D., Olkin, I., et al. (1996). Improving the quality of reporting of randomized controlled trials: The CONSORT statement. *Journal of the American Medical Association, 276,* 637–639.

Dittman, M. (2004). Guidelines seek to prevent bias in reporting of randomized trials. *American Psychological Association Monitor, 35*(8), 20.

Hamburg, D. A., Elliott, G. R., & Parron, D. L. (Eds.). (1982). *Health and behavior: Frontiers of research in the biobehavioral sciences.* Washington, DC: National Academy Press.

McGinnes, J. M., & Foege, W. H. (1993). Actual causes of death in the United States. *Journal of the American Medical Association, 270*(18), 2207–2212.

Mokdad, A. H., Marks, J. S., Stroup, D. F., & Gerberding, J. L. (2004). Actual causes of death in the United States, 2000. *Journal of the American Medical Association, 291*(10), 1238–1245.

Ory, M. G., Abeles, R. P., & Lipman, P. D. (1992). Introduction: An overview of research on aging, health, and behavior. In M. G. Ory, R. P. Abeles, & P. D. Lipman (Eds.), *Aging, health, and behavior* (pp. 1–26). Newbury Park, CA: Sage.

National Institutes of Health. (1983). Health and effective functioning in the middle and later years. *NIH Guide to Grants and Contracts, 12*(6).

Riley, M. W. (1992). Foreword. In M. G. Ory, R. P. Abeles, & P. D. Lipman (Eds.), *Aging, health, and behavior* (pp. vii–xiii). Newbury Park, CA: Sage.

Riley, M. W., Matarazzo, J. D., & Baum, A. (Eds.). (1987). *Perspectives in behavioral medicine: The aging dimension.* Hillsdale, NJ: Erlbaum.

U.S. Department of Health, Education and Welfare. (1979). *Healthy people: The Surgeon General's report on health promotion and disease prevention* (Publication No. 79-55071). Washington, DC: U.S. Government Printing Office.

# Contents

## PART IV. CLINICAL ISSUES

# PART I

# THEORETICAL AND METHODOLOGICAL ISSUES

# CHAPTER I

# Health Psychology and Aging

## An Introduction

CAROLYN M. ALDWIN, CRYSTAL L. PARK,
*and* AVRON SPIRO III

The past century has witnessed a dramatic increase in both life expectancy and the number of older adults. This demographic trend will be greatly accelerated in the next 10 years, as the first wave of baby boomers reaches retirement age. This trend is seen even more strongly among the oldest-old. For example, the 85+ population increased by 38% in the 1990s, from 3.1 million in 1990 to 4.2 million in 2000 (Hetzel & Smith, 2001). This number is expected to *quadruple* in the first half of this century, nearing a projected 18.9 million by the year 2050 (Hobbs & Damon, 1996). This "graying of America" is by no means unique to America—or even to the developed world. According to the World Health Organization, the number of older adults will increase dramatically in the next 20–40 years—nearly doubling in the developed world, but quadrupling in the developing world (Kalache, 2001). This demographic transition has immense implications for both the economy and the social structure, as governments, businesses, and individuals try to determine how best to pay for health care and pension costs.

With aging of the population has come a dramatic shift in causes of death, from acute illnesses at the beginning of the 20th century to chronic illnesses at the end of it. Indeed, most of the illnesses in later life are chronic rather than acute and reflect cumulative lifestyle choices such as smoking, drinking, being sedentary, and overeating. These diseases, such as hypertension, diabetes, and cancer, often require long treatment regimens and major changes in health behaviors. Both the psychosocial etiology of disease and

3

treatment compliance are the province of health psychology. However, many health psychologists do not have sufficient background in issues of aging, and age is often treated as a covariate rather than a *Ding an Sich*. Although gerontologists do study issues that are specific to aging, their ways of conceptualizing and assessing health outcomes are often less sophisticated than those used in behavioral medicine and health psychology. Thus, communication across the two disciplines is critical, and a major purpose of the book is to foster this interdisciplinary communication.

The specific focus of this book is on aging and vulnerability to *psychosocial* risk factors. It has long been known that older adults are more likely than younger adults to be affected by *physical* risk factors. For example, in times of major population upheavals such as wars or famines, both infants and aged adults are most likely to die. Furthermore, older people are particularly vulnerable to factors such as heat stress, as witnessed by the death of several hundred older adults during a heat wave in Chicago a few years ago or the more recent, tragic events with Hurricane Katrina.

However, it is unclear whether older adults are more or less vulnerable to *psychosocial risk factors,* with some arguing that elders are more vulnerable and others that they are less (for reviews, see Aldwin & Gilmer, 2004; Kaplan, Haan, & Wallace, 1999). In a book edited by Manuck, Jennings, Rabin, and Baum (2000), three chapters demonstrated this complexity. The first argued that older people are more vulnerable to psychosocial effects, especially vis-à-vis immune functioning (Solomon & Benton, 2000). The second showed that psychosocial factors had *weaker* effects in late life due to survivor effects (Williams, 2000). That is, people who are biologically vulnerable to particular types of risk factors are more likely to die in midlife; thus, the people surviving to late life may be less affected by psychosocial risk factors. For example, hostility, a risk factor for heart disease in midlife, may be associated with greater longevity in late life. The third chapter examined cardiovascular risk factors and cognitive functioning, and found no age-related differences in vulnerability (Elias, Elias, D'Agostino, & Wolf, 2000). In this otherwise excellent book, there was little attempt to integrate across the chapters and important issues were left unresolved.

We organized a conference on Health Psychology and Aging as part of the University of California Series on Health Psychology. Generous funding was provided for this conference by the Retirement Research Foundation, Divisions 20 and 38 of the American Psychological Association, and the College of Agriculture and Environmental Sciences at the University of California, Davis. The purpose of this conference was to examine the interface between health psychology and aging, with a specific focus on age differences in vulnerability to risk factors, although other aspects of aging and health psychology were also addressed. In particular, we were interested in understanding and promoting successful aging on the biological, psychological, and social levels.

This book grew out of this conference. Although many of the presenters have provided chapters, not all did, and, with encouragement from Jim Nageotte at The Guilford Press, we sought to expand the scope of this book. Thus, we asked a number of individuals to contribute chapters to increase comprehensiveness, so this could truly be a handbook.

This handbook is divided into four sections. The first serves as a general introduction to theory and method in the fields of health psychology and adult development and aging. Golub and Langer (Chapter 2) make a cogent argument that the assumptions of our theories of adult development and aging have practical implications for the well-being of older adults. By focusing so much on loss and its management, and neglecting the positive changes that occur in later life, we promote ageist stereotypes not only among providers but also among older adults themselves, resulting in self-handicapping. From a health psychology perspective, Berg, Smith, Henry, and Pearce (Chapter 3) seek to create a developmental framework for understanding risk and resilience by examining the interplay between physical health, cognitive, and social function.

The section next turns to methods. Young and Vitaliano (Chapter 4) review methods in health psychology, focusing on the assessment of physiological indicators of dysregulation in the neuroendocrine, cardiovascular, and immune systems, and how they mediate between psychosocial factors and disease outcomes. They extend this to examine these function systems in primary and secondary aging, using illustrations from the caregiving literature. In contrast, Spiro (Chapter 5) outlines the importance of taking a lifespan developmental approach to health, and reviews the different statistical analyses at the heart of lifespan developmental methods.

The second section reviews basic issues in psychoneuroimmunology. Gruenewald and Kemeny (Chapter 6) provide a very thorough description of how aging affects the immune system, as well as a comprehensive overview of the ways in which behavioral, social, and psychological factors can affect this functioning. Like many of the other chapters in this book, they also point out the many gaps in our knowledge of the intersection between aging, psychosocial processes, and immune functioning. Epel, Burke, and Wolkowitz (Chapter 7) address aging and neuroendocrinology. By delineating an innovative model that examines aging as a process involving the development of catabolic–anabolic imbalances, they sought to show how psychosocial factors affect the rate of development of these imbalances. Finally, cardiovascular disease remains the leading cause of death in America. Although the last three decades have seen a great deal of research demonstrating the importance of psychosocial factors in the development and course of this disease, Cooper, Katzel, and Waldstein (Chapter 8) identify cardiovascular reactivity as a linchpin linking psychosocial factors and the development of disease. Whereas some preliminary work on changes in cardiovascular reactivity with age exists, Cooper et al. point out the need for longitudinal studies to examine the interplay between psychosocial factors, cardiovascular reactivity, and the development of cardiovascular disease across the lifespan.

The third section addresses psychosocial vulnerability and protective factors. Friedman and Martin (Chapter 9) review the extensive literature on how personality affects health in later life, focusing on conscientiousness as a key construct. A sense of control has long held center stage in health psychology as a key construct, and Skaff (Chapter 10) provides a highly interesting lifespan development perspective that shows how both the sociocultural and development contexts influence control beliefs and thus health in later life.

Aldwin, Yancura, and Boeninger (Chapter 11) examine coping strategies as the process through which older adults can maintain both emotional and physical regulation in later life. Fortinsky, Tennen, Frank, and Affleck (Chapter 12) examine disease processes from the perspective of the caregiver, and the psychological, social, and health consequences of caregiving. Given the somewhat contradictory literature, they argue that contextual variables, including gender and the caregivers' own health moderate the effect of caregiving or health outcomes. They also review coping and benefit finding in the context of caregiving, ending with a discussion of intervention programs to protect the health of the caregivers.

Davis, Zautra, Johnson, Murray, and Okvat (Chapter 13) address the issue of individual differences in the aging process, and how some individuals are able to maintain a positive aging process in the face of increasing disabilities and loss. They argue that the propensity of older adults to focus on positive emotions is a way of sustaining health in later life. Rook, Mavandadi, Sorkin, and Zettel (Chapter 14) review not only the benefits of social support and health in the context of disability but also the importance of negative social interactions. They also discuss some quite interesting ways of optimizing social support to help maintain health in later life.

Yee and Chiriboga (Chapter 15) identify and define key constructs in race, ethnicity, and culture, and explain why they are important in understanding health disparities in aging. They also examine the role that gender plays in these disparities, centering the issue around differences in power relationships, social status, and social identity. Park (Chapter 16) reminds us that religiousness and spirituality can have both positive and negative effects in later life for a variety of health and well-being outcomes. Specifically, she examines whether religiousness and spirituality become more important in later life, and identifies a number of theoretical and empirical gaps that future research needs to address.

The fourth section specifically addresses clinical and health care issues. Leventhal, Forster, and Leventhal (Chapter 17) address self-regulation in the context of illess. They present a highly complex model showing the interplay between symptoms, heuristics used to interpret symptoms, illness representations, coping strategies, emotional reactions, and symptom monitoring processes. Thus, illness in late life is firmly embedded in a complex socioemotional context, the understanding of which is crucial in adequate treatment planning and adherence regiments. Qualls and Benight begin their chapter (Chapter 18) on clinical geropsychology and health psychology with an overview of interventions in medical settings for common diseases in late life. They discuss the impact of changes in recent Medicare legislation, as well as the importance of engaging the family in various aspects of health care. A truism in health psychology and geriatrics is that early diagnosis and prevention should play a critical role in the prevention of illness and promotion of longevity in late life. Kaplan (Chapter 19) presents some rather disturbing data that challenge this widespread assumption. He raises serious ethical and financial implications of changing thresholds of diagnosis, resulting in the "medicalization" of not only late life but also midlife. He presents data showing that early interventions may reduce disease-specific mortality rates but have little effect on all-cause mortality. Thus, he urges greater caution in considering aggressive interventions in late life.

We end with a final chapter integrating the different points of view expressed in this book. As we shall see, nearly all of the authors point to the lack of studies specifically examining aging issues within the context of health psychology. Thus, the final chapter provides a blueprint for future research, highlighting the gaps in our knowledge and helping to set the research agenda for the next few years.

We would like to thank our spouses, Rick Levenson, Craig Esposito, and Margie Lachman, for their support in the editing of this book. Their patience in our series of meetings (often during supposed "vacations") and many conference calls is greatly appreciated! We also thank the conference participants and the authors of this book, especially those who contributed to both, for their adherence to our repeated requests for revisions . . . and for their patience as well.

## REFERENCES

Aldwin, C. M., & Gilmer, D. F. (2004). *Health, illness, and optimal aging: Biological and psychosocial perspectives*. Thousand Oaks, CA: Sage.

Elias, M. F., Elias, P. K., D'Agostino, R. B., & Wolf, P. A. (2000). Comparative effects of age and blood pressure on neuropsychological test performance: The Framingham Study. In S. B. Manuck, R. Jennings, B. S. Rabin, & A. Baum (Eds.), *Behavior, health, and aging* (pp. 199–244). Mahwah, NJ: Erlbaum.

Hetzel, L., & Smith, A. (2001). *The 65 years and older population: 2000* (Department of Commerce Publication No. C2KBR/-1-10). Washington, DC: U.S. Government Printing Office.

Hobbs, B., & Damon, B. L. (1996). *65+ in the United States* (Current Population Reports: Special Studies Publication No. P23-190). Washington, DC: U.S. Government Printing Office.

Kalache, A. (2001). Rural aging: Reduction of existing inequities—Keynote address, June 10, 2000. *Journal of Rural Health, 17,* 312–313.

Kaplan, G., Haan, M. N., & Wallace, R. B. (1999). Understanding changing risk factor associations with increasing age in adults. *Annual Review of Public Health, 20,* 89–108.

Manuck, S. B., Jennings, R., Rabin, B. S., & Baum, A. (Eds.). (2000). *Behavior, health, and aging.* Mahwah, NJ: Erlbaum.

Solomon, G. F., & Benton, D. (2000). Immune functions, their psychological correlates, and health. In S. B. Manuck, R. Jennings, B. S. Rabin, & A. Baum (Eds.), *Behavior, health, and aging* (pp. 109–117). Mahwah, NJ: Erlbaum.

Williams, R. B. (2000). Psychological factors, health, and disease: The impact of aging and the life cycle. In S. B. Manuck, R. Jennings, B. S. Rabin, & A. Baum (Eds.), *Behavior, health, and aging* (pp. 135–151). Mahwah, NJ: Erlbaum.

# CHAPTER 2

# Challenging Assumptions about Adult Development

## Implications for the Health of Older Adults

SARIT A. GOLUB *and* ELLEN J. LANGER

Kurt Lewin was right—there is nothing so practical as a good theory. Theories provide the frame within which we pose questions, design research, and interpret findings. Theories also provide a means by which to communicate scientific data to the general public. The best theories have resonance and utility to a lay audience, with clear applications to everyday lives. At the same time, theories may serve as a vehicle for supporting past conclusions and instantiating biases. As they become widely accepted and applied, theories have the potential to shape our approach to the issues they address and limit the development of alternative hypotheses. For this reason, it is important to continuously assess and reevaluate existing theories, examining the ways in which they affect our understanding of the world and the assumptions inherent in them.

This chapter focuses on two assumptions that are reflected in many theories of adult development and examines their implications for psychosocial factors that influence the health of older adults. The first assumption is the unconditional equation of aging with physical and cognitive decline. The second assumption is the identification of coping with loss as the central task of aging. We argue that although both assumptions may have empirical bases and utility for understanding some issues facing the elderly, their broad application—especially as they are embedded within theories of adult development—has the potential to increase psychosocial risk factors for ill health. We discuss three mechanisms through which these psychosocial risk factors may operate: (1) the creation and perpetuation of negative stereotypes about aging and older adults; (2) the internalization of these negative stereotypes by older adults themselves; and (3) the creation of suboptimal environments within which older adults are provided care. Although we and others have written extensively about the negative consequences of ageism (Golub, Filipowitz, & Langer, 2002; Langer, 1981; Langer & Avorn, 1985; Levy, 2003), this chapter focuses specifically on (1) the link between assumptions about adult development and the roots of aging stereotypes; (2) a detailed explanation of the potential health risks associated with these stereotypes; and (3) a reconsideration of these two assumptions, rooted in mindfulness theory (Langer, 1989), that stresses practical implications of care and treatment for older persons.

## TWO ASSUMPTIONS IN THEORIES OF ADULT DEVELOPMENT

Central to almost all theories of development as they relate to later life is the idea that old age is a period characterized by physical and cognitive decline (see Langer, Rodin, Beck, Weinman, & Spitzer, 1979). To the extent that theories of development focus on a biological metaphor—the so-called "ontogenic" models–change over the lifespan is conceptualized as a series of sequential steps that shift from development to decline toward an "end state" (Alexander & Langer, 1990; Levenson, Aldwin, & Cupertino, 2001). Aging is often equated with illness and disability (Becker, 1994; Ory, Hoffman, Hawkins, Sanner, & Mockenhaupt, 2003), and many theories appear to regard aging as a "catastrophe" and discuss older adults as if they are "damaged goods" or "incapable of growth" (Guttmann, 1994, p. 9).

Not surprisingly, given this emphasis, psychosocial theories that discuss the developmental tasks salient to older adults focus primarily on coping with loss and decline (Gatz, 1998; Dixon & Bäckman, 1995; Staudinger, Marsiske, & Baltes, 1995). For Erikson (1959), the last stage of ego development negotiates the conflict between integrity and despair, primarily through coming to terms with loss and individual mortality. Sociogenic models, which stress change in social roles over the lifespan, emphasize the roles that must be *relinquished* by older adults as they age (Levenson et al., 2001). According to lifespan theory (Baltes, Staudinger, & Lindenberger, 1999), as we age, our goals shift from growth (behaviors aimed at attaining higher levels of function and capacity) toward regulation of loss (behaviors that accommodate functioning at lower levels). Self-development models, which consider developmental tasks in term of personal goals and self-determination, also define the central tasks of aging in terms of loss. In BŸhler's model (1968), late life is characterized by the "self-maintaining self," whose goal is compensating for developmental decrements.

Even when theories acknowledge that coping with loss does not preclude the possibility of growth, this "growth" is defined in terms of compensation for emerging deficits (Baltes et al., 1999). Coping in later life is characterized by processes of assimilation and accommodation (Rothermund & Brandtstädter, 2003), in which older adults compensate for actual or anticipated losses, while also lowering personal performance standards and aspirations.

These two assumptions—that age is associated only with biological decline, and that the major developmental task of aging is coping with loss—are empirically based, and many of the theories that rely on them have made significant contributions to our understanding of the aging process. Why then are we arguing that these assumptions may be associated with health risks for older persons?

Although we do not entirely disagree with the theoretical models we just mentioned, we suggest that these assumptions may increase vulnerability to health problems among older adults to the extent to which they are unquestioningly applied to all older persons irrespective of context. Whereas many older adults, of course, do struggle with physical limitations and chronic illness, other older individuals live into advancing age with few health problems (Ory et al., 2003), and despite the aging of the population, disability rates have continued to decline (Manton, Corder, & Stallard, 1994; Manton & XiLiang, 2001). Although some studies show that aging results in reduction in consciously controlled processing in attention and memory tasks (Jennings & Jacoby, 1993), others suggests that age differences may be due to different learning styles among different age groups (Kramer & Larish, 1996), conservative response bias among older adults (Batsakes & Fisk, 2000), or unfamiliarity with the testing environment or instructions (Fisk & Rogers, 1991).

In making assumptions about decline and loss, researchers, practitioners, and laypeople often overlook several important factors. First, once such assumptions are accepted, the evidence that instantiates them receives less attention. Research suggests that individuals have a tendency to look for (Trope & Thompson, 1997), remember (Hirt, McDonald, & Erikson, 1995), or even create (Tesser, 1978) information that confirms an existing belief. Confirmation biases may also cause individuals to interpret ambiguous information in a way that is consistent with their expectations (Darley & Gross, 1983; Kelley, 1950). A focus on physical and cognitive decline in theories of adult development and aging may lead to interpretive biases about the behavior of older adults, even when this behavior is due to other causes. For example, memory failure among older adults is likely to be attributed to their age, regardless of the availability of competing explanations (Langer et al., 1979). In one study (Bieman-Copland & Ryan, 1998), subjects were presented with scenarios that described memory successes and failures in both young and older adults. The scenarios included situational factors that could account for the given memory outcome, and that were chosen to minimize the potential for age-related differences. However, regardless of situational cues, memory success was seen as less typical for old compared to young targets, and memory failure among older adults was seen as more strongly associated with loss of ability and control than among younger adults.

Second, the behavior of older adults and their performance on tests of cognitive ability are often evaluated outside their developmental context. Theories of adult development acknowledge that individuals are motivated by different goals across their lifespan, but often fail to take into account how these differences in motivation may manifest in terms of behavior, interest, or attention. Although researchers acknowledge limitations in cross-cultural generalizability of stimuli and measures, little, if any, attention has been given to creating developmentally appropriate stimuli or measures. As a result, differences between younger and older adults may be interpreted as deficits when they were not experienced as such by the older adults themselves.

Third, regardless of the veracity or utility of these assumptions, their broad application has contributed to the development of many negative stereotypes about older adults. Aging stereotypes center on loss of health and decline of both physical and cognitive function (Levy, Hausdorff, Hencke, & Wei, 2000; Levy, Slade, Kunkel, & Kasl, 2002). By extension, the older adults are also believed to be physically unattractive (Kite & Johnson, 1988), mentally incompetent, slow, forgetful, weak, timid, and set in their ways (Langer, 1982; Levy & Langer, 1994).

Stereotypes about older adults may be even more insidious than stereotypes about other groups, because they are likely to be encoded as "premature cognitive commitments" (Chanowitz & Langer, 1981), a term used to describe information that is accepted and encoded without question, because the individual is not motivated to evaluate it critically. Unlike stereotypes about race or gender, we learn negative information about older adults before this information is self-relevant, that is, before we become a member of the stereotyped group. Research suggests that children develop negative stereotypes about aging by about 6 years of age, around the same time that they develop negative stereotypes about race and gender (Isaacs & Bearison, 1986). Because stereotypes about aging are learned when they do not apply to us, we are more likely to internalize them without questioning their veracity; thus, we form premature cognitive commitments that are extremely resistant to change, even in the face of disconfirming evidence (Giles, Fox, & Smith, 1993; Levy & Langer, 1994). As a result, older adults' negative feelings about being old are as strong, if not stronger, than those held by younger people (Shlesinger & Kronebusch, 1994; Nosek, Banaji, & Greenwald, 2002). Research on stereotype threat (Steele, 1997), self-fulfilling prophecies, learned helplessness (Seligman & Maier, 1976), and self-induced dependence (Langer & Benevento, 1978) suggests that the presence of these stereotypes can engender psychosocial processes that lead to their confirmation. Throughout our discussion, we refocus attention on these three factors—confirmation biases, lack of attention to developmental perspective, and interactive self-fulfilling prophecies—to suggest ways the experience of aging need not be characterized by inevitable loss and decline.

## PSYCHOSOCIAL HEALTH RISKS ASSOCIATED WITH NEGATIVE STEREOTYPES

Whereas the prevalence of these two assumptions in theories of adult development and aging does not in itself increase health risks for older adults, the negative stereotypes they engender and reinforce may be associated with a series of direct and indirect health risks. We outline mechanisms through which negative stereotypes can increase psychological vulnerability to ill health in three dimensions: (1) primary health risks associated with direct effects of discrimination, (2) secondary health risks associated with the internalization of negative stereotypes by older adults, and (3) tertiary health risks posed by the environments within which older adults receive treatment and care.

### Primary Health Risks: Discrimination

In a recent survey of adults over 50 in the United States and Canada, 85% reported experiencing at least one incident of ageism, and over 50% reported experiencing multiple incidents (Palmore, 2004). Incidents of ageism ranged from being told a joke that made fun of older people to being ignored, being called an insulting name, or being denied access to services, employment, or promotion. The experience of discrimination has been demonstrated to pose specific health risks to targeted populations. For African Americans, perceived racism can act as a physical stressor, inducing psychophsiological reactions that increase risk of cardiovascular disease. (Wyatt et al., 2003). There have been similar findings in response to the discrimination associated with ageism. In one study (Levy, Hausdorff, et al., 2000), older adults were subliminally primed with either positive or negative aging stereotypes. Participants exposed to negative stereotypes experienced a heightened cardiovascular response, including elevated systolic and diastolic blood pressure and increased heart rate. At the most basic level, the negative stereotypes related to assumptions of decline and loss may place stressors on the elderly that increase health risks.

The negative effects of stereotypes about aging may be even more strongly associated with psychosocial health risks among older adults, because they are so likely to accept these stereotypes as true. In several large-scale longitudinal studies, an individual's attitudes toward aging were significant predictors of mortality, having a greater impact than gender, socio-economic status, life satisfaction, or physical health (Levy Slade, et al., 2002; Maier & Smith, 1999). In one large-scale study, individuals with negative self-perceptions of aging (e.g., believing themselves to be worse off or less useful than when they were younger) died an average of 7.5 years earlier than did individuals with more positive self-perceptions, and evidence suggests that this relationship may in part be due to more adaptive cardiovascular responses to stress among individuals with more positive attitudes toward aging (Levy et al., 2000). The relationship between positive self-perceptions of aging and longevity may be partially mediated by the will to live, suggesting that the acceptance of negative stereotypes of aging may be associated with placing less value on life (Levy et al., 2002). This hypothesis is supported by a study that primed old and young subjects with negative or positive stereotypes of old age. Subjects were then asked to make a medical decision involving the acceptance or rejection of life-prolonging treatment. Positively primed older subjects were more likely to accept the treatment, whereas negatively primed older subjects were more likely to reject it (Levy, Ashman, & Dror, 1999–2000). At their most extreme, aging stereotypes may be internalized to the extent that they increase health risks by interfering with the value that older adults place on their own lives.

## Secondary Health Risks: Internalization

We have discussed the extent to which acceptance of themes of decline and loss may lead to an emphasis on confirmatory evidence and a dismissal of contradictory findings. Perhaps even more insidious, research suggests that the internalization of this information by older adults may lead to the *creation* of evidence that supports it, by activating unconscious processes of stereotype confirmation (Wheeler & Petty, 2001). According to the concept of stereotype threat (Steele, 1997), individuals experience increased anxiety about conforming to the stereotype, and this anxiety has a detrimental effect on performance in a given area. To the extent that older people believe that their own physical or cognitive decline is inevitable, they may begin to exhibit signs of this decline prematurely. Automaticity theory (see Bargh, Chen, & Burrows, 1996) explains similar behavior changes in terms of behavioral priming. When older adults think about aging, they may reflect internalized stereotypes in their physical movement or patterns of cognition. Regardless of the mechanism, research suggests that older adults modify their behavior in response to being primed with negative stereotypes. Older adults exposed to negative stereotypes demonstrate subsequent decrements in performance on tests of memory, mathematics, and handwriting (Levy, 1996; Stein, Blanchard-Fields, & Hertzog, 2002). Negative primes have similar detrimental effects on self-efficacy and general views of old people (Levy et al., 1999–2000). As a result, negative stereotypes pose a health risk to older adults by increasing vulnerability to the very decrements in physical or cognitive functioning that they assume.

The unconscious enactment of negative stereotypes is linked to three other processes that can lead to negative health outcomes among older adults. The first process is a self-fulfilling prophecy of decline. To the extent that older adults expect aging to be associated with physical or cognitive detriments, these expectations may be confirmed through conscious pressures on behavior. In a study by Chanowitz and Langer (1981), individuals were presented information about a (fictional) perceptual disorder and were later led to believe that they had it. Subjects who had been led to form stereotypical beliefs about the behavior of individuals with the disorder conformed to the stereotype and showed greater decrements in performance compared to subjects who had not formed such stereotypical beliefs. This study suggests that older adults who have internalized a theory of aging that stresses physical and cognitive decline may be more likely to experience these deficits, even if there is no biological reason for them to do so.

Another aspect of such a self-fulfilling prophecy relates to the interpretation of ambiguous information. Because they expect to experience deficits, older adults may be more likely to interpret their own behavior and experience as evidence for their physical decline. Consider a situation in which an older man spends the day working with his granddaughter in the garden and wakes up the next morning with a sore back. Because he knows that older people are likely to have aches and pains, he attributes his sore back to his advanced age. This association, "My back hurts; it must be because I'm old," can act as a self-generated prime, causing the grandfather to walk more slowly than the sore back would dictate, which in turn confirms additional, age-related stereotypes. Because of the grandfather's association between age and physical decline, it never occurs to him to discover that his granddaughter awoke with an equally sore back, which she attributed to four hours of weeding. Older adults are vulnerable to health risks to the extent that they overassimilate acute symptoms to the more chronic and global category "old." This assimilation may impact physical health by causing older adults to ignore symptoms that are actually attributable to other health problems, and may impact psychological well-being by increasing individuals' sense that they are already experiencing the limitations of age.

An individual's negative expectations about aging can also interact with the expectations of others, creating an *interactionally* fulfilling prophecy. Imagine that both George (age 83) and Martha (age 45) believe that aging is associated with cognitive decline. When Martha tries to explain a concept to George, she attempts to simplify her explanation, but this oversimplification leaves out certain details. George notices the simplified way in which Martha is speaking, and her omission of certain details leaves him confused. Research suggests that George will not only worry that his confusion is a result of his age (rather than attribute it to a deficiency in Martha's explanation) but also his behavior will change to confirm the expectations of both conversation partners. For example, students whose teachers who were told that they were on the verge of an intellectual growth spurt were not only more likely than their peers to be evaluated more favorably by their teachers, but they also exhibited actual increases in IQ compared with students assigned to a control group (Rosenthal & Jacobson, 1968). Many investigations of self-fulfilling prophecies have demonstrated similar effects on the attitudes and behavior of both partners in a given interaction (Ickes, Patterson, Rajecki, & Tanford, 1982; Snyder, Tanke, & Berscheid, 1977). Similarly, age stereotypes have been found to bias the interpretation of everyday memory failures. Compared to their younger counterparts, memory successes among older adults are considered less typical, and their memory failures are considered more worrisome and more likely due to lack of ability (Bieman-Copland & Ryan, 1998). Interactionally fulfilling prophecies present health risks to older adults to the extent that they contribute to decreased feelings of control, self-esteem, or self-efficacy. They may directly contribute to social isolation experienced by older persons, which is also associated with negative health effects.

Another cycle that increases health risks by promoting stereotype confirmation, "self-induced dependence" (Langer & Benevento, 1978), is a process through which an individual erroneously infers his or her own incompetence as a result of situational cues. Research has shown that self-induced dependence can result from seemingly innocuous factors, such as being (randomly) assigned a label that connotes inferiority or accepting unnecessary assistance (Langer & Imber, 1979). Self-induced dependence may lead to decrements in performance, which in turn confirms feelings of dependence. For example, individuals who are given a label that connotes inferiority demonstrate a decline in their own performance on a given task, despite evidence of superior past performance (Langer & Benevento, 1978). In a more recent study of hospitalized older adults (Faulkner, 2001), patients exposed to uncontrollable and disempowering care developed a learned helplessness style that generalized to other domains of their hospital stay, including performance on psychomotor tasks. If older adults are led to believe that they are no longer able to perform cognitive tasks requiring focused attention, they may accept unnecessary assistance, which confirms their belief in their own incompetence. The next time they are faced with a similar task, they may not even attempt it, providing further confirmation of their lost ability (Avorn & Langer, 1982).

A cycle of self-induced dependence may increase psychosocial vulnerability to health risks among the elderly by exacerbating a loss of control. Research demonstrates that often it is not the exercise of control that is important, but the belief (be it veridical or not) regarding one's ability to exercise control in a given situation. If environmental constraints or physical limitations deny individuals the opportunity to exercise control, the may experience a type of "learned helplessness," in which they continue to abdicate control once environmental constraints are no longer present (Seligman, 1975; Seligman & Maier, 1976). This loss translates directly into the exercise of control in health care settings; individuals over age 60 often report that they desire less control over health-related decisions, preferring less information and asking health care professionals to make decisions for them (Woodward & Wallston, 1987). However, research has demonstrated that the relationship between age and decreased desire for control is mediated by perceived self-efficacy, such that individuals who perceive themselves to be less able to make decisions report less desire for control (Christensen, Wiebe, Benotsch, & Lawton, 1996; Woodward & Wallston, 1987). Low levels of self-efficacy have been found to be associated with psychological maladjustment and distress in older adults, especially those living with chronic illness (Wu, Tang, & Kwok, 2002, 2004) Self-induced dependence places older persons at risk for abdicating control over medical decisions, which in turn gives them less control over their physical health.

To the extent that systemic or environmental factors limit older adults' control over their everyday lives, even the perception of control over small decisions becomes increasingly important (Aldwin, 1991; Perlmuter & Eads, 1998). In a study by Perlmuter and Eads, older adult males who sought assistance from a memory clinic were presented with a memory test in which they were given either a degree of control over the task (operationalized as increased choice) or no control. Subjects in the enhanced-control condition showed improved performance on the test compared to subjects who were not given control. In a second study, these improvements extended to subsequent memory tasks, suggesting that small increases in control go a long way for older adults, perhaps even motivating performance in the same way that loss of control impedes it. These findings are consistent with some of our own research on the impact of small increases in control for institutionalized adults (Langer & Rodin, 1979); the implication of these findings are discussed in greater detail below.

## Tertiary Health Risks: Environmental Influences

The third mechanism through which the negative stereotypes of aging related to the themes of biological decline and coping with loss may increase psychosocial risk factors for ill health in older adults is through the very institutions created to ensure their care. First, health care professionals are not immune to the impact of negative stereotypes about aging and may be subject to biases that increase health risks for older individuals. Nurses report more negative attributions about older adults than any other age group (Goebel, 1984), and misconceptions about older adults and their concerns have been identified as barriers to providing care by health care professionals (Meck-Higgins & Barkley, 2004). Physicians have been observed to offer less aggressive treatment to older patients, without considering other medical factors that might impact the treatment's success or illness course (Giugliano, Camargo, Lloyd-Jones, Zagrodsky, et al., 1998; Lewis et al., 2003). In a survey of adults over 50 in the United States and Canada, over 50% of respondents reported instances in which their health care provider attributed a health complaint to their age or told them that they were "too old" for a particular ailment or health concern (Palmore, 2004). In these ways, negative stereotypes about older adults have the potential to affect health outcomes directly by limiting access to medical care, disrupting patient–provider communication, and reducing treatment options.

Second, as alluded to earlier, many of the care systems created to provide treatment for older adults perpetuate feelings of dependence and loss of control. Research conducted in nursing homes suggests that "overhelping" can lead individuals to infer their own helplessness and incompetence, causing them to do poorly at a task that they had previously been able to accomplish (Avorn & Langer, 1982). A series of research studies conducted by Margret Baltes (1994) demonstrates that a "dependence support script" defines many social interactions between older adults and social partners, such that dependent behavior is reinforced through helping, while independent behaviors are ignored. These studies demonstrate that dependence support scripts are more pronounced and prevalent in institutional settings (Baltes & Wahl, 1992). Interestingly, the behavioral particulars need not change to bring about a reversal of these effects. Consider a nursing home program that has children "adopt a grandparent" versus one that has the residents "adopt a grandchild." In the latter scenario, the elder is implicitly active and in control.

Third, older adults often lack institutional structures that help them engage their social world. Many authors have noted the difficulty in finding social norms, roles, and social structure, role structure of society responsibilities for the elderly (Riley, Kahn, & Foner, 1994; Rosow, 1974) As a result, older adults may experience a lack of fit between their needs, aspirations, and abilities, and the opportunities provided by existing social structures (Kahn, 1994).

## TOWARD A MINDFUL
## RECONSIDERATION OF AGING

Let us return now to the ideas with which we began this chapter. Many theories of adult development and aging rest on two assumptions: an equation of aging with physical and cognitive decline, and an emphasis on coping with loss as the central developmental task of old age. We have argued that even though ideas and information related to these assumptions can make important contributions to understanding the experience of aging, the assumptions themselves may be inextricably linked to stereotypical processes that increase psychosocial health risks among the elderly. What then might counteract the effects of these stereotypes and help us decrease the risks associated with them?

As we stated earlier, theories—and the assumptions on which they are based—instantiate biases to the extent that they cease to be questioned and reexamined. In contrast, a "mindful approach" (Langer, 1989) to themes of decline and coping with loss allows us to consider alternative interpretations of the experience of aging. Mindfulness is a complex construct that may be best understood as a mode of engagement with the world. (For further reading on the construct, see Langer [1989]; for a more recent review, see Langer & Moldoveanu [2000].) Mindful engagement involves actively drawing novel distinctions, questioning new information and its implications, and considering new information from multiple perspectives. A mindful reconsideration of these themes would focus on two components: (1) reinterpreting the experience of aging in a way that recognizes the pitfalls of stereotype confirmation and stresses competencies rather than deficits; and (2) creating strategies for counteracting stereotypes and improving older adults' views of themselves as individuals.

## Alternative Interpretations of "Decline"

As mentioned earlier, evidence of cognitive decline among older adults may be subject to external biases and environmental influences. Whereas some researchers have argued that age-related decline in memory is inevitable and have documented consistent trends in memory loss (Baddeley, 1986; Johansson, Zarit, & Berg, 1992; Light & Burke, 1988), others believe that some aspects of the deterioration of memory may be environmentally determined, shaped by expectations and social contexts (Holland & Rabbit, 1992; Langer et al., 1979; Sinnett & Holen, 1999). A recent review of cross-cultural research about aging suggests that the context in which cognition occurs can shape cognitive-behavioral functioning (Park & Gutchess, 2002), and that environmental and social pressures may also play a role in exacerbating memory loss (Levy & Langer, 1994). When considering memory loss as a feature of the aging process, it might be useful to analyze what *categories* of memory are most subject to decline, and examine the developmental context in which older adults are asked to remember things. Older adults' mental capacities are often evaluated as though their desires, intentions, and interests are equivalent to those of younger people. When a child's parents calls a beloved muppet by the wrong name or cannot understand the lyrics to a popular song, the child does not conclude that her parents have decreased abilities in memory or comprehension. Rather, they conclude (correctly) that their parents do not care enough about Grover or Jay-Z. In some instances, older adults may appear more forgetful simply because they do not care enough about the information to encode it in memory. If this information cannot be retrieved, has it truly been forgotten?

Similarly, social gerontologists such as Tornstam have argued that some older individuals' decreased interest in social interaction should not be interpreted as disengagement due to attentional deficits. In his theory of gerotranscendence, a reinterpretation of disengagement theory (Cumming & Henry, 1961), Tornstam (1994) argues that aging is characterized by a shift in perspective away from a materialistic and rational view of the world toward a more holistic view that focuses on maturation and wisdom. As older adults experience this shift in perspective, they may also become more selective in their choice of social activities and less interested in super-fluous social interaction, and more interested in solitary meditation. While signs of gerotranscendence are often attributed to pathology by profession-als treating the elderly, a mindful consideration of these processes would emphasize the extent to which older adults may have a new perspective on the world that allows them to be removed without being disengaged.

However, because some physical changes in later life are likely to oc-cur, how might they too be reconsidered to remove labels of "decline" or disability? Consider our evaluation of two individuals—a 35-year-old who is no longer able to ride a tricycle, and an 85-year-old who is no longer able to ride a bicycle. Few of us would view the 35-year-old as "impaired" in her ability to ride a tricycle, nor would we say that she has developed "en-larged limbs" or "lost the flexibility" required to bring her knees to her chest to work the pedals. Just as tricycles were not made with 35-year-olds in mind, bicycles were not designed to be ridden by 85-year-olds. We might do better by 85-year-olds, however, to view this fact as a deficit in the appa-ratus (or our mechanical imagination) rather than a loss of strength, flexi-bility, or balance on the part of the older adult. This hyperbolic analogy may be extended to many situations in which we infer decline, while older adults are forced to navigate an environment designed neither for or by them.

In the most extreme application of such a reconsideration, even senility may be considered an adaptive strategy for coping with an overroutinized environment. Many institutional facilities lack opportunities for creative thinking, and the complexity of seemingly senile fantasies may be the exer-cise of cognitive capacities that have no other outlet. Indeed, Langer et al. (1979) found that when disease is held constant, those diagnosed as "se-nile" actually live longer.

Many directors of nursing homes recognize the change in dexterity that accompanies aging. Their solution is to fill their recreation rooms with puzzles and toys designed for children who have not yet learned fine motor skills. Surely, the differences in the two age groups demand more sophisticated crafts for the older adults. These are not easily found. Resorting to the only available materials, these environments reinforce the fallacious belief that as we age, we regress.

Finally, there is an opportunity to redefine the "losses" of later life in a way that reveals the wisdom that life experience helps individuals to attain. According to McKee and Barber (1999), wisdom is often developed in response to loss, and research suggests that specific losses, such as bereavement, may provide individuals with gains in self-knowledge and development of coping strategies (Aldwin, 1994; Lieberman, 1996). To the extent that loss also decreases egocentricity and increases empathy, it is central to the development of wisdom (Baltes & Staudinger, 2000). Levenson et al. (2001) call this the "liberative approach" to development, stressing the independence of self-actualization and identity development from either physical or cognitive development.

## Alternative Interpretations of "Loss"

A mindful reconsideration of the developmental tasks of aging may also lead us to question whether older adults must focus on the regulation of loss. Is it not possible to conceptualize growth and regulation of loss as different interpretations of the same phenomena? The developmental tasks encountered by a 2-year-old can be understood as regulating his or her *lack* of speech, manual dexterity, and sense of spatial relations. Similarly, an older adult must grapple with developmental tasks that enable him or her to *grow* in the ability to walk with a cane or create innovative mnemonic aids. Facilitating mindful aging may be related to fostering the work of developing (i.e., understanding what it means to help someone continue to "grow" throughout the lifespan). When older adults make changes in their behavior or activities, these are likely to be seen as "concessions" to old age rather than developmental adaptations, or even growth in understanding or innovation to deal with the situation. For example, an 80-year-old man is frustrated by the fact that he can no longer play tennis the way he could when he was 50. But perhaps the problem is not that he can no longer play the same way, but that he is still trying to do so. Venus Williams, who is 6'3" and has one of the largest grip sizes in women's tennis, and Amanda Coetzer, who is 5'2" and has one of the smallest, cannot possibly play with comparable strategies, nor would it occur to them to do so. However, Coetzer is well aware that her small stature allows her to be quick on the court, and Williams understands that her height gives her stroke tremendous power. Because his social environment and mindless encoding of stereotypes have taught the 80-year-old tennis player that his game is declining, not developing, it may never occur to him to adapt his game based on the identification of new skills. Because differences between young and old people are taken not as differences, but as decrements, we are not likely to find ways that older people might metaphorically "change their game." If we do begin to notice such potential adaptations, we might still make the mistake of seeing these changes as compensatory, instead of looking for ways in which they might be advantageous to individuals of all ages.

Similarly, mindfulness theory allows us to reconsider processes of accommodation (Rothermund & Brandtstädter, 2003) by focusing on not only *lowering* performance standards but also redefining them. For many older adults, aging may be associated with a narrowing of self-definition. Changes in ability, opportunity, or perspective may cause older adults to focus on their current restrictions, comparing themselves with what they "used to do." An understanding of aging as a process of increasing limitation or loss may result from an equation of behavior with identity (i.e., defining an aspect of self in terms of only a limited and specific set of activities). For example, imagine an older adult with a strong identity as a painter, who develops arthritis in his hands to an extent that makes it difficult for him to hold a brush. A mindless assessment of this situation might result in encouraging this individual to come to terms with the fact that, at some point, he may no longer be able to be a painter. He might be assisted in developing a new hobby or asked to reflect on all the wonderful art he produced in his youth. Broadening both our understanding of identity-defining categories and the variety of environmental and motivational influences that shape behavior may allow older individuals to focus on continuity across the lifespan rather than loss. Instead of coming to terms with the end of his career as a painter, this individual might be encouraged to reconsider the way he paints—holding the brush in his teeth, experimenting with finger painting or spray cans, spilling paint on the canvas. If he still allows himself to paint with a brush, he may notice that he does different things with it than he did before developing arthritis. If he entertains the idea that this new technique is a difference, not a decrement, he may even develop a new style of painting. But even if this individual is not interested in or satisfied with these modifications to his painting style, a mindful reconsideration of his abilities would focus on broadening the concept of "painter" to include a host of activities in which the individual can still engage and excel. Being "a painter" can mean a particular way of seeing the world, a way of understanding and interpreting art, or a gift for matching color and tone with meaning. This individual does not have to give up those aspects of self, and he will always be a painter, even if he is not painting at the moment. Similarly, older adults can consider themselves athletes long after their physical stamina or agility may prevent them from engaging in their preferred sport. This idea of concept-broadening stands in contrast to recommendations of downward social comparison, in which older adults are encouraged to feel good about themselves as "an athlete" because they are still in excellent shape compared to people of their own age. In contrast, this framing of self-definition does not rely on social comparison; for that reason, it is both more satisfying and more enduring (Langer, 2002). These processes may be integrally related to reminiscence, rehearsing past experience and success in a manner that allows one to remain connected to them. In studies of nursing home residents, reminiscence was correlated with high ego integrity scores (Boylin, Gordon, & Nehrke, 1976), and the ability to reminisce seems to help people maintain self-concept under stress (Lewis, 1971).

Finally, whereas we have argued that certain environments can perpetuate stereotypes and stereotyped behavior, research also suggests that altering environments for older adults may allow individuals to break free from stereotypical attitudes and behavior. Research has demonstrated that presenting elderly subjects with positive stereotypes and information designed to enhance perceptions of old age is associated with improvements in walking speed and gait (Hausdorff, Levy, & Wei, 1999). These results suggest that creating environments in which positive views of aging are subtly reinforced may lead to significant improvements even in physical functioning. As we have shown (Langer & Rodin, 1976; Rodin & Langer, 1977), giving elderly patients in a nursing home autonomy to make decisions and responsibility over a plant resulted in significant differences on measures of alertness, happiness, active participation, and a general sense of well-being 3 weeks later. Eighteen months later, these differences had expanded not only to measures of physical and psychological health but also to mortality rates (4 of the 47 participants in the experimental group vs. 13 of the 44 in the control group). Subsequent studies with nursing home residents have found similar improvements in psychological and physical health measures as a result of increase autonomy and perceived control (Schulz, 1976; Alexander, Langer, Newman, Chandler, & Davies, 1989). More recent research has demonstrated that even modest interventions with a focus on mastery or goal-setting to counteract learned helplessness can improve self-care performance (Faulkner, 2001) and improve older adults' performance on memory tasks (West, 2004). Among adults ages 65–95, the cognitive-perceptual factor of health self-determinism is associated with better psychological well-being, coping with aging, and engagement in healthful behaviors, such as physical activity and better nutrition (Lucas, 2000). Environments that combat stereotypes by increasing older adults' perceptions of control over their physical and mental health may lead to improvements that allow these individuals to overcome self-perpetuating cycles of detriment and dependence.

## CONCLUSION

This chapter focuses on two assumptions intrinsic to many theories of adult development—an equation of aging with physical and cognitive decline, and an emphasis on coping, with loss as the central developmental task of old age. We argue that these assumptions may lead to the evaluation of older adults based on invalid or irrelevant criteria and create deterministic expectations for deficiency and deterioration. In turn, such evaluations and expectations may be internalized by older adults, limiting their sense of their own abilities and ultimately impacting negatively on their health status and ability to engage in health-seeking behavior. In contrast, we suggest a mindful approach to adult development that focuses on the emerging competencies inherent in aging. A focus on continued growth and change throughout the lifespan may have positive implications not only for older adults' affect and cognition but also their health-related quality of life and experience of the aging process.

## REFERENCES

Aldwin, C. M. (1991). Does age affect the stress and coping process?: Implication of age differences in perceived control. *Journal of Gerontology*, 174–180.

Aldwin, C. M. (1994). *Stress, coping, and development: An integrative approach.* New York: Guilford Press.

Alexander, C. N., & Langer, E. J. (Eds.). (1990). *Higher stages of human development: Perspectives on adult growth.* London: Oxford University Press.

Alexander, C., Langer, E. J., Newman, R., Chandler, H., & Davies, J. (1989). Aging, mindfulness, and meditation. *Journal of Personality and Social Psychology, 57,* 950–964.

Avorn, J., & Langer, E. (1982). Induced disability in nursing home patients: A controlled trial. *Journal of the American Geriatrics Society, 30*(6), 397–400.

Baddeley, A. (1986). *Working memory.* New York: Oxford University Press.

Baltes, M. M. (1994). *The many faces of dependency in old age.* Cambridge: Cambridge, UK: University Press.

Baltes, M. M., & Wahl, H.W. (1992). The dependency–support script in institutions: Generalization to community settings. *Psychology and Aging, 9,* 179–188.

Baltes, P. B., & Staudinger, U. M. (2000). Wisdom: A metaheuristic (pragmatic) to orchestrate mind and virtue toward excellence. *American Psychologist, 55,* 122–136.

Baltes, P. B., Staudinger, U. M., & Lindenberger, U. (1999). Lifespan psychology: Theory and application to intellectual functioning. *Annual Review of Psychology, 50,* 471–507.

Bargh, J. A., Chen, M., & Burrows, L. (1996). Automaticity of social behavior: Direct effects of trait construct and stereotype activation on action. *Journal of Personality and Social Psychology, 71,* 230–244.

Batsakes, P. J., & Fisk, A. D. (2000). Age and dual task performance: Are performance gains retained? *Journals of Gerontology: Psychological Sciences and Social Sciences, Series D, 55,* P332–P342.

Becker, G. (1994). The oldest old: Autonomy in the face of frailty. *Journal of Aging Studies, 8,* 59–76.

Bieman-Copland, S., & Ryan, E. B. (1998). Age-biased interpretation of memory successes and failures in adulthood. *Journals of Gerontology: Psychological Sciences and Social Sciences, Series B, 53*(2), 105–111.

Boylin, W., Gordon, S. K., & Nehrke, M. F. (1976). Reminiscing and ego integrity in institutionalized elderly males. *Gerontologist, 16,* 118–124.

Bühler, C. (1968). The general structure of the human life cycle. In C. Buhler & F. Massarik (Eds.), *The course of human life: A study of goals in the humanistic perspective* (pp. 12–16). New York: Springer.

Chanowitz, B., & Langer, E. J. (1981). Premature cognitive commitment. *Journal of Personality and Social Psychology, 41,* 1051–1063.

Christensen, A. J., Wiebe, J. S., Benotsch, E. G., & Lawton, W. J. (1996). Perceived health competence, health locus of control, and patient adherence in renal dialysis. *Cognitive Therapy and Research, 20,* 411–421.

Cumming, E., & Henry, W. (1961). *Growing old: The process of disengagement.* New York: Basic Books.

Darley, J. M., & Gross, P. H. (1983). A hypothesis-confirming bias in labeling effects. *Journal of Personality and Social Psychology, 44,* 20–33.

Dixon, R. A., & Bäckman, L. (1995). Concepts of compensation: Integrated, differentiated, and Janus-faced. *Compentation for psychological deficits and declines: Managing losses and promoting gains* (pp. 3–19). Hillsdale, NJ: Erlbaum.

Erikson, E. (1959). *Identity and the life cycle: Psychological issues.* New York: New York University Press.

Faulkner, M. (2001). The onset and alleviation of learned helplessness in older hospitalized people. *Aging and Mental Health, 5,* 379–386.

Fisk, A. D., & Rogers, W. A. (1991). Toward an understanding of age-related memory and visual search effects. *Journal of Experimental Psychology: General, 120,* 131–149.

Gatz, M. (1998). Toward a developmentally informed theory of mental disorder in older adults. In J. Lomranz (Ed.), *Handbook of aging and mental health: An integrative approach* (pp. 101–120). New York: Plenum.

Giles, H., Fox, S., & Smith, E. (1993). Patronizing the elderly: Intergenerational evaluations. *Research on Language and Social Interaction, 26,* 129–149.

Goebel, B. L. (1984). Age stereotypes held by student nurses. *Journal of Psychology, 116,* 249–254.

Golub, S. A., Filipowicz, A., & Langer, E. J. (2002). Acting your age. In T. Nelson (Ed.), *Ageism: Stereotyping and prejudice against older persons* (pp. 277–294). Cambridge, MA: MIT Press.

Giugliano, R. P., Camargo, C. A., Lloyd-Jones, D. M., Zagrodsky, J. D., Alexis, J. D., Eagle, K. A., Fuster, V., & O'Donnell, C. G. (1998). Elderly patients receive less aggressive medical and invasive management of unstable angina: Potential impact of clinical guidelines. *Archives of Internal Medicine, 158,* 1113–1120.

Guttmann, D. (1994). *Reclaimed powers.* Evanston, IL: Northwestern University Press.

Hausdorff, J., Levy, B. R., & Wei, J. Y. (1999). The power of ageism on physical function of older persons: Reversibility of age-related gait changes. *Journal of the American Geriatrics Society, 47*(11), 1346–1349.

Hirt, E. R., McDonald, H. E., & Erikson, G. A. (1995). How do I remember thee?: The role of encoding set and delay in reconstructive memory processes. *Journal of Experimental Social Psychology, 31,* 379–409.

Holland, C., & Rabbit, P. (1992). Effects of age-related reductions in processing resources on text recall. *Journal of Gerontology, 47,* 129–137.

Ickes, W., Patterson, M. L., Rajecki, D. W., & Tanford, S. (1982). Behavioral and cognitive consequences of reciprocal versus compensatory responses to preinteractional expectancies. *Social Cognition, 1,* 160–190.

Isaacs, L., & Bearison, D. (1986). The development of children's prejudice against the aged. *International Journal of Aging and Human Development, 23,* 175–194.

Jennings, J. M., & Jacoby, L. L. (1993). Automatic versus intentional uses of memory: Aging, attention, and control. *Psychology and Aging, 8,* 283–293.

Johansson, B., Zarit, S., & Berg, S. (1992). Changed in cognitive functioning of the oldest old. *Journal of Gerontology, 47,* 75–80.

Kahn, R. (1994). Opportunities, aspirations, and goodness of fit. In M. Riley, R. Kahn, & A. Foner (Eds.), *Age and structural lag* (pp. 37–53). New York: Wiley.

Kelley, H. H. (1950). The warm–cold variable in first impressions of persons. *Journal of Personality, 18,* 431–439.

Kite, M. E., & Johnson, B. T. (1988). Attitudes toward older and younger adults: A meta-analysis. *Psychology and Aging, 3*(3), 233–244.

Kramer, A. F., & Larish, J. F. (1996). Aging and dual-task performance. In W. A. Rogers, A. D. Fisk, & N. Walker (Eds.), *Aging and skilled performance: Advances in theory and application* (pp. 83–112). Hillsdale, NJ: Erlbaum.

Langer, E. J. (1981). Old age: An artifact? In J. L. McGaugh & S. B. Kiesler (Eds.), *Aging: Biology and behavior* (pp. 255–282). New York: Academic Press.

Langer, E. J. (1989). *Mindfulness.* Reading, MA: Addison-Wesley.

Langer, E. J. (2002). Well-being: Mindfullness versus positive evaluation. In C. R. Snyder & S. J. Lopez (Eds.), *Handbook of positive psychology* (pp. 214–230). London: Oxford University Press.

Langer, E. J., & Avorn, J. (1985). Impact of the psychosocial environment of the elderly on behavioral and health outcomes. In B. Beth & E. W. Markson (Eds.), *Growing old in America: New perspectives no old age* (3rd ed., pp. 462–473). New Brunswick, NJ: Transaction.

Langer, E. J., & Benevento, A. (1978). Self-induced dependence. *Journal of Personality and Social Psychology, 36,* 886–893.

Langer, E. J., & Imber, L. (1979). When practice makes perfect: Debilitating effects of overlearning. *Journal of Personality and Social Psychology, 37,* 2014–2025.

Langer, E. J., & Moldoveanu, M. (2000). The construct of mindfulness. *Journal of Social Issues, 56,* 1–9.

Langer, E. J., & Rodin, J. (1976). The effects of choice and enhanced personal responsibility for the aged: A field experiment in an institutional setting. *Journal of Personality and Social Psychology, 34*(2), 191–198.

Langer, E. J., & Rodin, J. (1979). The effects of enhanced personal responsibility for the aged: A field experiment in an institutional setting. *Journal of Personality and Social Psychology, 34,* 191–198.

Langer, E., Rodin, J., Beck, P., Weinman, C., & Spitzer, L. (1979). Environmental determinants of memory improvement in late adulthood. *Journal of Personality and Social Psychology, 37,* 2003–2013.

Levenson, M. R., Aldwin, C. M., & Cupertino, A. P. (2001). Adult development as self-transcendence: Extending the liberative model. In A. L. Neri (Ed.), *Maturidade and Velhice: Um enfoque multidiciplinar* (pp. 99–116). Sao Paolo, Brazil: Papirus.

Levy, B. R. (1996). Improving memory in old age through implicit self-stereotyping. *Journal of Personality and Social Psychology, 71*(6), 1092–1107.

Levy, B. R. (2003). Mind matters: Cognitive and physical effects of aging self-stereotypes. *Journals of Gerontology: Psychological Sciences and Social Sciences, Series B, 58,* P203–P211.

Levy, B. R., Ashman, O., & Dror, I. (2000). To be or not to be: The effects of aging stereotypes on the will to live. *Omega, 40*(3), 409–420.

Levy, B. R., Hausdorff, J., Hencke, R., & Wei, J. Y. (2000). Reducing cardiovascular stress with positive self-stereotypes of aging. *Journals of Gerontology: Psychological Sciences and Social Sciences, Series B, 55,* 205–213.

Levy, B. R., & Langer, E. J. (1994). Memory advantage for deaf and Chinese elders: Aging free from negative premature cognitive commitments. *Journal of Personality and Social Psychology, 66*(6), 989–997.

Levy, B. R., Slade, M. D., Kunkel, S. R., & Kasl, S. V. (2002). Longevity increased by positive self-perceptions of aging. *Journal of Personality and Social Psychology, 83,* 261–270.

Lewis, C. (1971). Reminiscing and self-concept in old age. *Journal of Gerontology, 26,* 240–243.

Lewis, J. H., Kilgore, M. L., Goldman, D. P., Trimble, E. L., Kaplan, R., Montello, M. J., et al. (2003). Participation of patients 65 years of age or older in cancer clinical trials. *Journal of Clinical Oncology, 21,* 1383–1389.

Lieberman, M. (1996). *Doors close, doors open: Widows, grieving and growing.* New York: Putnam.

Light, L., & Burke, D. (1988). Patterns of language and memory in old age. In L. Light & D. Burke (Eds.), *Language, memory, and aging* (pp. 241–271). New York: Cambridge University Press.

Lucas, J. A. (2000). Determinants of health-promoting behavior among women ages 65 and above living in the community. *Scholarly Inquiry for Nursing Practice, 14,* 77–100.

Maier, H., & Smith, J. (1999). Psychological predictors of mortality in old age. *Journals of Gerontology: Psychological Sciences and Social Sciences, Series B, 54,* 44–54.

Manton, K. G., Corder, L., & Stallard, E. (1994). Chronic disability trends in elderly United States populations: 1982–1994. *Proceedings of the National Academy of Sciences of the Unites States of America, 94,* 2593–2598.

Manton, K. G., & XiLiang, G. (2001). Changes in the prevalence of chronic disability in the United States black and nonblack population above age 65 from 1982 to 1999. *Proceedings of the National Academy of Science of the Unites States of America, 98,* 6354–6359.

McKee, P., & Barber, C. (1999). On defining wisdom. *International Journal of Aging and Human Development, 249,* 149–164.

Meck-Higgins, M., & Barkley, M. C. (2004). Barriers to nutrition education for older adults, and nutrition and aging training opportunities for educators, healthcare providers, volunteers and caregivers. *Journal of Nutrition for the Elderly, 23*(4), 99–121.

Nosek, B. A., Banaji, M. R., & Greenwald, A. G. (2002). Harvesting implicit group attitudes and beliefs from a demonstration website. *Group Dynamics, 6,* 101–115.

Ory, M., Hoffman, M. K., Hawkins, M., Sanner, B., & Mockenhaupt, R. (2003). Challenging aging stereotypes: Strategies for creating a more active society. *American Journal of Preventive Medicine, 25,* 164–171.

Palmore, E. B. (2004). Research note: Ageism in Canada and the United States. *Journal of Cross-Cultural Gerontology, 19,* 41–46.

Park, D. C., & Gutchess, A. H. (2002). Aging, cognition, and culture: A neuroscience perspective. *Neuroscience and Biobehavioral Reviews, 26,* 859–867.

Perlmuter, L. C., & Eads, A. S. (1998). Control: Cognitive and motivational implications. In J. Lomranz (Ed.), *Handbook of aging and mental health: An integrative approach* (pp. 45–67). New York: Plenum.

Riley, M., Kahn, R., & Foner, A. (Eds.). (1994). *Age and structural lag.* New York: Wiley.

Rodin, J., & Langer, E. J. (1977). Long-term effects of a control-relevant intervention with the institutionalized aged. *Journal of Personality and Social Psychology, 35*(12), 897–902.

Rosenthal, R., & Jacobson, L. (1968). *Pygmalion in the classroom: Teacher expectation and student intellectual development.* New York: Holt, Rinehart & Winston.

Rosow, I. (1974). *Socialization to old age.* Berkeley: University of California Press.

Rothermund, K., & Brandtstädter, J. (2003). Coping with deficits and losses in later life: From compensatory action to accommodation. *Psychology and Aging, 18,* 896–205.

Schulz, R. (1976). Effects of control and predictability on the psychological well-being of the institutionalized aged. *Journal of Personality and Social Psychology, 33,* 563–575.

Seligman, M. E. P. (1975). *Helplessness.* San Francisco: Freeman.

Seligman, M. E. P., & Maier, S. F. (1976). Learned helplessness: Theory and evidence. *Journal of Experimental Social Psychology, 103,* 3–46.

Shlesinger, M., & Kronebusch, K. (1994). Intergenerational tensions and conflict: Attitudes and perceptions about social justice and age-related needs. In V. L. Bengston & R. A. Harootyan (Eds.), *Intergenerational linkages: Hidden connections in American society* (pp. 152–184). New York: Springer.

Sinnett, E. R., & Holen, M. C. (1999). Assessment of memory functioning among an aging sample. *Psychological Reports, 84,* 339–350.

Snyder, M., Tanke, E. D., & Berscheid, E. (1977). Social perception and interpersonal behavior: On the self-fulfilling nature of social stereotypes. *Journal of Personality and Social Psychology, 35,* 656–666.

Staudinger U. M., Marsiske, M., & Baltes, P. B. (1995). Resilience and reserve capacity in later adulthood: Potentials and limits of development across the life span. In D. Cicchetti & D. Cohen (Eds.), *Developmental psychopathology: Vol. 2. Risk, disorder, and adaptation* (pp. 801–847). New York: Wiley.

Steele, C. M. (1997). A threat in the air: How stereotypes shape the intellectual identities and performance of women and African-Americans. *American Psychologist, 52,* 613–629.

Stein, R., Blanchard-Fields, F., & Hertzog, C. (2002). The effects of age-stereotype priming on the memory performance of older adults. *Experimental Aging Research, 28*(2), 169–181.

Tesser, A. (1978). Self-generated attitude change. In L. Berkowitz (Ed.), *Advances in experimental social psychology* (Vol. 11, pp. 288–338). New York: Academic Press.

Tornstam, L. (1994). Gero-transcendence: A theoretical and empirical exploration. In L. E. Thomas & S. A. Eisenhandler (Eds.), *Aging and the religious dimension* (pp. 203–225). Westport, CT: Auburn House.

Trope, Y., & Thompson, E. P. (1997). Looking for truth in all the wrong places?: Asymmetric search of individuating information about stereotyped group members. *Journal of Personality and Social Psychology, 73,* 229–241.

West, R. L. (2004). Aging and memory control beliefs: Performance in relation to goal setting and memory self-evaluation. *Journals of Genrontology: Psychological Sciences and Social Sciences, Series B, 59,* 56–65.

Wheeler, S. C., & Petty, R. E. (2001). The effects of stereotype activation on behavior: A review of possible mechanisms. *Psychological Bulletin, 127,* 797–826.

Woodward, N. J., & Wallston, B. S. (1987). Age and health care beliefs: Self-efficacy as a mediator of low desire for control. *Psychology and Aging, 2*(1), 3–8.

Wu, A., Tang, C., & Kwok, T. (2002). Death anxiety among Chinese elderly people in Hong Kong. *Journal of Aging and Health, 14,* 42–56.

Wu, A., Tang, C., & Kwok, T. (2004). Self-efficacy, health locus of control, and psychological distress in elderly Chinese women with chronic illnesses. *Aging and Mental Health, 8,* 21–28.

Wyatt, S. B., Williams, D. R., Calvin, R., Henderson, F. C., Walker, E. R., & Winters, K. (2003). Racism and cardiovascular disease in African Americans. *American Journal of Medical Science, 325*(6), 315–331.

# CHAPTER 3

# A Developmental Approach to Psychosocial Risk Factors and Successful Aging

CYNTHIA A. BERG, TIMOTHY W. SMITH,
NANCY J. M. HENRY, *and* GALE E. PEARCE

Successful aging has been characterized as maintaining physical health (avoiding disease), sustaining good cognitive function, and having active engagement with other people and productive activities (Rowe & Kahn, 1998). Although these three factors are known to be interrelated, the field has largely examined physical health outcomes as primary and separate from cognitive outcomes, with active social engagement as a predictor of physical health and occasionally cognitive functioning. In this chapter we take a more transactional perspective to these factors of successful aging, understanding how they interact throughout the lifespan to create developmental trajectories of varying levels of success. In addition, we utilize the extensive evidence from health psychology that personality characteristics such as hostility and neuroticism also place individuals at risk for aging unsuccessfully (Krantz & McCeney, 2002; Smith & Ruiz, 2004). The associations among physical health, cognitive functioning, social functioning, and personality (Elias, Elias, Robbins, Wolf, & D'Agostino, 2001; Seeman, Lusignolo, Albert, & Berkman, 2001; Smith & Ruiz, 2004; Waldstein & Katzel, 2001) are suggestive of a lifetime connection among these factors of successful aging. From a developmental perspective, the important question is "What are the processes whereby risk factors operate over the course of a lifespan to affect successful aging?"

In this chapter we provide a lifespan developmental approach to understand how individuals, with their early personality predispositions and ways of interacting with their social world, can age successfully (or unsuccessfully) physically, cognitively, and socially. First, we begin by briefly reviewing existing work within health and aging that focuses on two types of psychosocial risk factors for physical health: personality characteristics and the quality of the social environment (social support, active engagement with others, and productive activities). Next we present a transactional developmental model that explores how early individual differences in personality may provide a way of interacting with one's environment that affects the quality of one's social interactions and has implications for both physical health and cognitive outcomes. This model proposes that personality and social support are not separate risk factors, but that they aggregate in their potential for risk and coexist with cognitive and physical health in the lifespan experience of individuals (Smith, Glazer, Ruiz, & Gallo, 2004; Smith & Spiro, 2002). Finally, we provide a window into this developmental process as we explore how specific aspects of personality (namely, hostility) may place individuals at risk for poor physical, cognitive, and social functioning in the context of marriage. The transactional quality of this developmental framework holds promise for understanding the intricate connection among the elements of successful aging (physical health, cognitive health, and social health) identified by Rowe and Kahn (1998) that often are examined separately in the literature.

## TRADITIONAL PSYCHOSOCIAL RISK FACTORS AND AGING

The study of psychosocial risk factors for disease and reduced longevity has typically included a conceptual distinction between characteristics of persons—notably, personality variables—and characteristics of their social circumstances (e.g., social isolation, support, conflict). Decades of research have produced compelling evidence that personality characteristics predict the onset and course of serious and often fatal illness (Friedman & Martin, Chapter 9, this volume; Smith & Ruiz, 2004), and social isolation and other characteristics of the social environment are similarly well-established as risk factors (Uchino, 2004). In what follows here we briefly review major observations in this literature and describe how these associations between psychosocial risk factors and health outcomes may change with age. We focus in this section on traditional physical health outcomes and address in the next section how these risk factors can also affect cognitive and social outcomes.

## Personality as Risk

Among the wide variety of personality characteristics studied as risk factors, hostility, neuroticism, and optimism are among those with the greatest empirical support. "Hostility" refers to a set of cognitive, affective, and behavioral characteristics (Smith, 1992). Cognitively, hostility refers to "a devaluation of the worth and motives of others, an expectation that others are likely sources of wrong-doing, a relational view of being in opposition toward others, and a desire to inflict harm or see others harmed" (Smith, 1994, p. 26). Affectively, "anger" refers to the tendency to experience frequent and pronounced episodes of this emotion, which varies from irritation or annoyance to fury and rage. Aggressiveness includes a variety of behaviors involving attacking, destructive, or hurtful actions, though behaviors associated with trait hostility also include a cold, disagreeable, quarrelsome, and antagonistic interpersonal style.

Recent interest in hostility as a risk factor for cardiovascular disease and premature mortality stems from efforts to identify the specific unhealthy elements within the broader Type A behavior pattern (Siegman, 1994). A prior quantitative review indicated that across a variety of measures of hostility, trait anger, and aggressiveness, this set of characteristics is associated with increased risk of coronary heart disease (CHD) and reduced longevity (Miller, Smith, Turner, Guijarro, & Hallet, 1996). Although not all subsequent studies have produced positive findings (Eng, Fitzmaurice, Kubansky, Rimm, & Kawochi, 2003; Sykes et al., 2002), several large and well-controlled prospective studies have produced positive results (see Smith, Orleans, & Jenkins, 2004, for a review). Various measures of hostility have been associated with concurrent levels and progression of atherosclerosis in otherwise healthy samples (Harris, Matthews, Sutton-Tyrell, & Kuller, 2003; Iribarren et al., 2000; Matthews, Owens, Kuller, Sutton-Tyrell, & Jansen-McWilliams, 1998), and with the progression of atherosclerosis and susceptibility to myocardial ischemia acute coronary events among persons with established cardiovascular disease (Angerer et al., 2000; Mendes de Leon, Kop, de Swart, Bar, & Appels, 1996). This suggests that hostility may influence multiple processes within the decades-long changing etiology of CHD (Smith, Glazer, et al., 2004).

Individual differences in the tendency to experience sadness, anxiety, and other negative emotions have long been suspected as leading to poor health (Smith & Ruiz, 2004). Negative affectivity (Watson & Clark, 1984) and neuroticism (Costa & McCrae, 1987) reflect the disposition to experience negative emotions and related cognitions (e.g., low self-esteem, worry) within the range of normal adjustment, but they also confer vulnerability to the development of clinically diagnosable mood and anxiety disorders (Zonderman, Herbst, Schmidt, Costa, & McCrae, 1993). Neuroticism and negative affectivity are associated with symptom reporting and other illness behaviors that are in excess of independently confirmed physical illness (Costa & McCrae, 1987; Watson & Pennebaker, 1989). However, a large and growing body of evidence suggests that these traits are also associated with increased risk of objectively verified cardiovascular disease and reduced longevity (Smith & Ruiz, 2004). For example, various measures of negative affectivity have been associated with the development of high blood pressure (Jones, Frank, & Ingram, 1997), and among persons with hypertension, the incidence of stroke and death from CHD (Simonsick, Wallace, Blaser, & Gerkman, 1995). Among initially healthy individuals, these traits have been found to predict the development of CHD (Barefoot & Schroll, 1996; Kubzansky et al., 1997), premature mortality (Hermann et al., 1998), and reduced survival among persons with established CHD (Barefoot et al., 1996; Januzzi, Stern, Pasternak, & DeSanctis, 2000; Smith & Ruiz, 2002).

Individual differences in optimistic and pessimistic expectations about future events have also been found to predict important health outcomes (Smith & Ruiz, 2004). Compared to persons endorsing pessimistic expectations or hopelessness, optimists experience fewer medical complications following cardiac surgery or angioplasty (Helgeson & Fritz, 1999; Scheier et al., 1999) and survive longer following a diagnosis of breast cancer (Schulz, Bookwala, Knapp, Scheier, & Williamson, 1996). Optimism is also associated with longevity and reduced incidence of cardiovascular disease and death (Kubzansky et al., 1997; Maruta, Colligan, Malinchoc, & Offord, 2000). Optimism is closely (i.e., inversely) associated with neuroticism and negative affectivity (Smith, Pope, Rhodewalt, & Poulton, 1989), and this overlap is often not controlled in studies of the health consequences of optimism. Hence, the unique predictive utility of this trait relative to the broader dimension of neuroticism and negative affectivity has not been clearly established.

## Mechanisms Involved in the Association between Personality and Physical Health

Several mechanisms could account for the association between these characteristics and the development of disease. The association between hostility and health may reflect an underlying biological factor that both promotes the development of these behavioral characteristics and confers vulnerability to disease (Williams, 1994). Furthermore, potential psychophysiological mechanisms include heightened cardiovascular and neuroendocrine responses to potentially stressful events during daily life. Hostile persons evidence heightened physiological reactivity across a variety of methodologies (for a review, see Smith, Glazer, et al., 2004). Chronic symptoms of anxiety and depression are associated with suppressed immune functioning (Cohen & Herbert, 1996; McGuire, Kiecolt-Glaser, & Glaser, 2002), increasing the likelihood of infectious illness and cancer (Rabin, 1999); whereas optimism is associated with better immune functioning (Segerstrom, Taylor, Kemeny, & Fahey, 1998) and lower levels of ambulatory blood pressure (Raikkonen, Katainen, Keskivaara, & Keltikangas-Jarvinen, 2000). Heightened sympathetically mediated physiological stress responses and decreased parasympathetic activity associated with anxiety and depression could contribute to the development and progression of atherosclerosis, as well as the later emergence of manifestations of CHD (Kop, 1999).

These traits are also associated with differential exposure to interpersonal conflict and social support. Hostility is associated with increased exposure to unhealthy social contexts (i.e., low support, high conflict), which could contribute to the health consequences of hostility (Smith, Glazer, et al., 2004) and also reflect the interpersonal or transactional consequences of the hostile person's cynical thinking and antagonistic actions (Smith, 1992; Smith, Glazer, et al., 2004). Similarly neuroticism and negative affect are also associated with low levels of support and high levels of interpersonal conflict, and this psychosocial vulnerability could reflect transactional processes through which chronically dysphoric persons create stress and undermine support in their social networks (Smith & Ruiz, 2004). In contrast, optimists experience greater social support (Brissette, Scheier, & Carver, 2002).

Finally, these characteristics may operate through negative or positive health behaviors (Carney, Freedland, Rich, & Jaffe, 1995). For instance, hostility is associated with negative health behaviors such as smoking, excessive alcohol intake, and physical inactivity, and some studies have indicated that these health behaviors account for the association between hostility and subsequent cardiovascular disease (Everson et al., 1997). Optimism is associated with more effective participation in medical care (Strack, Carver, & Blaney, 1987).

### Personality and Health Risk across Adult Development

Across these three personality risk factors, developmental processes could moderate the strength of their associations with health outcomes or the underlying mechanisms through which they influence health (Smith & Spiro, 2002). First, despite the considerable stability (Costa & McCrae, 1994) in personality traits, there are also differences across development. For instance, declines are seen from young to middle adulthood in hostility, with potential increases in late adulthood (Barefoot, Beckham, Haney, Siegler, & Lipkus, 1993). There is a potential curvilinear relationship between negative affect and depression, with the highest scores occurring during young and late adulthood (Gatz, Kasl-Godley, & Karel, 1996). In addition to these age patterns in personality across individuals, there is also considerable intraindividual change in personality traits (Mroczek & Spiro, 2003). Second, even traditional risk factors have a changing pattern of association with health outcomes with increasing age (Kaplan, Haan, & Wallace, 1999). Several important diseases (e.g., cancer, CHD) have complex etiologies that involve multiple mechanisms that differ as they progress (Cohen, Kaplan, & Manuck, 1994; Rabin, 1999). Hence, the association of age with stage of disease virtually guarantees changing levels of association between personality characteristics and disease outcomes and mechanisms with increasing age. For example, pathophysiological processes involved in the initiation and progression of atherosclerosis differ from those involved in the emergence of CHD or ischemic stroke among persons with advanced atherosclerosis, and the medical course of CHD and stroke involves still other mechanisms. Any given personality trait could influence these stages of disease differently if they are distinctly related to the varying mechanisms.

Third, if a psychosocial risk factor influences the initial development and progression of a potentially fatal disease, then with increasing age of a study sample, survivor effects may weaken the association between the trait and health outcomes (Williams, 2000); that is, a risk factor may contribute to the elimination of vulnerable persons from the potential sample through mortality. Those persons scoring high on this risk factor who survive without developing disease may be resilient in some way that is not typical of the general population. This general issue of changing effects and mechanisms with increasing age has only recently been studied, and initial results suggest that such effects are important (Aldwin, Spiro, Levenson, & Cupertino, 2001; Duberstein et al., 2003).

## Social Functioning as Risk

Social functioning, as assessed via a wide variety of measures, is associated with a multitude of positive health outcomes, including reduced risk for cardiovascular disease, cancer, infectious illness, functional decline, and lower risk of mortality (see Rook, Mavandadi, Sorkin, & Zettel, Chapter 14, this volume; Berkman, 1995; House, Landis, & Umberson, 1988; Uchino, Cacioppo, & Keicolt-Glaser, 1996). Social functioning represents many facets of the social environment, including both the amount of interaction within the network, the structure of an individual's social network (i.e., group membership or familial ties), as well as the function served by the network (i.e., emotional vs. instrumental support; Krause, 2001; Uchino, 2004). Although studies have examined the separate contribution of these facets to understanding health, they clearly coexist in daily life. For instance, individuals who are more socially active are likely to experience a larger social network and to derive multiple functions from the support provided (Krause, 2001). In fact, older individuals who experience the greatest physical health problems may be those who experience risk across the different facets of social support (Bosworth & Schaie, 1997). The literature has traditionally conceptualized social functioning as a risk factor leading to poorer health. However, poorer physical health could also limit one's ability to engage in productive social activities, reflecting a more transactional nature of the relationship. In this chapter we allude to these transactional relationships in the next section; a full treatment of social functioning and aging is beyond the space limitations in this chapter.

"Social activity" refers to the frequency of one's social contacts or interactions, and has been associated with positive emotional and physical outcomes (Uchino et al., 1996). In a longitudinal study, Menec (2003) found that participation in social and productive activities was associated with happiness, reduced physical and cognitive functional decline, and reduced mortality over a 6-year time span, whereas participation in several solitary activities was associated with happiness only. A social activation program aimed at increasing activity levels in the elderly was associated with improved neuroendocrine responses and maintenance of height (Arnetz, Theorell, Levi, & Kallner, 1983). Carstensen (1987) suggested that because physical activity and social activity go hand in hand in daily life, it is impossible to attribute findings linking social activity with successful aging to psychosocial variables alone.

Studies of the structure of the social network examine the existence, extensiveness, and interconnections of social ties, assessing the existence of a spouse, parents, siblings, other family relationships, and friends among the most common social network members (Uchino, 2004). In a meta-analysis of the relationship between physiological processes and social support Uchino and colleagues (1996) found that structural measures of support were associated as strongly with health outcomes as were functional measures of support, suggesting that the structure of the social network is as important to physical health as the actual functional support received from social ties.

Literature examining the relationship between social support and health also relies heavily on the quality or function of social relationships. A high amount of perceived support is seen as a positive aspect of a relationship and is associated with positive health outcomes (Uchino, 2004). Functional social support, such as emotional support, is related to lower cardiovascular mortality (Case, Moss, Case, McDermott, & Eberly, 1992; Orth-Gomer & Johnson, 1987), as well as all cause mortality (Uchino, 2004). In older adults, Blazer (1982) and Berkman and Syme (1979) found that low levels of perceived social support predicted negative health outcomes, whereas the level of social activity did not, suggesting that quality of relationships may be more important than quantity of contacts.

## Mechanisms of the Association between Social Functioning and Health

Several mechanisms may operate to account for the relationship between social support and physical health. First, social support may reduce the pathological effects of stress through appraisal processes that dampen the sympathetic–adrenomedullary (SAM) and hypothalamic–pituitary–adrenocortical (HPA) responses to stress (Lepore, 1998; Uchino et al., 1996). The amount of perceived emotional support may be a key feature in understanding reduced cardiovascular reactivity and immune function (Lepore, 1995). Although social support may also provide individuals with the encouragement to engage in less risky behaviors and seek treatment earlier (Berkman, 1995), such mechanisms do not seem to be largely responsible for the link between social support and physical health (Uchino et al., 1996).

## Social Functioning and Health Risk across Adult Development

The findings we have reviewed linking social support and measures of health must be understood in the context of normative developmental changes in the social network of adults across the lifespan. Multiple theories have been advanced to account for the general finding that as individuals age, both the frequency of social activity and size of the social network decline (Antonnuci, 2001). Disengagement theory describes the narrowing of the social world as a normative process whereby elders and society jointly disengage as a preparatory response to death (Cumming & Henry, 1961). In contrast, activity theory (Lemon, Bengston, & Peterson, 1972) asserts that optimal aging involves continued social engagement in late life, and that a reduction in social interaction is a result of declining health, reduction in the number of social roles, and the death of friends and relatives. Most current accounts rely on Carstensen's socioemotional selectivity theory (1987, 1991), which posits that the reduction in social interactions is an adaptive effort to control physiological and psychological reactivity by retaining energy for the most significant and emotionally satisfying relationships in late life. Research indicates that although social network sizes are reduced in very old age, individuals retain contact with persons to whom they are emotionally close in the network (Lang, Staudinger, & Carstensen, 1998). Therefore, quality of social relationships may be even more salient for healthy aging. As the social environment is actively narrowed, emotional closeness in significant relationships increases.

In this section we have reviewed the evidence linking personality and social support to indicators of physical health across the lifespan. We have alluded to a transactional process whereby these factors are not separate, but are inextricably connected (Smith, Glazer, et al., 2004; Smith & Spiro, 2002). For instance, hostile individuals and those displaying high neuroticism were described as being at risk because of not only their individual difference characteristics but also of the poor social support systems (high in conflict and small in number) that they experience. Recent risk profile analyses have revealed that individuals at greatest risk for aging unsuccessfully experience multiple psychosocial risk factors (Lang, Rieckmann, & Baltes, 2002; Smith & Baltes, 1999). In addition to personality and social functioning, these profile analyses indicate that cognitive function is a crucial variable in understanding risk and resilience (see also Gottfredson & Deary, 2004; Seeman et al., 2001). We now present a developmental framework that links these multiple risk factors together to understand the process whereby individuals can age successfully or unsuccessfully in terms of physical, cognitive, and social function.

## DEVELOPMENTAL FRAMEWORK FOR UNDERSTANDING RISK AND RESILIENCE IN PHYSICAL, COGNITIVE, AND SOCIAL FUNCTION

The developmental framework advanced here is consistent with broad theoretical lifespan principles put forth by Baltes, Lindenberger, and Staudinger (1998). Development is viewed as a lifelong process whereby events in child development are important in informing trajectories of physical health, cognitive functioning, and social integration across the lifespan. Although early temperamental predispositions and family systems provide the foundation for understanding trajectories of resilience versus risk for health (Repetti, Taylor, & Seeman, 2002), there is plasticity across lifespan development in terms of alterations in these trajectories (Aldwin et al., 2001; Siegler, Costa, et al., 2003). Furthermore, lifespan development occurs through age-graded (e.g., puberty, parenthood, menopause), history-graded (e.g., obesity epidemic, rise in divorce rate), and non-normative (e.g., development of chronic illness, early death of spouse) events.

### Successful Aging Begins Early in Life

Our framework traces the traditional risk factors associated with poor health in late adulthood to early personality predispositions, ways of interacting with the social world, and physiological stress responses that occur early in childhood. The view that successful aging begins early in life is consistent with recent biobehavioral models of the social and emotional processes that occur in risky families that may contribute to disruptions in stress regulatory systems, social competence, and negative health behaviors (Repetti et al., 2002; Ryff, Singer, Wing, & Love, 2001). Repetti et al. (2002) argue that in families characterized by anger and aggression, children who may already be predisposed for risk in social competence and physiological stress responses (because of the genetic predisposition for these same personality characteristics) may experience a cascade of risk. These families provide a context in which the development of normal emotion regulation (Eisenberg & Morris, 2002) and social skills (Coie & Dodge, 1998) may not occur and may lead to disruptions in SAM and HPA reactivity leading to the development of major chronic illness (e.g., hypertension, CHD) and death. Our framework traces how these early vulnerabilities may place individuals on particular trajectories of risk across the lifespan (Smith & Spiro, 2002), and how plasticity in these trajectories may also occur.

As reviewed earlier, personality is one important factor in understanding the trajectory of health that occurs across the lifespan (Aldwin et al., 2001; Siegler, Costa, et al., 2003). Neuroticism and hostility have been implicated in the incidence of illness such as CHD disease, coping with illness, and adherence to specific medical regimens (Smith & Ruiz, 2004; Spiro, Aldwin, Ward, & Mroczek, 1995). These personality characteristics can be traced in part to early patterns of temperament displayed in infancy and childhood that reflect relatively stable patterns of the quality and intensity of one's emotional reactions to events (Caspi & Silva, 1995; Räiikkönen et al., 2000). Räiikkönen et al. found that child's temperament and mother's child-rearing practices predicted hostile attitudes during preadolescence 9 years later. Furthermore, Keltikanagas-Jarvinen and Heinonen (2003) found that components of Type A behavior (i.e., impatience, aggression) predicted cognitive (cynicism and paranoid ideation) and emotional (irritation) components of hostility in adulthood 15 years later. Thus, evidence is accumulating that early childhood temperament and personality may be a precursor to the display of personality traits in adulthood that place individuals at risk for poor physical and health outcomes.

These early temperamental and personality characteristics hold important implications for the social and academic competence of children, and the types of social support networks on which children can draw to deal with stressful life events. Aggressive children process social situations with a hostile attribution bias that contributes to these hostile strategies in social problem-solving settings, leading to reduced quality and size of social networks (Coie & Dodge, 1998). These children experience difficulties at school due to numerous concomitant factors (attention difficulties, behavior problems, etc.) that compromise their cognitive functioning as well (Huesmann, Eron, & Yarmel, 1987). Such children enter a developmental trajectory toward poor social functioning, cognitive abilities, and physical health (Grunbaum, Vernon, & Clasen, 1997; Repetti et al., 2002).

## Developmental Trajectories of Successful and Unsuccessful Aging

An extensive literature demonstrates high relative stability (rank-order stability estimates average around .60 across many longitudinal studies) of personality characteristics from young adulthood through late adulthood (Costa & McCrae, 1994; Roberts & DelVecchio, 2000). Normative changes have been found such that during young adulthood, mean-level declines occur for neuroticism, extraversion, and openness to experience and increases for conscientiousness and agreeableness (Caspi & Roberts, 1999; Srivastava, John, Gosling, & Potter, 2003), whereas declines are seen later in middle-adulthood for hostility, with potential increases in late adulthood (Barefoot et al., 1993). Developmental trajectories that go against these normative trends appear to be particularly damaging to health outcomes. For instance, Siegler, Costa, et al. (2003) found that an increase in hostility from young to middle adulthood was particularly detrimental for a range of health risk factors.

Personality characteristics and social support have been associated with both cognitive and health outcomes. Results from several longitudinal studies (Arbuckle, Moag, Pushkar, & Chaikelson, 1998; Field, Schaie, & Leino, 1998; Gold et al., 1995; Schaie, 1996) suggest that early adulthood neuroticism and rigidity are associated with poorer cognitive function in late life, whereas introversion is associated with better cognitive function. The role of personality in understanding lifetime intellectual development is typically interpreted by understanding how personality may provide a characteristic way of adapting to the environment and selecting intellectual environments. For instance, introverts are thought to show better cognitive function in late life through a lifetime of greater reflection and processing of information (Gold et al., 1995). Neuroticism is thought to affect cognitive functioning through anxiety, and the resources that anxiety may draw from central working memory as individuals process information (Wetherell, Reynolds, Gatz, & Pedersen, 2002). Hostility may affect cognitive function through the effect of elevations in blood pressure on cognitive performance (Elias et al., 2001; Waldstein & Katzel, 2001) or the effect of development of CHD on cognitive function (Hertzog, Schaie, & Gribbin, 1978). Although little work has explicitly examined the link between social support and cognitive function, recent work indicates that the amount of social support, and particularly emotional support received predicts less longitudinal decline in cognitive function (Seeman et al., 2001).

Numerous critical events may provide further impetus for promoting an individual's trajectory toward successful or unsuccessful aging, or changes in this trajectory. One important event, marriage, promises to be particularly influential, because the vast majority of adults enter marriage at some point during adulthood (Fields & Cesper, 2001). Individuals choose mates that are more like them in physical characteristics, cognitive abilities, and personality traits (Epstein & Guttman, 1984). Furthermore, shared experiences within the marriage may play an important role in maintaining similarities in personality across time for spouses (Caspi, Herbener, & Ozer, 1992). Shared experiences within the marriage also may be responsible for the finding that couples become more similar across time in their cognitive functioning (Gruber-Baldini, Schaie, & Willis, 1995) and are at increased risk of having the same disease (Hippisley-Cox, Coupland, Pringle, Crown, & Hammersley, 2002). Disruptions in marriage, such as experiencing marital difficulties, divorce, or widowhood, may be associated with changes in these trajectories. For example, divorce is associated with personality changes in both men and women (Costa, Herbst, McCrae, & Siegler, 2000; Mroczek & Spiro, 2003) and reductions in health. Other non-normative events such as chronic illness and job loss may also be associated with changes in developmental trajectories (Aldwin et al., 2001).

These personality-based differences in adulthood continue to be associated with particular patterns of social interaction, social skills, and social support, as was true during childhood (Gallo & Smith, 1999; Mischel & Shoda, 1995). Perceived social support is associated with several personality characteristics, important in understanding health outcomes such as neuroticism and hostility (Costa, Zonderman, McCrae, & Williams, 1986). Similar to the literature we mentioned earlier on aggressive children, hostile individuals perceive other individuals with a hostile lens (Allred & Smith, 1991) and are perceived by others as less socially skilled. Thus, hostile or emotionally unstable individuals may perpetuate social environments that are unhealthy during adulthood, because they are unable to interact skillfully with others (Smith, 1992; Smith, Glazer, et al., 2004). Experiencing difficult interpersonal relationships may cross social relationships (e.g., family, friends), leaving the older adult with fewer social resources (Krause & Rook, 2003).

In late life, the frequency and chronicity of health and cognitive losses may potentially boost the predictive utility of psychosocial risk factors in understanding successful physical and cognitive functioning. Social support may be particularly important for older adults experiencing serious, chronic health conditions (Seeman & Chen, 2002) and cognitive dysfunction (Gurung, Taylor, & Seeman, 2003). The size and activity of one's social network may protect against physical and cognitive decline, because such ties may facilitate engaging in productive activities that may prevent such decline (i.e., "Use it or lose it"; Hultsch, Hertzog, Small, & Dixon, 1999), and boost self-efficacy and reduce depression (Seeman et al., 1996). Consistent with the transactional quality of our model, the ability to maintain an active social network may be affected by one's lifelong pattern of interacting with the world that has been linked to basic personality characteristics (e.g., hostility, neuroticism). This means that individuals experiencing depression and/or hostility may interpret their social world more negatively and receive less benefit from it (Krause & Rook, 2003). The tight connections among physical health, cognitive function, and social support in late life may allow for more distinct clusters or profiles of "successful" or "unsuccessful" aging, illuminating the role of the aggregation of a lifetime of psychosocial risk (Smith & Baltes, 1999).

## A Window into the Developmental Process: Physical and Cognitive Function in the Context of Marriage

The most direct support for the developmental processes outlined in this chapter has been with respect to the links between hostility, social support, and physical health (Repetti et al., 2002; Smith, Gallo, & Ruiz, 2002). As mentioned previously, hostility, which encompasses chronic anger, hostile beliefs and attitudes, and aggressive interpersonal behavior, is associated with increased risk of CHD, decreased longevity (see Friedman & Martin, Chapter 9, this volume; Smith, Orleans, et al., 2004), and death. One of the mechanisms underlying the poorer health outcomes of hostile individuals is a decrease in the quality of their social interactions (Smith, 1992). Hostile individuals experience more frequent and severe interpersonal stressors, such as conflicts at work and home, and they respond to related stressors (e.g., disagreement, provocation) with more reactive cardiovascular and neuroendocrine responses (Smith, Glazer, et al., 2004). The cumulative effects of more frequent and severe reactivity displayed by hostile persons is believed to contribute to the development of CHD and other threats to health and longevity (Williams, Barefoot, & Shekelle, 1985).

As mentioned previously, marriage is an important context for lifespan development and a particularly relevant social context for hostile individuals, who experience more marital distress and greater cardiovascular responses to stressful marital interactions (Newton & Kiecolt-Glaser, 1995; Smith, Pope, Sanders, Allred, & O'Keefe, 1988) than less hostile individuals. Marriage generally has beneficial effects on cardiovascular risk and longevity, but marital distress and disruption can have negative impacts (see Kiecolt-Glaser & Newton, 2001). Furthermore, unlike their more agreeable counterparts, hostile persons do not display attenuated physiological stress responses when they receive social support (Lepore, 1995; Smith, Uno, Uchino, & Ruiz, 2000). Thus, hostile individuals are likely to experience greater interpersonal distress in the marriage, greater cardiovascular reactivity when distressed, and are less likely to receive the positive benefits of being married.

Hostile persons may also not experience the socially productive activities that are important for maintaining cognitive function in late life, particularly within the context of the marital relationship. Collaboration during everyday problem solving (e.g., how to complete one's taxes, decisions regarding supplemental insurance, running errands) becomes increasingly important in later life, because it allows individuals to adapt to new demands and compensate for changes in cognitive functioning (Dixon & Gould, 1996). The spouse is a particularly important collaborator in daily problem solving among older adults (Berg, Johnson, Meegan, & Strough, 2003; Meegan & Berg, 2002). Compared to working alone, collaboration with the spouse can produce increased memory and problem-solving performance among older adults (Meegan & Berg, 2002). Effective collaboration requires cooperation, guidance, and mutual understanding. Critical or controlling behavior can impede progress and produce poorer cognitive outcomes (Berg et al., 2003). Given the increased marital distress and antagonistic marital interactions associated with hostility, collaborative interactions are likely to be both more stressful and less effective for hostile persons—and for those married to hostile persons. Chronically hostile individuals may be somewhat less likely to engage in such collaboration, because the necessary interactions would be emotionally negative and antagonistic. Thus, hostility may undermine everyday cognitive performance by disrupting interactions that are most conducive to cognitive adaptation among older adults. This represents a secondary cost of hostility that is particularly relevant to later life.

A developmental perspective is critical to understanding the social-psychophysiological mechanisms linking hostility and health in marital interactions, because of both the negative health effects of hostility that likely accrue over the course of many years, and the nature of marital interaction and adjustment changes across middle and late adulthood (Levenson, Carstensen, & Gottman, 1993). Compared to marriages of middle-aged couples, older couples' marriages involve less potential for conflict (Levenson et al., 1993), less negative and more affectionate behavior during conflict discussions (Carstensen, Gottman, & Levenson, 1995), and less reactive physiological responses to conflict. The increased affectionate behavior of long-term marriages in late life may be due to many factors, including cohort, the exit of children from the home, the attrition of older adults who divorced and were unsatisfied from the pool, and so on. Whatever the reason, these changes suggest "conflict" may not be as important an interpersonal stress for chronically hostile older adults as opposed to middle-aged adults. Instead, interpersonal stress may occur in the context of everyday problem solving that involves daily decisions and stressors (e.g., regarding health, finances, and interpersonal conflicts). To the extent that everyday problem solving revolves around problems with other people and involvement with others (Berg, Strough, Calderone, Samsone, & Weir, 1998; Strough, Berg, & Sansone, 1996), these collaborative interactions may be particularly stressful for chronically hostile individuals.

In summary, within the marital context we can see the effects of the traditional risk factors (e.g., hostility, social support) on physical and cognitive functioning. The cumulative effects of less satisfying social interactions and heightened reactivity displayed by hostile persons contribute to the development of CHD and other threats to health and longevity (Williams et al., 1985). In addition, chronically hostile individuals may be less likely to benefit from collaborative problem solving as an adaptation to cognitive demands in late adulthood (Dixon & Gould, 1996). Through disrupted social interactions and less frequent productive collaboration with the spouse, hostility may undermine cognitive performance and physical functioning among older adults.

## SUMMARY AND CONCLUSIONS

The developmental approach to psychosocial risk and successful aging illustrates the lifetime connection among personality, social support, and cognitive and physical functioning. The model indicates that successful aging may begin early in life as individuals, with their various temperamental predispositions, adapt to and shape their cognitive and social environments. This inextricable link between psychosocial risk and successful aging is maintained during adult development as individuals enter new social relationships such as marriage and adapt to changing cognitive demands. These psychosocial risk factors may become particularly important during late adulthood, when the balance is tipped toward adapting to losses as opposed to gains across the lifespan (Baltes et al., 1998).

We began this chapter with the question, "What are the processes whereby risk factors operate over the course of a lifespan to affect physical and cognitive outcomes?" This question assumes that physical health and cognition are outcomes, and personality and social support are risk factors that predict these end points. However, the transactional nature of our framework for successful aging breaks down the traditional assignment of risk factors as antecedents, and cognitive and physical functioning as end points. Rather than focusing only on the linear effects of risk factors predicting outcomes, the developmental process is likely to be much more dynamic and recursive. Adequate physical health may be needed in order for older adults to engage in the types of social activities that may be important in maintaining cognitive function. High cognitive function may allow for a lifetime of greater skills in handling difficult social and health situations that promote positive health practices and adherence to difficult medical regimens (Gottfredson & Deary, 2004). A greater understanding of the dynamic relations among these variables drawn from recent systems and transactional theories of human development is needed and will advance the construct of successful aging.

The lifespan nature of our developmental approach assumes greater importance as work in behavioral medicine begins to acknowledge the early precursors to poor health in late adulthood (Keltikangas-Jarvinen & Heinonen, 2003; Repetti et al., 2002; Siegler, Bosworth, & Merrill, 2003; Smith, Orleans, et al., 2004). The long-standing nature of the characteristic ways that individuals interact with their social world and the intricate connections among cognitive, physical, and social factors may pose challenges to beginning the process to change adaptations. Change may be more likely at particular transition points across the adult lifespan (e.g., marriage, divorce, serious health incidents). The importance of the marital relationship as a context for development may suggest that marriage could be targeted for change that may affect health, social engagement, and cognitive functioning (Ewart, Taylor, Kraemer, & Agras, 1984). Assisting individuals in aging successfully is important because an ever-increasing number of adults are expected to live into advanced old age (85+). It is likely that the answer to the question "How does one age successfully?" has its roots in early development and occurs via a complex transactional process.

## ACKNOWLEDGMENT

Preparation of this chapter was supported by Grant No. R01 AG 18903 from the National Institute on Aging.

## REFERENCES

Aldwin, C. M., Spiro, A., Levenson, M., & Cupertino, A. P. (2001). Longitudinal findings from the normative aging study: III. Personality, individual health trajectories, and mortality. *Psychology and Aging, 16*, 450–465.

Allred, K. D., & Smith, T. W. (1991). Social cognition in cynical hostility. *Cognitive Therapy and Research, 15*, 399–412.

Angerer, P., Siebert, U., Kothny, W., Muhlbauer, D., Mudra, H., & von Schacky, C. (2000). Impact of social support, cynical hostility and anger expression on progression of coronary atherosclerosis. *Journal of the American College of Cardiology, 15*, 1781–1788.

Antonucci, T. C. (2001). Social relations: An examination of social networks, social support, and sense of control. In J. E. Birren & K. W. Schaie (Eds.), *Handbook of the psychology of aging* (5th ed., pp. 427–453). New York: Academic Press.

Arnetz, B. B., Teorell, T., Levi, L., Kallner, A., & Eneroth, P. (1983). An experimental study of social isolation of elderly people: Psychoendocrine and metabolic effects. *Psychosomatic Medicine, 45*, 395–406.

Arbuckle, T. Y., Maag, U., Pushkar, D., & Chaikelson, J. S. (1998). Individual differences in trajectory of intellectual development over 45 years of adulthood. *Psychology and Aging, 13*(4), 663–675.

Baltes, P. B., Lindenberger, U., & Staudinger, U. M. (1998). Life-span theory in developmental psychology. In W. Damon (Series Ed.), R. M. Lerner (Vol. Ed.), *Handbook of child psychology* (Vol. 1, pp. 1029–1143). New York: Wiley.

Barefoot, J. C., Beckham, J. C., Haney, T. L., Siegler, I. C., & Lipkus, I. M. (1993). Age differences in hostility among middle-aged and older adults. *Psychology and Aging, 8*(1), 3–9.

Barefoot, J. C., Helms, M. S., Mark, D. B., Blumenthal, J. A., Califf, R. M., Haney, T.

L., et al. (1996). Depression and long term mortality risk in patients with coronary artery disease. *American Journal of Cardiology, 78,* 613–617.

Barefoot, J. C., & Schroll, M. (1996). Symptoms of depression, acute myocardial infarction, and total mortality in a community sample. *Circulation, 93,* 1976–1980.

Berg, C. A., Johnson, M. M. S., Meegan, S. P., & Strough, J. (2003). Collaborative problem-solving interactions in young and old married couples. *Discourse Processes, 35,* 33–58.

Berg, C. A., Strough, J., Calderone, K. S., Sansone, C., & Weir, C. (1998). The role of problem definitions in understanding age and context effects on strategies for solving everyday problems. *Psychology and Aging, 5,* 334–370.

Berkman, L. F. (1995). The role of social relations in health promotion. *Psychosomatic Medicine, 57,* 245–254.

Berkman, L. F., & Syme, S. L. (1979). Social networks, host resistance, and mortality: A nine-year follow-up study of Alameda County residents. *American Journal of Epidemiology, 109,* 186–204.

Blazer, D. G. (1982). Social support and mortality in an elderly community population. *American Journal of Epidemiology, 115,* 684–694.

Bosworth, H. B., & Schaie, K. W. (1997). The relationship of social environment, social networks, and health outcomes in the Seattle Longitudinal Study: Two analytical approaches. *Journals of Gerontology: Psychological Sciences, and Social Sciences, Series B, 52,* 197–205.

Brissette, I., Scheier, M. F., & Carver, C. S. (2002). The role of optimism in social network development, coping, and psychological adjustment during a life transition. *Journal of Personality and Social Psychology, 82*(1), 102–111.

Carney, R. M., Freedland, K., Rich, M., & Jaffe, A. S. (1995). Depression as a risk factor for cardiac events in established coronary heart disease: A review of possible mechanisms. *Annals of Behavioral Medicine, 17,* 142–149.

Carstensen, L. L. (1987). Age-related changes in social activity. In L. L. Carstensen & B. A. Edelstein (Eds.), *Handbook of clinical gerontology* (pp. 222–237). New York: Pergamon Press.

Carstensen, L. L. (1991). Socioemotional selectivity theory: Social activity in life-span context. *Annual Review of Gerontology and Geriatrics, 11,* 195–217.

Carstensen, L. L., Gottman, J. M., & Levenson, R. W. (1995). Emotional behavior in long-term marriage. *Psychology and Aging, 10*(1), 140–149.

Case, R. B., Moss, A. J., Case, N., McDermott, M., & Eberly, S. (1992). Living alone after myocardial infarction: Impact on prognosis. *Journal of the American Medical Association, 267,* 515–519.

Caspi, A., Herbener, E. S., & Ozer, D. J. (1992). Shared experiences and the similarity of personalities: A longitudinal study of married couples. *Journal of Personality and Social Psychology, 62*(2), 281–291.

Caspi, A., & Roberts, B. W. (1999). Personality continuity and change across the life course. In L. A. Pervin & O. P. John (Eds.), *Handbook of personality: Theory and research* (2nd ed., pp. 300–326). New York: Guilford Press.

Caspi, A., & Silva, P. A. (1995). Temperamental qualities at age three predict personality traits in young adulthood: Longitudinal evidence from a birth cohort. *Child Development, 66,* 486–498.

Cohen, S., & Herbert, T. (1996). Health psychology: Psychological factors and disease from the perspective of human psychoneuroimmunology. *Annual Review of Psychology, 47*, 113–142.

Cohen, S., Kaplan, J. R., & Manuck, S. B. (1994). Social support and coronary heart disease: Underlying psychological and biological mechanisms. In S. A. Schumaker & S. M. Czajkowski (Eds.), *Social support and cardiovascular disease* (pp. 195–222). New York: Plenum.

Coie, J. D., & Dodge, K. A. (1998). Aggression and antisocial behavior. In W. Damon (Series Ed.), & N. Eisenberg (Vol. Ed.), *Handbook of child psychology* (Vol. 3, pp. 779–862). New York: Wiley.

Costa, P. T., Jr., Herbst, J. H., McCrae, R. R., & Siegler, I. C. (2000). Personality at midlife: Stability, intrinsic maturation, and response to life events. *Assessment, 7*, 365–378.

Costa, P. T., Jr., & McCrae, R. R. (1987). Neuroticism, somatic complaints, and disease: Is the bark worse than the bite? *Journal of Personality, 55*, 299–316.

Costa, P. T., Jr., & McCrae, R. R. (1994). Set like plaster: Evidence for the stability of adult personality. In T. F. Heatherton & J. L. Weinberger (Eds.), *Can personality change?* (pp. 21–40). Washington, DC: American Psychological Association.

Costa, P. T., Jr., Zonderman, A. B., MacCrae, R. R., & Williams, R. B. (1986). Cynicism and paranoid alienation in the Cook and Medley HO Scale. *Psychosomatic Medicine, 48*, 283–285.

Cumming, E., & Henry, W. H. (1961). *Growing old: The process of disengagement.* New York: Basic Books.

Dixon, R. A., & Gould, O. N. (1996). Adults telling and retelling stories collaboratively. In P. B. Baltes & U. M. Staudinger (Eds.), *Interactive minds: Life-span perspective on the social foundation of cognition* (pp. 221–241). New York: Cambridge University Press.

Duberstein, P. R., Sorensen, S., Lyness, J. M., King, D. A., Conwell, Y., Seidlitz, L., et al. (2003). Personality is associated with perceived health and functional status in older primary care patients. *Personality and Aging, 18*, 25–37.

Eisenberg, N., & Morris, A. S. (2002). Children's emotion-related regulation. In R. V. Kail (Ed.), *Advances in child development and behavior* (Vol. 30, pp. 189–229). San Diego: Academic Press.

Elias, M. F., Elias, P. K., Robbins, M. A., Wolf, P. A., & D'Agostino, R. B. (2001). Cardiovascular risk factors and cognitive functioning: An epidemiological perspective. In S. R. Waldstein & M. F. Elias (Eds.), *Neuropsychology of cardiovascular disease* (pp. 83–104). Mahwah, NJ: Erlbaum.

Eng, P. M., Fitzmaurice, G., Kubzansky, L. D., Rimm, E. B., & Kawachi, I. (2003). Anger expression and risk of stroke and coronary heart diseases among male health professionals. *Psychosomatic Medicine, 65*, 100–110.

Epstein, E., & Guttman, R. (1984). Mate selection in man: Evidence, theory, and outcome. *Social Biology, 31*, 243–278.

Everson, S. A., Kauhanen, J., Kaplan, G., Goldberg, D., Julkunen, J., Tuomilehto, J., et al. (1997). Hostility and increased risk of mortality and myocardial infarction: The mediating role of behavioral risk factors. *American Journal of Epidemiology, 146*, 142–152.

Ewart, C. K., Taylor, C. B., Kraemer, H. C., & Agras, W. S. (1984). Reducing blood pressure reactivity during interpersonal conflict: Effects of marital communication training. *Behavior Therapy, 15*, 473–484.

Field, D., Schaie, K. W., & Leino, E. V. (1998). Continuity in intellectual functioning: The role of self-reported health. *Psychology and Aging, 3*(4), 385–392.

Fields, J., & Cesper, L. M. (2001). *America's families and living arrangements, March 2000.* (Current Population Reports, P20-537). Washington, DC: U.S. Census Bureau.

Gallo, L. C., & Smith, T. W. (1999). Patterns of hostility and social support: Conceptualizing psychosocial risk as a characteristic of the person and the environment. *Journal of Research in Personality, 33,* 281–310.

Gatz, M., Kasl-Godley, J. E., & Karel, M. J. (1996). Aging and mental disorders. In J. E. Birren & K. W. Schaie (Eds.), *Handbook of the psychology of aging* (4th ed., pp. 365–382). New York: Academic Press.

Gold, D. P., Andres, D., Etezadi, J., Arbuckle, T., Schwartzman, A., & Chaikelson, J. (1995). Structural equation model of intellectual change and continuity and predictors of intelligence in older men. *Psychology and Aging, 10,* 294–303.

Gottfredson, L. S., & Deary, I. J. (2004). Intelligence predicts health and longevity, but why? *Current Directions in Psychological Science, 13*(1), 1–4.

Gruber-Baldini, A. L., Schaie, K. W., & Willis, S. L. (1995). Similarity in married couples: A longitudinal study of mental abilities and rigidity flexibility. *Journal of Personality and Social Psychology, 69*(1), 191–203.

Grunbaum, J. A., Vernon, S. W., & Clasen, C. M. (1997). The association between anger and hostility and risk factors for coronary heart disease in children and adolescents: A review. *Annals of Behavioral Medicine, 19*(2), 179–189.

Gurung, R.A. R., Taylor, S. E., & Seeman, T. E. (2003). Accounting for changes in social support among married older adults: Insights from the MacArthur Studies of Successful Aging. *Psychology and Aging, 18*(3), 487–496.

Harris, K. F., Matthews, K. A., Sutton-Tyrell, K., & Kuller, L. H. (2003). Associations between psychological traits and endothelial function in postmenopausal women. *Psychosomatic Medicine, 65*(3), 402–409.

Helgeson, V. S., & Fritz, H. L. (1999). Cognitive adaptation as a predictor of new coronary events after percutaneous transluminal coronary angioplasty. *Psychosomatic Medicine, 61,* 488–495.

Hermann, C., Brano-Driehorst, S., Kaminsky, B., Leibring, E., Staats, H., & Ruger, U. (1998). Diagnostic groups and depressed mood as predictors of 22-month mortality in medical inpatients. *Archives of General Psychiatry, 46,* 345–350.

Hertzog, C., Schaie, K. W., & Gribbin, K. (1978). Cardiovascular disease and changes in intellectual functioning from meddle to old age. *Journal of Gerontology, 33,* 872–883.

Hippisley-Cox, J., Coupland, C., Pringle, M., Crown, N., & Hammersley, V. (2002). Married couples' risk of same disease: Cross sectional study. *British Medical Journal, 325*(7365), 636–640.

House, J. S., Landis, K. R., & Umberson, D. (1988). Social relationships and health. *Science, 241,* 540–545.

Huesmann, L. R., Eron, L. D., & Yarmel, P. W. (1987). Intellectual functioning and aggression. *Journal of Personality and Social Psychology, 52*(1), 232–240.

Hultsch D. F., Hertzog, C., Small, B. J., & Dixon, R. A. (1999). Use it or lose it: Engaged lifestyle as a buffer of cognitive decline in aging? *Psychology and Aging, 14,* 245–263.

Iribarren, C., Sidney, S., Bild, D. E., Liu, K., Markovitz, J. H., Roseman, J. M., et al.

(2000). Association of hostility with coronary artery calcification in young adults: The CARDIA study. *Journal of the American Medical Association, 283,* 2546–2551.

Januzzi, J. L., Stern, T. A., Pasternak, R. C., & DeSanctis, R. W. (2000). The influence of anxiety and depression on outcomes of patients with coronary artery disease. *Archives of Internal Medicine, 160,* 1913–1921.

Jones, B. S., Franks, P., & Ingram, D. D. (1997). Are symptoms of anxiety and depression risk factors for hypertension? *Archives of Family Medicine, 6,* 43–49.

Kaplan, G. A., Haan, M. N., & Wallace, R. B. (1999). Understanding changing risk factor associations with increasing age in adults. *Annual Review of Public Health, 20,* 89–108.

Keltikangas-Jarvinen, L., & Heinonen, K. (2003). Childhood roots of adulthood hostility: Family factors as predictors of cognitive and affective hostility. *Child Development, 74,* 1751–1768.

Kiecolt-Glaser, J. K., & Newton, T. L. (2001). Marriage and health: His and hers. *Psychological Bulletin, 27,* 472–503.

Kop, W. J. (1999). Chronic and acute psychological risk factors for clinical manifestations of coronary artery disease. *Psychosomatic Medicine, 61,* 476–487.

Krantz, D. S., & McCeney, M. K. (2002). Effects of psychological and social factors on organic disease. *Annual Review of Psychology, 53,* 341–369.

Krause, N. (2001). Social support. In R. H. Binstock & L. K. George (Eds.), *Handbook of aging and the social sciences* (5th ed., pp. 272–294). New York: Academic Press.

Krause, N., & Rook, K. S. (2003). Negative interaction in late life: Issues in the stability and generalizability of conflict across relationships. *Journals of Gerontology: Psychological Sciences and Social Sciences, Series B, 58,* 88–99.

Kubzansky, L. D., Kawachi, I., Spiro, A., Weiss, A. T., Vokanas, P. S., & Sparrow, D. (1997). Is worrying bad for your heart: A prospective study of worry and coronary heart disease in the Normative Aging Study. *Circulation, 95,* 818–824.

Lang, F. R., Rieckmann, N., & Baltes, M. M. (2002). Adapting to aging losses: Do resources facilitate strategies of selection, compensation, and optimization in everyday functioning? *Journals of Gerontology: Psychological Sciences and Social Sciences, Series B, 57,* 501–509.

Lang, F. R., Staudinger, U. M., & Carstensen, L. L. (1998). Perspectives on socioemotional selectivity in late life: How personality and social context do (and do not) make a difference. *Journals of Gerontology: Psychological Sciences and Social Sciences, Series B, 53,* 21–30.

Lemon, B. W., Bengston, V. L., & Peterson, J. A. (1972). An exploration of the activity theory of aging: Activity types and life satisfactions among in movers to a retirement community. *Journal of Gerontology, 27,* 511–523.

Lepore, S. J. (1995). Cynicism, social support, and cardiovascular reactivity. *Health Psychology, 14,* 210–216.

Lepore, S. J. (1998). Problems and prospects for the social support–reactivity hypothesis. *Annuals of Behavioral Medicine, 20,* 257–269.

Levenson, R. W., Carstensen, L. L., & Gottman, J. M. (1993). Long-term marriage: Age, gender, and satisfaction. *Psychology and Aging, 8*(2), 301–313.

Maruta, T., Colligan, R. C., Malinchoc, M., & Offord, K. P. (2000). Optimists vs. pessimists: Survival rate among medical patients over a 30-year period. *Mayo Clinic Proceedings, 75,* 140–143.

Matthews, K. A., Owens, J. F., Kuller, L. H., Sutton-Tyrell, K., & Jansen-McWilliams, L. (1998). Are hostility and anxiety associated with carotid atherosclerosis in healthy postmenopausal women? *Psychosomatic Medicine, 60,* 633–638.

McGuire, L., Kiecolt-Glaser, J. K., & Glaser, R. (2002). Depressive symptoms and lymphocyte proliferation in older adults. *Journal of Abnormal Psychology, 111,* 192–197.

Meegan, S. P., & Berg, C. A. (2002). Contexts, functions, forms, and processes of collaborative everyday problem solving in older adulthood. *International Journal of Behavioural Development, 26*(1), 6–15.

Mendes de Leon, C. F., Kop, W. J., de Swart, H. B., Bar, F. W., & Appels, A. P. (1996). Psychosocial characteristics and recurrent events after percutaneous transluminal coronary angioplasty. *American Journal of Cardiology, 77,* 252–255.

Menec, V. H. (2003). The relation between everyday activities and successful aging: A 6-year longitudinal study. *Journal of Gerontology: Social Sciences and Social Sciences, Series B, 58,* S74–S82.

Miller, T. Q., Smith, T. W., Turner, C. W., Guijarro, M. L., & Hallet, A. J. (1996). A meta-analytic review of research on hostility and physical health. *Psychological Bulletin, 119,* 322–348.

Mischel, W., & Shoda, Y. (1995). A cognitive-affective system theory of personality: Reconceptualizing situations, dispositions, dynamic, and invariance in personality structure. *Psychological Review, 102,* 246–268.

Mroczek, D. K., & Spiro, A. (2003). Modeling intraindividual change in personality traits: Findings from the normative aging study. *Journal of Gerontology: Psychological Sciences and Social Sciences, Series B, 58,* P153–P165.

Newton, T. L., & Kiecolt-Glaser, J. K. (1995). Hostility and erosion of marital quality during early marriage. *Journal of Behavioral Medicine, 18,* 601–619.

Orth-Gomer, K., & Johnson, J. V. (1987). Social network interaction and mortality: A six year follow-up study of a random sample of the Swedish population. *Journal of Chronic Diseases, 40,* 949–957.

Rabin, B. S. (1999). *Stress, immune function, and health: The connection.* New York: Wiley-Liss.

Räiikkönen, K., Katainen, S., Keskivaara, P., & Keltikangas-Jarvinen, L. (2000). Temperament, mothering, and hostile attitudes: A 12-year longitudinal study. *Personality and Social Psychology Bulletin, 26,* 3–12.

Repetti, R. L., Taylor, S. E., & Seeman, T. E. (2002). Risky families: Family social environments and the mental and physical health of offspring. *Psychological Bulletin, 128,* 330–366.

Roberts, B. W., & DelVecchio, W. F. (2000). The rank-order consistency of personality traits from childhood to old age: A quantitative review of longitudinal studies. *Psychological Bulletin, 126,* 3–25.

Rowe, J. W., & Kahn, R. L. (1998). *Successful aging.* New York: Pantheon Books.

Ryff, C. D., & Singer, B. H. (2003). The role of emotion on pathways to positive health. In R. J. Davidson & K. R. Scherer (Eds.), *Handbook of affective sciences* (pp. 1083–1104). London: Sage.

Ryff, C. D., Singer, B. H., Wing, E., & Love, G. D. (2001). Elective affinities and uninvited agonies: Mapping emotion with significant others onto health. In C. D.

Ryff & B. H. Singer (Eds.), *Relationship experiences and emotional well-being* (pp. 133–174). New York: Oxford University Press.

Schaie, K. W. (1996). *Intellectual development in adulthood: The Seattle Longitudinal Study.* New York: Cambridge University Press.

Scheier, M. F., Matthews, K. A., Owens, J. F., Schulz, R., Bridges, M. W., Magovern, G. J., & Carver, C. S. (1999). Optimism and rehospitalization after coronary artery bypass graft surgery. *Archives of Internal Medicine, 159,* 829–835.

Schulz, R., Bookwala, J., Knapp, J. E., Scheier, M., & Williamson, G. M. (1996). Pessimism, age, and cancer mortality. *Psychology and Aging, 11,* 304–309.

Seeman, T., & Chen, X. (2002). Risk and protective factors for physical functioning in older adults with and without chronic conditions: MacArthur Studies of Successful Aging. *Journals of Gerontology: Psychological Sciences and Social Sciences, Series B, 57*(3), S135–S144.

Seeman, T., McAvay, G., Merrill, S., Albert, M., & Rodin, J. (1996). Self-efficacy beliefs and change in cognitive performance: MacArthur Studies on Successful Aging. *Psychology and Aging, 11*(3), 538–551.

Seeman, T. E., Lusignolo, T. M., Albert, M., & Berkman, L. (2001). Social relationships, social support, and patterns of cognitive aging in healthy, high-functioning older adults: MacArthur Studies of Successful Aging. *Health Psychology, 20,* 243–255.

Segerstrom, S. C., Taylor, S. E., Kemeny, M. E., & Fahey, J. L. (1998). Optimism is associated with mood, coping, and immune change in response to stress. *Journal of Personality and Social Psychology, 74,* 1646–1655.

Siegler, I. C., Bosworth, H. B., & Merrill, F. (2003). Adult development and aging. In A. M. Nezu (Series Ed.), C. M. Nezu, et. al. (Vol. Eds.), *Handbook of psychology: Health psychology* (Vol. 9, pp. 487–510). New York: Wiley.

Siegler, I. C., Costa, P. T., Brummett, B. H., Helms, M. J., Barefoot, J. C., Williams, R. B., et. al. (2003). Patterns of change in hostility from college to midlife in the UNC Alumni Heart Study predict high-risk status. *Psychosomatic Medicine, 65,* 738–745.

Siegman, A. W. (1994). From Type A to hostility to anger: Reflections on the history of coronary-prone behavior. In A. W. Siegman & T. W. Smith (Eds.), *Anger, hostility, and the heart* (pp. 1–21). Hillsdale, NJ: Erlbaum.

Simonsick, E. M., Wallace, R. B., Blaser, D. G., & Gerkman, L. F. (1995). Depressive symptomatology and hypertension-associated morbidity and mortality in older adults. *Psychosomatic Medicine, 57,* 427–435.

Smith, J., & Baltes, P. B. (1999). Trends and profiles of psychological functioning in very old age. In P. B. Baltes & K. U. Mayer (Eds.), *The Berlin Aging Study: Aging from 70 to 100* (pp. 197–226). New York: Cambridge University Press.

Smith, T. W. (1992). Hostility and health: Current status of a psychosomatic hypothesis. *Health Psychology, 11,* 139–150.

Smith, T. W. (1994). Concepts and methods in the study of anger, hostility, and health. In A. W. Siegman & T. W. Smith (Eds.), *Anger, hostility, and the heart* (pp. 23–42). Hillsdale, NJ: Erlbaum.

Smith, T. W., Gallo, L. C., & Ruiz, J. M. (2002). Toward a social psychophysiology of cardiovascular reactivity: Interpersonal concepts and methods in the study of stress and coronary disease. In J. Suls & K. A. Wallston (Eds.), *Social psychological foundations of health and illness* (pp. 335–366). Blackwell.

Smith, T. W., Glazer, K., Ruiz, J. M., & Gallo, L. C. (2004). Hostility, anger, aggres-siveness and coronary heart disease: An interpersonal perspective on personality, emotion and health. *Journal of Personality, 72,* 1217–1270.

Smith, T. W., Orleans, C. T., & Jenkins, C. D. (2004). Prevention and health promo-tion: Decades of progress, new challenges, and an emerging agenda. *Health Psy-chology, 23,* 126–131.

Smith, T. W., Pope, M. K., Rhodewalt, F., & Poulton, J. L. (1989). Optimism, neuroticism, coping, and symptom reports: An alternative interpretation of the Life Orientation Test. *Journal of Personality and Social Psychology, 56,* 640–648.

Smith, T. W., Pope, M. K., Sanders, J. D., Allred, K. D., & O'Keefe, J. L. (1988). Cyni-cal hostility at home and work: Psychosocial vulnerability across domains. *Jour-nal of Research in Personality, 22,* 525–548.

Smith, T. W., & Ruiz, J. M. (2002). Psychosocial issues in the management of coro-nary heart disease. In A. J. Christensen & M. Antoni (Eds.), *Chronic physical disorders: Behavioral medicine's perspective.* Oxford, UK: Blackwell.

Smith, T. W., & Ruiz, J. M. (2004). Personality theory and research in the study of health and behavior. In T. Boll (Series Ed.) & R. Frank, J. Wallender, & A. Baum (Vol. Eds.), *Handbook of clinical health psychology: Models and perspectives in health psychology* (pp. 143–199). Washington, DC: American Psychological As-sociation.

Smith, T. W., & Spiro, A., III. (2002). Personality, health and aging: Prolegomenon for the next generation. *Journal of Research in Personality, 36,* 363–394.

Smith, T. W., Uno, D., Uchino, B. N., & Ruiz, J. M. (2000, October). *Hostility, social support from friends, and blood pressure reactivity in young women.* Paper pre-sented at the annual meeting of the Society for Psychophysiological Research, San Diego.

Spiro, A., Aldwin, C. M., Ward, K. D., & Mroczek, D. K. (1995). Personality and the incidence of hypertension among older men: Longitudinal findings from the nor-mative aging study. *Health Psychology, 14,* 563–569.

Srivastava, S., John, O. P., Gosling, S. D., & Potter, J. (2003). Development of person-ality in early and middle adulthood: Set like plaster or persistent change. *Journal of Personality and Social Psychology, 84,* 1041–1053.

Strack, S., Carver, C., & Blaney, P. (1987). Predicting successful completion of an af-tercare program following treatment for alcoholism: The role of dispositional optimism. *Journal of Personality and Social Psychology, 53,* 579–584.

Strough, J., Berg, C. A., & Sansone, C. (1996) The interpersonal context of everyday problem solving: The role of age, gender, and the problem context in understand-ing goals. *Developmental Psychology, 32,* 1106–1115.

Sykes, D. H., Arveiler, D., Salters, C. P., Ferrieres, J., McCrum, E., Amouyel, P., et al. (2002). Hostility, race, and glucose metabolism in nondiabetic individuals. *Dia-betes Care, 25,* 835–839.

Uchino, B. N. (2004). *Social support and physical health.* New Haven, CT: Yale Uni-versity Press.

Uchino, B. N., Cacioppo, J. R., & Kiecolt-Glaser, J. K. (1996). The relationship between social support and physiological processes: A review with emphasis on underlying mechanisms and implications for health. *Psychological Bulletin, 119,* 488–531.

Waldstein, S. R., & Katzel, L. I. (2001). Hypertension and cognitive function. In S. R.

Waldstein & M. F. Elias (Eds.), *Neuropsychology of cardiovascular disease* (pp. 15–36). Mahwah, NJ: Erlbaum.

Watson, D., & Clark, L. A. (1984). Negative affectivity: The disposition to experience aversive emotional states. *Psychological Bulletin, 96,* 465–490.

Watson, D., & Pennebaker, J. W. (1989). Health complaints, stress, and distress: Exploring the central role of negative affectivity. *Psychological Review, 96,* 234–254.

Wetherell, J. L., Reynolds, C. A., Gatz, M., & Pedersen, N. L. (2002). Anxiety, cognitive performance, and cognitive decline in normal aging. *Journal of Gerontology: Psychological Sciences and Social Sciences, Series B, 57*(3), 246–255.

Williams, R. B., Jr. (1994). Basic biological mechanisms. In A. W. Siegman & T. W. Smith (Eds.), *Anger, hostility, and the heart* (pp. 117–125). Hillsdale, NJ: Erlbaum.

Williams, R. B., Jr. (2000). Psychological factors, health, and disease: The impact of aging and the life cycle. In S. B. Manuck, R. Jennings, B. S. Rabin, & A. Baum (Eds.), *Behavior, health and aging* (pp. 135–151). Mahwah, NJ: Erlbaum.

Williams, R. B., Jr., Barefoot, J. C., & Shekelle, R. B. (1985). The health consequences of hostility. In M. A. Chesney & R. H. Rosenmann (Eds.), *Anger and hostility in cardiovascular and behavioral disorders* (pp. 173–185). New York: Hemisphere.

Zonderman, A. B., Herbst, J., Schmidt, C., Costa, P., & McCrae, R. R. (1993). Depressive symptoms as a non-specific graded risk for psychiatric diagnoses. *Journal of Abnormal Psychology, 102,* 544–552.

# CHAPTER 4

# Methods in Health Psychology

*Relevance to Aging*

HEATHER YOUNG
*and* PETER VITALIANO

The disciplines of gerontology and health psychology are natural complements of one another. Gerontology encompasses biopsychosocial aspects of aging from the cellular to the societal levels, and health psychology focuses on the study of interrelationships of biopsychosocial and behavioral processes with mental and physical health. Not surprisingly, more and more attempts have been made to integrate these two disciplines into what we refer to as "lifespan health psychology." Although such research has seen many advances, there are design and measurement issues that should be considered when applying methods in health psychology to research on aging.

In this chapter we present a paradigm for studying one area of great relevance to lifespan health psychology, namely, the influences of psychosocial and behavioral factors on both illness and disease. In the process we discuss common physiological measures used in health psychology to link psychosocial/behavioral factors with illness. In addition to explaining why such measures have been examined as mediating variables, we also discuss how these measures vary with age in the absence of illness (primary aging), and how they may be used to assess dysregulation and disease risk and presage disease (secondary aging). Finally, we discuss problems in measures (e.g., confounds in older adults) and designs in lifespan health psychology and offer possible solutions by providing recommendations for future research.

## PARADIGM FOR STUDYING
## PSYCHOSOCIAL/BEHAVIORAL FACTORS AND ILLNESS

Although health psychologists are interested in associations of illness with many types of psychosocial constructs and behavioral factors, one of the most highly studied is acute and chronic stress, probably because it is pervasive in world societies. The study of chronic stress is particularly important, because it is enduring and long term and, as such, is expected to influence illness outcomes. Many theoretical models have been proposed to explain complex relationships of chronic stress, psychosocial and behavioral responses, physiological responses, and illness outcomes. Figure 4.1 illustrates the pathways of a model that has been studied in various forms among health psychologists. These include associations among chronic stress, psychosocial factors (e.g., depression, anxiety), risky health habits, physiological dysregulation/risk, and subsequent health problems.

This model includes individual differences, such as vulnerabilities, that moderate relationships of stressors with illness and disease processes. As we discuss below, the model posits that the main effect latent constructs—exposures (here, chronic stress), vulnerabilities (e.g., gender, state anger), and resources (e.g., social support, positive coping)—are directly associated with latent constructs for psychosocial distress (e.g., depression or anxiety) and risky health habits (e.g., sedentary behavior, excessive alcohol use). Moreover, interactions among these constructs influence illness, over and above their main effects (Vitaliano, Maiuro, Bolton, & Armsden, 1987). This assertion is consistent with the stress–diathesis model (Mechanic, 1967). For example, two-way interactions of exposures and vulnerabilities predict distress and poorer health habits, which influence physiological dysregulation (discussed below), then illness. Vulnerabilities are therefore

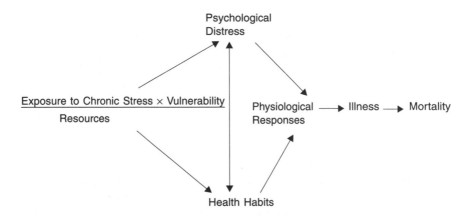

**FIGURE 4.1.** Model of the relationship between chronic stress and illness.

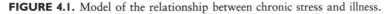

expected to moderate the relationship of chronic stress with health outcomes.

This model has been tested extensively in the context of the chronic stress of caregiving for a partner with Alzheimer's disease. Table 4.1 presents a proposed design that would allow examination of interactions between chronic stress (here, caregiving) and one type of vulnerability, namely, comorbid illness. By sampling persons with and without chronic stress and comorbid illness, one can use the resulting four groups (e.g., A, B, C, D) to test important hypotheses. These include the relative associations of chronic stress, chronic disease, and their interactions with psychosocial/behavioral constructs and physiological variables and the exacerbation/progression of illness or prediction of new cases of illness. As noted below, such a design allows one to assess the influences of chronic stress on physiological risk for severity of disease or the influence of disease on physiological risk for chronic stress. We conclude this chapter with a discussion of future directions in lifespan health psychology.

## COMMON PHYSIOLOGICAL MEASURES

Physiological measures in health psychology are commonly used to indicate stress responses and/or physiological dysregulation that may presage illness. Given that a major focus of health psychology is the study of relationships of psychosocial factors (e.g., stressors, distress), behavioral factors, and illness, physiological measures related to both stress and illness can be used to examine mediating processes. Indeed, many of these same measures are used in clinical medicine to diagnose illnesses and to plan treatment regimens. The rationale used here is that specific physiological pathways provide connections from chronic stressors to psychosocial distress/risky behaviors to stress hormones to subsequent physiological dysregulation downstream, then to physical health problems.

The predominant physiological response to stress occurs via the hypothalamic-pituitary-adrenal axis, from which corticotropic hormone–adrenocorticotropic hormone and cortisol are secreted, and the sympathetic adrenomedullary axis, from which norepinephrine and epinephrine are secreted (Steptoe, Cropley, Griffith, & Kirschbaum, 2000; also discussed by Eppel, Burke, & Wolkowitz, Chapter 7, this volume). These hormones stimulate peripheral activity, intended to respond to acute stress. In the context of chronic stress; however, consistent stimulation of this response can lead to "allostatic load" or wear and tear from repeated arousal and inefficient control of physiological responses (McEwen, 2000). Distress may also trigger risky health behaviors, such as poor diet, sedentary behavior, and substance abuse. These pathways may contribute to illness by increasing cardiovascular, metabolic, or immunological dysregulation (also discussed

TABLE 4.1. Stress, Aging, Health Habits, Psychological Distress, and Physiological Dysregulation among Four Groups

|  | Noncaregivers | Caregivers (exposure to chronic stress) |
|---|---|---|
| No chronic disease | Group A<br>• No chronic caregiving stress, no chronic disease, life stress<br>• Primary aging<br>• Likely to have good health habits<br>• Minimal psychological distress<br>• No physiological dysregulation | Group B<br>• Caregiving, no chronic disease, life stress<br>• Primary aging<br>• Likely to have good health habits<br>• Psychological distress<br>• No physiological dysregulation |
| Chronic disease | Group C<br>• No chronic caregiving stress, life stress, chronic disease<br>• Primary and secondary aging<br>• Likely to have good health habits<br>• Psychological distress<br>• Physiological dysregulation | Group D<br>• Caregiving, life stress, chronic disease<br>• Primary and secondary aging<br>• Unlikely to have good health habits<br>• Psychological distress<br>• Increased physiological dysregulation |

in this volume by Cooper, Katzel, & Waldstein, Chapter 8; Epel et al., Chapter 7; and Gruenewald & Kemeny, Chapter 6). As such, they should help to explain why psychosocial/mental health problems and risky behaviors are associated with physical illnesses (Fischer & Raschke, 1997; Musselman, Evans, & Nemeroff, 1998).

Physiological measures may be used several ways to examine physiological functioning in the absence of stressors, physiological functioning in response to stress, physiological functioning in response to age (primary aging), physiological dysregulation as a response to distress and health habits and/or as predictors/indicators of illness (what we later refer to as secondary aging). The difference between primary and secondary aging is expected to result from psychosocial distress and health behaviors.

Several categories of measures have been used to study physiological functioning in health psychology. The categories include stress hormones/ neurotransmitters, cardiovascular measures, metabolic measures, and immunological measures. Here we briefly discuss each type of measure and provide its description and references that support its relationships with stressors and illness. We assume that stressors negatively affect physiological risk, which in turn increases illness risks. Stressors increase stress hormone levels, which increase blood pressure and glucose; hypertension increases cardiovascular disease (CVD) risk; and high glucose and obesity increase risk for Type II diabetes. Also, indicators of immune function such as wound healing, and antibodies to vaccinations and Epstein–Barr virus

(EBV) herpes simplex virus (HSV), have strong links with health outcomes. Physiological indicators that are most proximal to the stress response show the greatest effect size. For example, measures that are immediately responsive to central nervous system arousal, such as stress hormones (e.g., cortisol, epinephrine, norepinephrine), are expected be more related to chronic stress than more peripheral cardiovascular (e.g., elevated blood pressure) and metabolic responses (e.g., increased blood glucose levels; Lovallo & Thomas, 2000). Variations also exist in the associations of psychosocial variables and immunity. Meta-analyses of studies examining the effect of stress and depression on immune measures have reported that mean effect sizes for antibodies generated in response to viral stimulation are larger than T-cell counts and natural killer cell activity in similar studies that examine immune outcomes (Herbert & Cohen, 1993a, 1993b).

## Stress Hormones and Neurotransmitters

The autonomic system consists of the sympathetic and parasympathetic systems, complementary negative feedback systems needed to maintain homeostasis. The sympathetic system, characterized by the "fight–flight" response to acute stress, generally stimulates the body, whereas the parasympathetic inhibits or relaxes the body after the threat has passed. During the fight–flight response, heart rate, blood pressure, and perspiration increase and airways dilate. At the same time, the parasympathetic "rest and digest" phase becomes inhibited, readying the body for anticipated danger. Cortisol and catecholamines, such as epinephrine and norepinephrine, are secreted in response to stress, and increase cardiac function and blood pressure (BP). These are commonly used physiological indicators of the stress response.

Other stress hormones and neurotransmitters that have been examined by health psychologists include ACTH (adrenocorticotropic hormone), prolactin, neuropeptide Y, beta-receptor function, and gamma-aminobutyric acid (GABA). ACTH stimulates cortisol release, whereas prolactin has an immune stimulating effect in response to stress. Neuropeptide Y increases catecholamine activities and influences feeding behaviors. Beta receptors mediate relationships between catecholamines, cardiac function, and BP. The neurotransmitter GABA counters certain stress responses.

## Cardiovascular Measures

Common cardiovascular measures are systolic and diastolic blood pressure and heart rate. Blood pressure fluctuates as the heart beats, from the highest pressure, or systolic blood pressure (SBP) to the lowest pressure, or diastolic blood pressure (DBP). Blood pressure is reported as SBP/DBP. A SBP greater than 140 or a DBP greater than 90 at rest define hypertension, which is associated with CHD and mortality. Heart rate reflects the work of the heart. An elevated rate occurs in response to stress; at rest, an elevated rate is an indication of compensation for reduced heart function. (See Cooper et al., Chapter 8, this volume for a discussion of age and heart rate variability.)

## Metabolic Measures

An overall indicator of metabolic balance, the body mass index (BMI), is calculated as weight (in kilograms) divided by height (in meters squared). Values of BMI over 30 usually reflect obesity. Metabolic function is also assessed through blood levels of hormones and chemicals. The endocrine system relies on homeostasis, a process of negative feedback, to control chemical levels. If the level of a substance rises or drops beyond the normal limits of the body, the corrective homeostatic influence reverses the process. Examples of metabolic indicators in the blood include cholesterol, insulin, glucose, and transferrin.

Low-density lipoprotein (LDL) cholesterol and triglycerides are measures of blood lipid levels, and are associated with obesity and CHD risk. High-density lipoprotein (HDL) cholesterol, another blood lipid, is associated with physical fitness and reduced CHD risk. Insulin increases after meals to promote glucose storage. Glucose is necessary for muscular activity and proper brain function, but a high fasting glucose (110+) suggests glucose intolerance and possible diabetes, conditions associated with CHD risk. Finally, transferrin is an index of stored iron in the body. Low iron levels may be associated with anemia.

## Immunological Measures

The ability of the body to remain healthy is dependent on whether it can defend against infections, diseases, and cancers. The lymphatic system, the primary system responsible for immunity against microorganisms or pathogens, consists of many different specialized cells, such as lymphocytes, lymph fluid for transportation, and lymphoid organs that produce lymphocytes. T-cells account for 80% of all lymphocytes and are responsible for attacking foreign microorganisms or cells that have been infected by them. Helper T-cells call other T-cells and β-cells into the attack, whereas suppressor T-cells send a signal to stop the attack. Immune measures include absolute counts of immune factors (enumerative cellular immunity) and measure of immune function. In general, increases in immune indices suggest an active process of fighting off disease, and immune suppression suggests compromised immune function.

Enumerative cellular immunity is examined by lymphocyte counts and percentages of different subsets (e.g., CD4, CD8, CD4/CD8 ratios, etc.). A high white blood cell (WBC) count is generally associated with active infections. High levels of some immune cells are generally associated with health and others, with infectious illness. CD4 cells are considered to be positively related to the capacity to defend against many illnesses, and a low CD4 count can be caused by severe disease (e.g., HIV infection) and can increase susceptibility to opportunistic infections. Higher natural killer cell (CD56) and B-cell counts are generally thought to reflect better immune reserves. In contrast, high CD8 (cytotoxic T-cells) counts may reflect an overactive immune system or a current illness the immune system has difficulty controlling. As such, the CD4:CD8 ratio is used as an immunological index, with higher ratios suggesting stronger immunity.

Functional immune measures include antibodies. β-cells are produced in the bone marrow. Their main role in fighting pathogens is to secrete antibodies that attach to the receptors of pathogens (e.g., antigens), making them inert. When the antigens are blocked, the pathogen cannot attach to healthy cells; therefore, it cannot spread its infection. Antibodies may be measured in response to vaccinations. Antibodies are assessed by immunoglobulin G (IgG) responses to HSV-1 and vaccination, EBV, viral capsid antigen (VCA) IgG titers, and immunoglobulin. High antibody responses reflect health. Although different diseases can result in increases or decreases in immunoglobulins, in the absence of disease, lower levels tend to reflect poorer immunity.

Other functional immune measures evaluate the response of the immune system to certain challenges. Lymphocyte proliferation is assessed in response to mitogens such as phytohemagglutinin (PHA), concanavalin A (Con A), and pokeweed (PW). Low levels may suggest illness susceptibility. Natural killer cell activity (NKA) and lymphokine-activated killing (LAK) are early defenses against tumor cells and viral infections, independent of prior exposure. NKA measures include unstimulated killing response to tumor cells and response to tumor cells after cytokine stimulation (e.g., interleukin-2 [IL-2] or interferon-gamma), which may better reflect *in vivo* NKA. Moderate/high NKA is consistent with good health; chronically low NKA may reflect disease susceptibility. Delayed-type hypersensitivity (DTH) response is the body's capacity to respond to multiple antigens (e.g., tuberculin, Tetanus, Streptococcus, Diptheria, Candida, Trichophyton, and Proteus), usually 48 hours after exposure. Two typical response measures are the number of positive antigen reactions and the diameter of the antigenic skin response (induration). Tumor necrosis factor (TNF) is an inflammatory cytokine. High levels promote loss of muscle tissue, aging, and poor general health. Cytokine secretion has complex effects on immunological responses and can affect cellular–immune responses (e.g., activating macrophages) and humoral immunity through β-cell activation.

As has been illustrated, a variety of neuroendocrine, cardiovascular, metabolic, and immune measures are available to examine physiological responses to stress across body systems. Specific selections are made according to study hypotheses and the sensitivity of the particular assay to the hypothesized psychological–physiological pathway.

## PHYSIOLOGICAL MEASURES AND AGING

Physiological measures vary with age in the absence of illness (primary aging), suggest disease risk in the presence of dysregulation, and presage disease (secondary aging). There are two types of physiological/physical changes with age: primary (normal age changes that are universal, progressive, and irreversible) and secondary (disease-related) changes (DiGiovanna, 2000). For this reason, aging is of great importance to health psychology, and interactions of psychological variables, and primary and secondary aging are all important areas of study.

### Primary Aging Processes

Primary aging processes refer to normative and universal changes that occur with aging and affect the physical structures and functioning of the body. In general, these changes affect homeostasis and the ability of the body to respond to physical and psychological stressors. The rate of aging and the time at which changes become apparent vary within the human body, with some organs showing age effects decades before others. The rate of aging also varies widely among individuals and is related both to genetic factors and to behaviors. This variability in the aging process results in increasing heterogeneity among older adults, and greater difficulty in creating normative values for physiological measures according to chronological age.

An important concept in understanding the effects of primary aging on physiological and psychological responses, reserve capacity, refers to the range of an individual's possible responses to physical and/or psychological challenges (Hoyer & Rybash, 1999). Under resting conditions, only a small proportion of healthy organ function is needed to maintain homeostasis; the unused fraction is called "reserve capacity." With age, the reserve capacity of several major organs and body systems diminishes. For example, age-related changes in kidney function, diminished skin elasticity, decreased cardiac and pulmonary reserve, decreased glucose tolerance, and decreased physical endurance, strength, and stamina all have the potential to affect the ability of an individual to respond physiologically to external stressors (DiGiovanna, 2000; Vandervoort, 2002). Reserve capacity is helpful in understanding the effects of age on risk for increased deleterious outcomes.

Several age-related changes are relevant to an individual's capacity to respond to stress. Although the ability of the heart to supply the body with blood under usual conditions remains essentially unchanged, maximum exercise capacity generally declines with age. The body adapts to reductions in maximum heart rate by increasing stroke volume, so that cardiac output remains unchanged. Myocardial muscles require more oxygen during strenuous activity to pump the same amount of blood, which results in efficiency decline when the body is under exertion. In the central nervous system, there are a loss of neurons, general atrophy, and a decline in the functioning of neurotransmitter and synaptic systems. Older adults have a natural rise of the sympathetic neurotransmitter norepinephrine (NE) in the body during the normal, day-to-day resting phase. Also, when a stressor is perceived as dangerous, NE levels increase more quickly, partly because of higher initial levels. Finally, once the stressor is controlled, NE levels take longer to decline. Moreover, as a by-product of greater NE levels, receptors of NE need higher quantities to be activated. This is known as habituation, and it results from the greater amount of NE already in the system. As part of primary aging, endocrine and other biochemical functions change, including decreases in the amount of estrogen in women and testosterone in men. Hormonal increases in glucose also occur.

The effectiveness of the immune system tends to be diminished in late life, with a reduction in the speed, strength, and duration of immune responses. Lymphocytes originate in the bone marrow, then migrate to different parts of the body to become specialized in fighting pathogens. Two types of lymphocytes that have adverse, age-related changes are T-cells and β-cells. Seventy-five percent of older adults show some decline in T-cell production/maturation, related to declining thymic hormone levels. The reduction in T-cells has adverse affects on the immune system, with a weaker and less coordinated response to pathogens. The production and maturation of β-cells are not affected by age. However, weak signals from helper T-cells mean that too few β-cells arrive to assist and may be outnumbered and overrun. For these reasons, older adults are at higher risk for influenza, and their response to vaccination is lower than that in younger adults (Bernstein, Gardner, Abrutyn, Gross, & Murasko, 1998).

## Secondary Aging Processes

In contrast to primary aging, the processes of secondary aging are pathological, including the negative effects of previous unhealthy behaviors (e.g., reduced glucose tolerance related to obesity), disuse (e.g., reduced muscle strength related to a sedentary lifestyle), or disease processes. There are three main reasons for higher rates of disease among older adults. The first is a reflection of a reduction in the ability to maintain homeostasis, resulting in the development of disease. The second reason is that it takes years for some diseases to develop, and they become apparent in late life. Finally, advanced age is associated with greater exposure over time to factors that promote disease, such as trauma, pathogens, environmental contaminants, and radiation.

Secondary aging further contributes to the variability in physiological functioning that exists among persons of the same chronological age. Disease-related changes with age increase one's relative risk of dying versus that of the population as a whole. For example, hypertension, a major player in accelerated aging, retards proper functioning of many systems of the body and advances the aging process. Aging of arteries is of great importance, because the amount of oxygen and nutrients that enter the cells is diminished. This not only affects the cardiovascular system, but it influences the entire body and causes aging to occur more quickly.

CVD, the leading cause of death for adult Americans, accounts for more than 40% of all deaths. It is the second most common chronic disease in individuals over 65 years of age. In coronary artery disease, arteries become less elastic and plaque lines the artery walls, decreasing their capacity to supply adequate blood to cardiac muscles, which reduces blood flow to vital organs and increases the risk for myocardial infarction. Arteries throughout the body are similarly affected by arteriosclerosis. Over time, this causes SBP to rise. During strenuous exertion, the plaque-lined arteries cannot expand properly. BP is a function of sympathetic and parasympathetic systems working together. Homeostasis ensures that if blood pressure is too high, the parasympathetic system will be activated to reduce blood pressure and if blood pressure is too low, the sympathetic system will increase blood pressure. With age, the ability to make adjustments in the autonomic system diminishes.

## PREVALENCE OF MORBIDITY AND COMORBIDITY IN OLDER ADULTS

More than 80% of persons over 70 years of age have at least one chronic physical illness, and many have multiple chronic conditions. According to 2004 statistics, among men over 65 years of age, 47% have hypertension, 37% have heart disease, 18% have diabetes, and 25% have cancer; among women over 65, 52% have hypertension, 27% have heart disease, 14% have diabetes, and 18% have cancer (Federal Interagency Forum on Aging Related Statistics, 2004). The prevalence of mental disorders among older community-dwelling adults varies from 15 to 25%, depending on the population and type of mental disorder (Hooyman & Kiyak, 2005). Although not stratified to identify older adults, two population studies have shown that the comorbidity of mental conditions is widespread (Reiger et al., 1990). The recent National Comorbidity Survey replication showed that psychiatric comorbidity is pervasive, with 45% of persons with a lifetime history of at least one DSM-IV disorder having a second diagnosis (Kessler,

Chiu, Demler, & Walters, 2005). Among persons in the National Comorbidity Survey, 46.4% had a lifetime history of any DSM-IV disorder, while 27.7% had two, and 17.3% had three or more disorders (Kessler, Berglund, et al., 2005). Although psychiatric disorders are widespread, the major burden of psychopathology is concentrated within the 14% of the population with severe symptoms (Kessler, Chin, et al., 2005).

## MEASUREMENT AND DESIGN ISSUES WITH OLDER ADULTS

The effects of aging on physiological measures are difficult to quantify in a general way for several reasons. Developmental norms for biological measures are well established for the young and middle years, but there is a tendency to combine all older adults into an "over 65 years of age" group. This is a significant problem considering that the heterogeneity among older adults increases with age as the complex interactions between primary aging and disease trajectories develop. In addition, there is considerable variability in the rate of change in specific body systems within and between individuals. The ages between 65 and 105 represent a full 40 years; physiologists would never consider a newborn and a person in middle age as being equivalent biologically. Therefore, biological and functional diversity among older adults is to be expected and must be considered when interpreting data.

Norms for many physiological measures have been established through extrapolation rather than empirical data, and therefore require further study to increase the reliability of the values by age group. Physiological measures are further confounded by polypharmacy and concurrent disease conditions. Medications can alter physiological values intentionally (e.g., in antihypertensive therapy to lower BP) or unintentionally as a side effect (e.g., in anti-inflammatory steroid therapy that increases blood glucose). One approach to assessing physiological measures in older adults is to compare their results both to existing norms and to their previous patterns and status, assessing intraindividual change rather than comparison to an absolute, extrapolated value.

### Cultural Differences

In addition to demographic trends favoring an aging population, older adults are becoming more ethnically diverse, a trend that has been called the "browning of the graying of America" (Hayes-Bautista, Hsu, Perez, & Gamboa, 2002). Health disparities based on ethnicity have received more attention in recent years. Of particular importance are data revealing different patterns of disease and mortality among different ethnic groups, with some subgroups exhibiting greater risk for certain diseases and others having protective factors. For example, Latino and Asian/Pacific Islander mortality is approximately 40% lower than that of non-Hispanic whites, whereas African American mortality is 7% higher (Hayes-Bautista et al., 2002). This discrepancy is not explained by the usual risk factors associated with mortality, such as education, income, and access to care. The important issue here is to consider relative risk and disease expression according to patterns exhibited by specific ethnic groups rather than combining minority elders into one group. Clearly, the model in Figure 4.1 suggests that in addition to genetic factors, psychosocial, behavioral, and physiological factors should help to explain such differences in mortality. For a more extensive discussion, please see Yee and Chiroboga, Chapter 15, this volume.

## Assessment Context

Ideally, physiological measures should be obtained in a context that most closely approximates normal life, and collected concurrently with survey data. Traveling to a clinic setting, being in an unfamiliar environment, and experiencing anxiety associated with physical examinations are all stressors in themselves that can alter physiological measures. However, clinic and laboratory settings potentially offer greater reliability in measurement, with more careful calibration of instruments, and ready storage and transportation of samples. Conducting measurements in the field, or in individuals' homes, requires careful protocols for collecting data and transporting biological samples. Older adults who have compromised cognitive or behavioral functioning may have greater difficulty following research protocols.

## Recruitment and Selection Bias

Studies of the effects of stress on psychophysiological functioning are most effective when conducted over time, because the influences of stress are expected to take time and to be reflected in changes among vulnerable, exposed individuals. Access to populations under stress is sometimes biased in favor of those who utilize health services, unless comprehensive community-based recruitment approaches are used. Further selection bias may be introduced by individuals who are under the greatest stress. Such persons may either feel that participating in a study is undesirable or that participation will be therapeutic. This introduces more variability in the samples studied than that found among general populations of persons under stress.

Changes with age, such as development of cognitive impairment, sensory loss (hearing or vision), and changes in mobility (the ability to walk or to drive) can further introduce selection bias, because these individuals may not elect to participate. In designing research with older adults, careful examination of the prevalence of common changes with age within the sample can promote recruitment and inclusion of participants who represent the range of functional ability and health status of the total population.

## DESIGN ISSUES IN LIFESPAN HEALTH PSYCHOLOGY: AN EXAMPLE FROM CAREGIVER RESEARCH

The goals of observational research in health psychology are to describe and manage illness by examining associations between variation and exposure to agents external to the individual, variations in vulnerabilities of individuals, and variations in resources of the person and environment (see Figure 4.1). Longitudinal studies are ideal for examining these relationships over time, yet funding cycles preclude optimal examination of the entire disease trajectory. For example, in a 5-year study, it would be difficult to design observations over more than 2 years. However, the inclusion of older adults (vs. young adults) increases the chance of observing dysregulation in physiology, by virtue of the acceleration of these changes with age.

Caregiving research exemplifies the methodological issues in examining psychosocial and physiological variables among an aging cohort and is presented here as an illustration of the most salient issues. We now discuss some studies that we have conducted to support the importance of examining interactions between individual vulnerabilities and chronic stress exposures. In contrast to the prediction of illness from chronic stress, this research focuses on the importance of exacerbations and progressions of illnesses in persons with chronic illnesses who are also under chronic stress. We believe that physiological dysregulation in persons with chronic illnesses who are exposed to chronic stress is just as important to the well-being of older adults as new cases of illnesses induced by stress. For this reason, studies of disease progression are just as meaningful as studies that predict incident illnesses: We illustrate this design using Groups D versus C and B versus A in Table 4.1.

### Comorbidity of Mental/Physical Health Problems and Chronic Stress

Epidemiologists have traditionally been much more concerned with the causes than with the consequences of the illnesses they study. In our previous work with older adults, and consistent with the diathesis–stress model, we found that 73% of caregivers with a history of diagnosed depression had a recurrence of depression while they were caregivers, but only 30% of noncaregivers with such a history had a recurrence during a similar time frame (Russo & Vitaliano, 1995; Russo, Vitaliano, Brewer, Katon, & Becker, 1995). Comorbid medical illnesses are important because many caregivers are middle-aged to older adults who may become ill before they become caregivers (Vitaliano, Zhang, & Scanlan, 2003). In other words, they are members of Group D (Table 4.1). In fact, medical illnesses may interact with caregiver status to explain variability in physiological measures that are relevant to these illnesses.

A history of cancer may predispose one to immunological risk (Fawzy et al., 1993), and caregivers with cancer histories (Group D) have been shown to have lower NKA than noncaregivers with cancer histories (members of Group C). In contrast, NKA did not differ in caregivers and noncaregivers free of cancer histories (Vitaliano, Scanlan, Ochs, et al., 1998; members of Groups A and B). This may be important, because a major function of NKA is to attack tumors (Herbert & Cohen, 1993b).

In another study, no effect was observed for normotensive caregivers (Group B) and normotensive noncaregivers (Group A) in SBP reactivity to a laboratory stressor, but hypertensive caregivers (Group D) showed greater reactivity than did hypertensive noncaregivers (Group C; Vitaliano, Bailey, Young, & McCann, 1993). This result may be significant because persons who are hypertensive are at higher risk for reactivity, and reactivity is a risk factor for hypertension (Pickering & Gerin, 1990). Hence, chronic stress and a comorbid condition may yield synergistic effects in physiological functioning. Finally, caregivers with coronary disease (Group D) have been shown to have higher levels of the metabolic syndrome, a linear combination of higher fasting glucose, insulin, lipid levels, mean arterial pressure, and obesity, than noncaregivers with coronary disease (Group C). However, no difference was observed for caregivers and noncaregivers free of such disease (Vitaliano, Scanlan, Siegler, McCormick, & Knopp, 1998; Group A vs. Group B).

Although research allows one to study whether caregivers with comorbid illnesses have more disease progression than noncaregivers with such illnesses, this paradigm can be extended to any combinations of comorbidities, such as mental illness (e.g., depression) and physical illness (e.g., coronary disease), or bereavement and diabetes, and so on. To be of concern to society, chronic stress does not have to cause illnesses; it only has to contribute to illness progression and symptoms that affect quality of life. These results may be important, because the metabolic syndrome is a risk factor for Type II diabetes and coronary disease (Schneiderman & Skyler, 1996) and caregivers with diabetes and/or coronary disease may be at higher risk than noncaregivers with coronary disease for severe complications from this disease. Given the work cited earlier, this may be especially true for caregivers who have heart disease/diabetes and depression.

## Caregiver and Care Recipient Trajectories and Reciprocal Dyadic Relationships

The studies we discussed for comorbidity and caregiving are cross-sectional analyses of longitudinal data. They do suggest, however, that caregivers with comorbid psychiatric and medical conditions should be studied for disease progression relative to noncaregivers with comorbid conditions. For example, the decline trajectories may be steeper in caregivers with coronary disease than in noncaregivers with coronary disease, because the former are more vulnerable to physiological risk and complications. Indeed, caregivers at highest risk for problems may be those with diabetes and comorbid depression. In addition to showing that caregiving predicts new illnesses in caregivers at higher rates than in noncaregivers, researchers should assess whether caregivers with comorbid conditions are at higher risk for exacerbation of their conditions than are noncaregivers with such conditions. By studying caregivers with comorbidity, one can assess relationships between health declines in vulnerable caregivers and health declines in care recipients, and assess whether care recipients of vulnerable caregivers decline faster than care recipients of less vulnerable caregivers (Vitaliano et al., 2003). Finally, the influences of primary and secondary aging on physiological measures should be considered when predicting new cases of physical illnesses from psychosocial factors, and when examining the exacerbation of and progression of a comorbid physical condition by the presence of a psychosocial condition.

The vast majority of research that has examined the health of caregivers has been cross-sectional case–control studies. Indeed, this is generally true of most research on stress and its sequelae. There have, however, been some prospective studies that predicted health problems and mortality from caregiving (Vitaliano et al., 2002). In a prospective cohort study, the researcher defines an exposure that may be associated with a given outcome, then selects exposed and unexposed subjects before the outcome of interest has occurred. Here, direct measurement of the incidence of a condition occurs.

It is rare to examine psychosocial, behavioral, and physiological mediators of caregiver status with disease outcomes (e.g., CHD) prospectively. One study followed caregivers and noncaregivers for coronary heart disease and evaluated mediators between caregiving and the prevalence/incidence of coronary disease (Vitaliano et al., 2002). Pathways were observed from a composite variable for chronic stress (e.g., care recipient cognitive functioning, activities, and behaviors). The model also included a vulnerability variable comprising of anger measures that predicted a distress composite (i.e., burden, sleep problems, low levels of positive experiences), a health habit composite (i.e., diet, exercise), and a physiological composite (i.e., metabolic syndrome). These pathways explained the greater incidence of coronary disease in male caregivers relative to male noncaregivers.

## RECOMMENDATIONS FOR FUTURE RESEARCH

Doubly prospective studies that examine participants prior to exposure to the stressor are needed to advance lifespan health psychology. This approach enables the researcher to test several important hypotheses, including whether high-risk persons self-select into caregiving more than low-risk persons, level of risk before becoming a caregiver, and whether persons who became caregivers were at greater risk for illness, independent of caregiving (Vitaliano et al., 2003). Relevant to this is a literature that has discussed the importance of shared risk factors within couples (Davis, Murphy, Neuhaus, Gee, & Quiroga, 2000). For example, the risks for cardiovascular illnesses may overlap with the risks for dementia, the illness of the caregiver's spouse (Rasgon & Jarvik, 2004). Indeed, caregivers and care recipients probably shared many of these risk factors (stress, high fat diets, and lack of exercise) before they adopted their current roles. If this is true, then persons who become caregivers may be at higher risk for cardiovascular problems independent of becoming caregivers (Vitaliano et al., 2003). In summary, prospective studies allow researchers to infer that caregiving precedes the outcomes studied, but they are only prospective for illness or mortality, not for caregiving. Hence, no information about experiences prior to caregiving is available.

There are several reasons why doubly-prospective studies should work well in lifespan health psychology. The first involves the higher prevalence of morbidities and comorbidities that exists in older versus younger adults. Such rates are an advantage if researchers wish to stratify persons with and without chronic stress, according to chronic disease, then follow them for disease exacerbation/progression prospectively to predict incident cases of physical illnesses from biopsychosocial and behavioral factors. Indeed, although illnesses take time to be detected, this might not pose as great a problem with older adults as it would with younger adults. Older adults would also have a greater likelihood than younger adults of becoming incident cases during the study period.

Yet another reason why doubly-prospective studies should work well is that psychosocial and behavioral factors have been shown to predict physical illness in prospective studies. Major depression disorder is known to increase the risk for heart disease (Rugulies, 2002) and diabetes (Kawakami, Takatsuka, Shimizu, & Ishibashi, 1999). Diabetics who do not have major depression have lower risk for obesity, sedentary lifestyle, and smoking than do diabetics who have major depression (Katon, Lin, & Russo, 2004). Importantly, the association between depression and mortality is influenced by physical health. In a 6-year follow-up of community-dwelling women over age 65, the risk of mortality increased with the number of depressive symptoms, but depressive symptoms were only associated with mortality among women in poor health (Fredman & Rosenbaum, 1998). Among post-myocardial infarction patients or those with Type II diabetes, depression has been shown in longitudinal studies to be a risk factor for mortality (Black, Markides, & Ray, 2003; Frasure-Smith, Lesperance, & Talajic, 1993). Hence, end organ damage secondary to ischemic heart disease or diabetes may make depressed caregivers more vulnerable to mortality in response to chronic stress. In a longitudinal study of over 6,000 older subjects free of disability, those who were depressed at baseline had a greater risk than nondepressed subjects for incident disability (6 years later) in both activities of daily living and mobility controlling for baseline chronic illnesses and sociodemographic factors (Pennix, Leveille, Ferrucci, van Eijk, & Guralnick, 1999).

Chronic stress has also been shown to predict illnesses/mortality and to exacerbate physical illnesses and disease progression in persons who are already ill. For example, bereavement is associated with greater physical illnesses (Kaprio, Koskenvuo, & Rita, 1987), health care utilization (Prigerson et al., 1997), and mortality (Goldman, Korenman, & Weinstein, 1995), and caregiving is associated with physiological risk/physical health problems, such as elevated stress hormones and reduced antibody production relative to age- and gender-matched noncaregivers (Vitaliano et al., 2003) and mortality (Schulz & Beach, 1999). Prolonged physiological reactions to elevated stress hormones, such as elevated BP and glucose, can increase one's risk for hypertension and diabetes.

## NEW DIRECTIONS FOR LIFESPAN HEALTH PSYCHOLOGY

Lifespan health psychology focuses on developmental mechanisms and person–environment interactions. Developmental epidemiology provides an interesting parallel to research in lifespan health psychology. The former is concerned with early risk factors for adult illnesses and the cumulative risk of illness over the lifespan (Susser, Brown, & Matte, 2000). The life course model incorporates elements such as cumulative insults over the lifespan, critical periods of susceptibility throughout life, and the interaction between early and late risk factors. Illnesses occur from a dynamic transactional relationship between the development of the individual and the changing demands of the environment. Hence, the same risk factor may lead to multiple possible outcomes. This has been referred to as "multifinality" (Cicchetti, 1990).

Obtaining data from childhood is especially relevant in lifespan health psychology, because it is now believed that early childhood, or even prenatal life, may "sensitize" individuals to develop subsequent illnesses. Longitudinal developmental research has shown that behavioral and temperamental characteristics in children as young as age 3 can predict adult psychiatric disorders (Caspi, Moffitt, Newman, & Silvia, 1996). One such example is posttraumatic stress disorder (PTSD) in response to later trauma in adulthood (Bramsen, Dirkzeager, & Van der Ploeg, 2000). In Vietnam veterans, the risk for PTSD is four times higher for those who had childhood abuse as for those who did not (Bremner, Southwick, Johnson, Yehuda, & Charney, 1993). Hence, the view that a traumatic event is a sufficient condition for PTSD is no longer preeminent. In contrast to the original definition of a traumatic stressor as one that "would evoke significant symptoms of distress in almost everyone" (American Association, 1987), it is now believed that PTSD is caused by interactions of individual vulnerabilities with the traumatic event (McNally, 2001). This observation supports the model in Figure 4.1.

## SUMMARY

Taylor and Repetti (1997) have argued that health psychology needs to be continually responsive to changes in health trends and medical practice. They cited Riley, Matarazzo, and Baum (1987), who noted that the graying of America poses a challenge for health psychologists to identify important lifestyle problems for this population and how they will influence the health of older adults. Health psychologists can play an important role in exploring the complex relationships among stress, and psychosocial and physiological responses. Understanding underlying mechanisms for chronic disease development and exacerbation is a critical step in designing interventions to promote health and prevent disability. The burden of chronic illness not only threatens the individual's quality of life, but it also has implications for family and friends involved in caregiving, and for society at large, where the financial costs of managing chronic disease are escalating at an alarming rate.

## REFERENCES

American Psychiatric Association (1987). *Diagnostic and Statistical Manual of Mental Disorders (Third Edition—Revised). DSM-III-R.* Washington: American Psychiatric Association.

Bernstein, E., Gardner, E., Abrutyn, E., Gross, P., & Murasko, D. (1998). Cytokine production after influenza vaccination in a healthy elderly population. *Vaccine, 16,* 1722–1731.

Black, S., Markides, K., & Ray, L. (2003). Depression predicts increased incidence of adverse health outcomes in older Mexican Americans with Type 2 diabetes. *Diabetes Care, 26,* 2822–2828.

Bramsen, I., Dirkzeager, A., & Van der Ploeg, H. (2000). Predeployment personality traits and exposure to trauma as predictors of posttraumatic stress symptoms: A prospective study of former peacekeepers. *American Journal of Psychiatry, 157,* 1115–1119.

Bremner, J., Southwick, S., Johnson, D., Yehuda, R., & Charney, D. (1993). Childhood physical abuse and combat-related posttraumatic stress disorder in Vietnam beterans. *American Journal of Psychiatry, 152,* 235–239.

Caspi, A., Moffitt, T., Newman, D., & Silvia, P. (1996). Behavior oberservations at age 3 years predict adult psychiatric disorders. *Archives of General Psychiatry, 53,* 1033–1039.

Cicchetti, D. (1990). An historical perspective on the discipline of developmental psychopathology. In A. Rolf, D. Masten, D. Cicchetti, K. Neuchterlein, & S. Weintraub (Eds.), *Risk and protective factors in the development of psychopathology* (pp. 2–28). New York: Cambridge University Press.

Davis, M., Murphy, S., Neuhaus, J., Gee, L., & Quiroga, S. (2000). Living arrangements affect dietary quality for U.S. adults aged 50 years and older: NHANES III 1988–1994. *Journal of Nutrition, 30,* 2256–2264.

DiGiovanna, A. (2000). *Human aging: Biological perspectives.* New York: McGraw-Hill.

Fawzy, F., Fawzy, N., Hyun, C., Elashoff, R., Guthrie, D., Fahey, J., et al. (1993). Malignant melanoma: Effects of an early structured psychiatric intervention, coping, and affective state on recurrence and survival 6 years later. *Archives of General Psychiatry, 50,* 681–690.

Federal Interagency Forum on Aging-Related Statistics. *Americans 2004: Key Indicators of Well Being. Federal Interagency Forum on Aging-Related Statistics.* Washington, DC: U.S. Government Printing Office.

Fischer, J., & Raschke, F. (1997). Economic and medical significance of sleep-related breathing. *Respiration, 64,* 39–44.

Frasure-Smith, N., Lesperance, F., & Talajic, M. (1993). Depression following myocardial infarction: Impact on 6-month survival. *Journal of the American Medical Association, 270,* 1819–1825.

Fredman, S., & Rosenbaum, J. (1998). Recurrent depression, resistant clinician? *Harvard Review of Psychiatry, 5*(5), 281–285.

Goldman, N., Korenman, S., & Weinstein, R. (1995). Marital status and health among the elderly. *Social Science and Medicine, 40,* 1717–1730.

Hayes-Bautista, D., Hsu, P., Perez, A., & Gamboa, C. (2002). The "browning" of the graying of America: Diversity in the elderly population and policy implications. *Generations, 26*(3), 15–24.

Herbert, T., & Cohen, S. (1993a). Depression and immunity: A meta-analytic review. *Psychological Bulletin, 113,* 472–486.

Herbert, T., & Cohen, S. (1993b). Stress and immunity in humans: A meta-analytic review. *Psychosomatic Medicine, 55,* 364–379.

Hooyman, N., & Kiyak, H. (2005). *Social gerontology: A multidisciplinary perspective.* Boston: Allyn & Bacon.

Hoyer, W., & Rybash, J. (1999). Life span theory. In J. Birren (Ed.), *Encyclopedia of gerontology: Age, aging and the aged* (pp. 65–71). New York: Academic Press.

Kaprio, J., Koskenvuo, M., & Rita, H. (1987). Mortality after bereavement: Prospective study of 95,647 widowed persons. *American Journal of Public Health, 77,* 283–287.

Katon, W., Lin, E., & Russo, J. (2004). Cardiac risk factors in patients with diabetes mellitus and major depression. *Journal of General Internal Medicine, 19*(12), 1192–1199.

Kawakami, N., Takatsuka, W., Shimizu, H., & Ishibashi, H. (1999). Depressive symptoms and occurrence of Type II diabetes among Japanese men. *Diabetes Care, 22,* 1071–1076.

Kessler, R., Berglund, P., Demler, O., Jin, R., Merikangas, K., & Walters, E. (2005). Lifetime prevalence and age-of-onset distributions of DSM-IV disorders in the National Comorbidity Survey Replication. *Archives of General Psychiatry, 62*(6), 593–602.

Kessler, R., Chiu, W., Demler, O., & Walters, E. (2005). Prevalence, severity, and comorbidity of 12-month DSM-IV disorders in the National Comorbidity Survey Replication. *Archives of General Psychiatry, 62*(6), 617–627.

Lovallo, W., & Thomas, T. (2000). Stress hormones in psychophysiological research: Emotional, behavioral, and cognitive implications. In J. T. Cacioppo, L. G. Tassinary, & G. Berntson (Ed.), *Handbook of psychophysiology* (pp. 342–367). New York: Cambridge University Press.

McEwen, B. S. (2000). The neurobiology of stress: From serendipity to clinical relevance. *Brain Research, 886*, 172–189.

McNally, R. J. (2001). Vulnerability to anxiety disorders in adulthood. In R. E. Ingram & J. M. Price (Eds.), *Vulnerability to psychopathology* (pp. 304–321). New York: Guilford Press.

Mechanic, D. (1967). Invited commentary on self, social environment and stress. In M. H. Appeley & R. Trumbull (Eds.), *Psychological stress* (pp. 123–150). New York: Appleton–Century–Crofts.

Musselman, D., Evans, D., & Nemeroff, C. (1998). The relationship of depression to cardiovascular disease. *Archives of General Psychiatry, 55*, 580–592.

Pennix, B., Leveille, S., Ferrucci, L., van Eijk, J., & Guralnick, J. M. (1999). Exploring the effect of depression on physical disability: Longitudinal evidence from the Established Populations for Epidemiologic Studies of the Elderly. *American Journal of Public Health, 89*, 1346–1352.

Pickering, T. G., & Gerin, W. (1990). Blood pressure reactivity: Cardiovascular reactivity in the laboratory and the role of behavioral factors in hypertension: A critical review. *Annals of Behavioral Medicine, 12*, 3–16.

Prigerson, H. G., Bierhals, A. J., Kasl, S. V., Reynolds, C. F., Shear, K., Day, N., et al. (1997). Traumatic grief as a risk factor for mental and physical morbidity. *American Journal of Psychiatry, 154*, 616–623.

Rasgon, N., & Jarvik, L. (2004). Insulin resistance, affective disorders, and Alzheimer's disease: Review and hypothesis. *Journals of Gerontology: Biological Sciences and Medical Sciences, Series A, 59*, 178–183.

Reiger, D. A., Farmer, M. E., Rae, D. S., Locke, B. Z., Keith, S. J., Judd, L. L., et al. (1990). Comorbidity of mental disorders with alcohol and other drug abuse. *Journal of the American Medical Association, 264*, 2511–2518.

Riley, M., Matarazzo, J., & Baum, A. (1987). *Perspectives in behavioral medicine: The aging dimension.* Hillsdale, NJ: Erlbaum.

Rugulies, R. (2002). Depression as a predictor for coronary heart disease: A review and meta-analysis. *American Journal of Preventive Medicine, 23*, 51–61.

Russo, J., & Vitaliano, P. (1995). Life events, caregiver status, and distress. *Experimental Aging Research, 21*, 273–294.

Russo, J., Vitaliano, P. P., Brewer, D., Katon, W., & Becker, J. (1995). Psychiatric disorders in spouse caregivers of care-recipients with Alzheimer's disease and matched controls: A diathesis–stress model of psychopathology. *Journal of Abnormal Psychology, 104*, 197–204.

Schneiderman, N., & Skyler, J. (1996). Insulin metabolism, sympathetic nervous system regulation, and coronary heart disease prevention. In K. Orth-Gomer & N. Schneiderman (Eds.), *Behavioral medicine approaches to cardiovascular disease prevention* (pp. 105–133). Hillsdale, NJ: Erlbaum.

Schulz, R., & Beach, S. (1999). Caregiving as a risk factor for morbidity: The Caregiver Health Effects Study. *Journal of the American Medical Association, 282,* 2215–2260.

Steptoe, A., Cropley, M., Griffith, J., & Kirschbaum, C. (2000). Job strain and anger expression predict early morning elevations in salivary cortisol. *Psychosomatic Medicine, 62,* 286–292.

Susser, E., Brown, A., & Matte, T. (2000). Prenatal antecedents of neuropsychiatric disorder over the life course: Collaborative studies of United States birth cohorts. In J. Rapoport (Ed.), *Childhood onset of adult psychopathology.* Washington, DC: American Psychiatric Press.

Taylor, S., & Repetti, R. (1997). Health psychology: What is an unhealthy environment and how does it get under the skin? *Annual Review of Psychology, 48,* 411–447.

Vandervoort, A. (2002). Aging of the human neuromuscular system. *Muscle and Nerve, 25,* 17–25.

Vitaliano, P., Maiuro, R., Bolton, P., & Armsden, G. (1987). A psychoepidemiologic approach to the study of disaster. *Journal of Community Psychology, 15,* 99–122.

Vitaliano, P., Scanlan, J., Zhang, J., Savage, M., Hirsch, I., & Siegler, I. (2002). A path model of chronic stress, the metabolic syndrome, and coronary heart disease. *Psychosomatic Medicine, 64,* 418–435.

Vitaliano, P., Zhang, J., & Scanlan, J. (2003). "Is caregiving hazardous to one's physical health?": A meta-analysis. *Psychological Bulletin, 129,* 946–972.

Vitaliano P. P., Russo, J., Bailey, S., Young, H., & McCann, B. (1993). Psychosocial factors associated with cardiovascular reactivity in older individuals. *Psychosomatic Medicine, 55,* 164–177.

Vitaliano, P. P., Scanlan, J. M., Ochs, H. D., Syrjala, K., Siegler, I. C., & Snyder, E. A. (1998). Psychosocial stress moderates the relationship of cancer history with natural killer cell activity. *Annals of Behavioral Medicine, 20,* 199–208.

Vitaliano, P. P., Scanlan, J. M., Siegler, I. C., McCormick, W. C., & Knopp, R. H. (1998). Coronary heart disease moderates the relationship of chronic stress with the metabolic syndrome. *Health Psychology, 17,* 520–529.

# CHAPTER 5

# The Relevance of a Lifespan Developmental Approach to Health

## AVRON SPIRO III

In this chapter, I use the lifespan developmental approach to integrate three topics: health, aging, and methodology. Elsewhere, my colleagues and I have discussed some aspects of a lifespan developmental approach (Aldwin, Spiro, & Park, 2006; Smith & Spiro, 2002; Spiro, 2001; Spiro, Schnurr, & Aldwin, 1997). Here, I summarize some aspects of these earlier works and extend them by focusing on two particular aspects: health as a developmental phenomenon of particular interest in the study of aging, and methodological implications of studying health from a lifespan developmental perspective. What I hope to accomplish is to suggest how this combination of substance and method will yield new avenues for the study of health and aging.

The lifespan developmental approach, although overlapping in some respects with the life course approach in sociology (e.g., Settersten, 2003) is nonetheless distinct. For example, the lifespan approach focuses primarily on issues of ontogenetic development of the individual, with less prominence given to the role of societal and social factors. In contrast, the life course approach tends to focus more on the role of social institutions and social interaction as constitutive of individual development, and is less concerned with intrapsychic developmental phenomena. The individual life course is seen more as a sequence of roles and statuses, structured by the social context, the transitions among them, and the extent to which individuals move along these sequences in more or less ordered fashion.

## PROPOSITIONS OF A LIFESPAN DEVELOPMENTAL APPROACH

The key theoretical propositions of a lifespan developmental approach have been elaborated previously (Baltes, 1987; Baltes, Staudinger, & Lindenberger, 1999). In the following, some aspects are elaborated more fully to serve as a motivation for the arguments below; others are discussed briefly, but this signifies simply that they are less relevant for this discussion regarding health, and not that they are unimportant more generally.

For our purposes, the lifespan perspective can be summarized with four key propositions. *First, development is lifelong, and not restricted to a given age.* Over the individual's lifespan, development occurs at all ages rather than being confined to one age, stage, or phase. Furthermore, development is subject to evolutionary, sociohistorical, and ontogenetic influences. *Second, a lifespan perspective is pluralistic.* It is multidisciplinary, drawing theoretical insights and methodological principles from multiple disciplines. A lifespan perspective recognizes that developmental phenomena are often multidimensional, are subject to a multitude of causal influences, and that they vary in the directionality of change. *Third, a lifespan developmental perspective is located within a contextual worldview* (Pepper, 1942). As such, it recognizes that human development is embedded within evolutionary and sociohistorical, as well as ontogenetic, contexts. Thus, a broader perspective on the causes and contexts of development results, which recognizes that human development is not universal, but contingent, subject to a broad range of sociohistorical influences. *Finally, a lifespan perspective recognizes that development is variable,* and that not all persons change in the same ways. Furthermore, an individual's development can vary across domains, as well as occasions. Thus, a lifespan perspective emphasizes both the universal and the particular in development, embodying Kluckhohn and Murray's (1948) dictum (paraphrased here) that every person is in some respects like all other persons, like some other persons, and like no other person.

### Corollaries of a Lifespan Developmental Approach

What does it mean, then, to take seriously the propositions of a lifespan developmental approach (e.g., that change happens, people differ, and context matters)? I propose that a number of corollaries follow from such an approach, and that they have conceptual and methodological implications that must be taken seriously in the study of health and aging, as well as more generally, in the examination of any developmental phenomenon.

First, *age is not a causal variable,* but a descriptive one. This point, made forcefully over 30 years ago by Wohlwill (1973), is seldom given its full due. In a gerontological context, and posed more strongly, does aging exist (Peto & Doll, 1997)? Is aging a disease (Smith, 2002), or is it what remains after extrinsic factors (e.g., disease) are taken into account (Grimley Evans, 1988; Fozard, Metter, & Brant, 1990)?

For example, in our work on cognitive change in later life, my colleagues and I are asking whether "cognitive aging" is a misnomer, and examining whether the effects of diseases during later life account for much of the cognitive declines observed in older adults (Spiro & Brady, in press). As we have shown, an index of stroke risk accounts for nearly as much variance in performance on a measure of executive functioning as does age (Brady, Spiro, McGlinchey-Berroth, Milberg, & Gaziano, 2001).

Related to the view that age is not causal, we must recognize that *age is only one of several potential temporal axes along which to organize our data.* Other relevant temporal metameters, some of which are discussed below, include time since (or until) an event (e.g., time since diagnosis of a disease, or time until death). Furthermore, findings differ depending on the temporal metameter (e.g., age vs. time since entry into a study) that is used, which can result in incorrect inferences regarding the phenomenon under study (Mehta & West, 2000; Thiebaut & Benichou, 2004). Time scales can range from milliseconds to millennia, depending on the phenomenon under study (e.g., reaction time vs. evolution), and should be selected according to a theory of the phenomenon under study (Mroczek, Spiro, & Almeida, 2003).

Second, from a lifespan perspective, *longitudinal data are necessary, not optional,* if we are to understand human development. To interpret cross-sectional differences as age changes is to commit the life course fallacy (Riley, 1994). Of course, the flip side of the coin is that longitudinal studies are often restricted to a given range of birth cohorts, and the conclusions about their aging should be tempered by knowledge of their unique historical circumstances. Much of what we know about aging is based on cohorts born during the first third of the 20th century, many of whom went on to experience the Depression as children, World War II or the Korean Conflict as young adults, and the prosperity of the 1950s and 1960s during midlife. Given that approximately 25% of men now in their 70s experienced combat during World War II or Korea, its entirely possible that their experiences have colored our knowledge of midlife and old age in ways we do not yet understand (Spiro et al., 1997; Settersten, 2006).

Third, given that longitudinal data are fundamental, as is a recognition that persons differ from one another, *we require methods that allow consideration of differences in change among persons and a focus on variation, as well as average trends.* Change and development are not universal across persons; heterogeneity exists among persons in various parameters of change (Nesselroade, 1991; Wohlwill, 1973). Vaupel and Yashin (1985) provided some fascinating illustrations of the mistaken inferences that can result from ignoring heterogeneity in mortality rates among subpopulations. When making inferences from aggregated data to individuals, we must exercise caution (Molenaar, 2004). One of the interesting tasks for psychology, and behavioral sciences more generally, is to map various developmental functions (Wohlwill, 1973) that characterize the population, yet also retain a sensitivity to variations around these "normative" trajectories; that is, some phenomena (e.g., physical growth) develop universally (although there are variations in level attained or in rate of growth, or timing of growth spurts), whereas others develop more individually, in form as well as in level or rate (e.g., personality or ego development).

Returning again to Kluckhohn and Murray (1948), we need to ask which developmental functions are similar for all persons, for some persons, and which are unique to an individual. A lifespan approach, while often emphasizing general or universal principles of development, also recognizes explicitly the exceptions and takes note of the diversity of development. In some ways, the time has indeed come, as Molenaar (2004) declared in his manifesto, to make psychology an idiographic science, because the lack of agreement between within-person change and between-person variation has long hampered behavioral sciences in both theory and methodology. Indeed, we must ask whether, as developmental scientists, we should collect cross-sectional (single occasion between-person) data at all, because they can tell us little about within-person changes that are, after all, the key phenomena of the developmental sciences (Hofer & Sliwinski, 2001; Kraemer, Yesavage, Taylor, & Kupfer, 2000). Developmental phenomena are best studied with developmental data obtained longitudinally at the person level by means of repeated observation. Between-person differences obtained from cross-sectional data are not generally a valid basis for inferences regarding within-person changes (Molenaar, 2004).

Given the primacy of longitudinal (repeated observational) data, it would seem appropriate to consider the trajectory as the foundational metaphor of developmental sciences, as suggested by Wohlwill (1973), who proposed a focus on the developmental function over 30 years ago (see also Raudenbush, 2001). In the past, when two-occasion (pretest and posttest) designs constituted the prototypical longitudinal study, the difference score was the basic building block (Harris, 1963). Although it has a checkered past, many of the limitations of the difference score were more perceived than real (Rogosa, 1995). With the advent of growth curve methodologies (e.g., Singer & Willett, 2003) for analyzing repeated measures, we have had the tools to consider trajectories. With the extension of these methods to the multivariate case (e.g., Sliwinski, Hofer, & Hall, 2003), as well as the development of latent class approaches (Muthén, 2001; Nagin, 1999) we can now weave together the trajectories of multiple measures over time to better examine how different trajectories are related to one another within persons, and how these within-person relations differ between persons.

In discussions of lifespan development and different approaches to it, it seems useful to propose a metaphor that can serve to capture key aspects in a more intuitive fashion. The metaphors that I consider next vary along two dimensions: the first, a dimension of determinism versus contingency, and the second, a dimension of universal versus particular. For example, strong (unidirectional) developmental theories (e.g., stage theories such as those proposed by Freud, Erikson, and Piaget) can be represented by an escalator, on which all persons ascend a single sequence of stages in the same order, although at different rates, and not all end at the same stage. Weaker conceptions of development, which allow more heterogeneous patterns of change (e.g., decline during old age), might be represented by a trajectory, such as that of a model rocket, which rises and then falls, according to relatively deterministic physical principles. Although such a trajectory is nearly as deterministic as the escalator, it does allow more variability, because various forces can modify the trajectory (e.g., its height), but due to gravity, what rises must also fall. By weaving together multiple trajectories, combining the warp and the woof (Nesselroade, 1991) as it were, we can study the *tapestry* of human development across the lifespan (or portions thereof), and examine whether it is universal, local, or particular (applying to all, to some, or only to a single individual). By adopting the trajectory rather than the difference score as the methodological metaphor for the study of change, we can begin to better understand human development in general, whether our focus is on health, personality, or intelligence.

## HEALTH: FROM A LIFESPAN DEVELOPMENTAL PERSPECTIVE

Although a lifespan perspective has long been accepted in adult development and aging, it has made few inroads in the study of health (but for some exceptions see National Public Health Partnership [NPHP], 2001; Office of Behavioral and Social Science Research [OBSSR], 2005; World Health Organization [WHO], 2000). Related approaches are just beginning to gain favor, for example, life course sociology (e.g., George, 2003), life course epidemiology (Kuh & Ben-Shlomo, 2004; Kuh & Hardy, 2002; Lynch & Davey Smith, 2005), and the life course health development model of Halfon and Hochstein (2002). Although these approaches have their origins in other behavioral sciences (e.g., sociology, epidemiology, child health policy), and are not completely consistent with the four propositions considered earlier, they nonetheless take a developmental stance toward health, thereby overlapping with a lifespan approach. Insofar as these approaches are united in viewing health as a developmental phenomenon, despite some differences, we consider them, for our purposes here, as consistent with a lifespan approach.

   In this section, I consider some aspects of health from lifespan developmental perspective. From this vantage point, health is viewed as a developmental construct, one that is in some sense not dissimilar from other constructs such as intelligence or personality. It should be noted that in the following, health is being considered as an individual attribute, although like personality or intelligence, it could be considered at the population level (Murray, Salomon, Mathers, & Lopez, 2002). By focusing on health as an individual attribute, I bracket for the most part discussion of both its determinants (e.g., genetics, socioeconomic circumstances, social capital) and its consequences (e.g., health care use), while recognizing that these are nonetheless related to the health of the individual (Evans & Stoddart, 2003).

Consider for example the WHO's (1946, p. 2) definition of health as "a state of complete physical, mental, and social well-being, and not merely the absence of disease or infirmity." Note that "health" is defined as a state and not a process; this ignores, or at least downplays, its developmental aspects. However, consistent with the lifespan developmental view, note that health is explicitly considered to be multidimensional, here encompassing three dimensions. Note also that health is defined as the positive end of the spectrum, as something more than the absence of disease or infirmity. As this definition, which has been widely cited if not utilized, makes clear, health and disease are part of the same continuum, and are more complex than binary states (e.g., healthy or not).

## Developmental Perspectives on Health

From a lifespan developmental perspective, health can be considered in an evolutionary context at the species level, in a sociohistorical context at a population level, and in an ontogenetic context at the individual level.

Over the last century, the developed world has witnessed a doubling in life expectancy. The causes of this increased lifespan are a matter of some debate. Whereas evolution is unlikely to have accounted for such a recent change, a number of sociohistorical circumstances may be relevant. Among these are shifts in the age composition of human societies, reduced impact of infectious diseases (although offset perhaps by the greater impact of chronic diseases), improved nutrition and public health, and better health care and greater access to it, all leading to an increase in physiological capital over successive generations (Finch & Crimmins, 2004; Fogel, 2003; Omran, 1971/2005).

Here, we focus on the individual level of analysis by applying the four lifespan developmental propositions I discussed earlier to health (cf. Aldwin et al., 2006; Smith & Spiro, 2002; Spiro, 2001). Health is a construct whose definition and relations to disease, illness, disability, and even to aging, remain the subject of active debate in medicine and behavioral sciences (Grimley Evans, 1988; Peto & Doll, 1997; Smith, 2002), as well as in philosophy (e.g., Boorse, 1997). However, rather than join that debate, I propose here only to add a developmental perspective to the many characterizations of health.

First, from a lifespan developmental perspective, *health is a lifelong process*. One's health is affected by not only one's genetic endowment but also one's intrauterine environment, maternal health, and socioeconomic circumstances subsequent to birth (Gluckman & Hanson, 2004; Kuh & Ben-Shlomo, 2004; Kuh & Hardy, 2002). Health is not fixed at birth, but it is determined at any given time by one's current behaviors and endowment, as well as by one's history to that point. In other words, health has both proximal and distal determinants, and whereas some proximal (e.g., behavioral) determinants might be more amenable to change, such changes may not offset more distal, upstream determinants (Lynch & Davey Smith, 2005).

From a lifespan developmental perspective, then, one may wonder whether health (and disease, which is also a process) in later life is determined more by one's previous life course and its cumulative risks than by one's current lifestyle (Kuh & Ben-Shlomo, 2004; Kuh & Hardy, 2002). To the extent that this is the case, it suggests that current societal emphases on reducing risky health behaviors (e.g., obesity, smoking, excessive alcohol use) may place undue emphasis on the individual, whereas the concern is perhaps more appropriately located within their early environment, and with risks cumulated from that point, or the pathways on which they were set during early life (Halfon & Hochstein, 2002). On the other hand, the neo-Freudian aspect of the "child as father to the man," or blaming later life problems on early life behaviors, can go too far to an extreme and lead to a *laissez-faire* attitude toward reducing current risk factors. Perhaps the message to take from a lifespan perspective is that our health is a function of *both* who we are now *and* what we have done in the past, and that the responsibilities for good health lie within the person, as well as within his or her current (and past) experiences. One implication of viewing health as a lifelong process is that health care services should be organized along the life course and focus more on prevention, especially early in life, rather than on treatment later in life (Halfon & Hochstein, 2002; NPHP, 2001). An ounce of prevention taken early may well be worth a pound of cure later in life.

Second, the study of *health is pluralistic*. The study of health is obviously multidisciplinary, involving both biomedical and behavioral science disciplines. Part of the motivation for this volume is to further multidisciplinary studies of health from an aging or developmental point of view by integrating gerontology and developmental sciences with health psychology. In addition to considering health as multidimensional, it is also useful to view it as hierarchical. Although we often speak of health (or personality, or intelligence) as a single thing (e.g., "He has a good personality";

"Her intelligence is amazing"), it is somewhat misleading to do so given the widespread acceptance by academics, if not laypersons, of such hierarchical models as the five-factor model of personality traits and facets (McCrae & Costa, 2003), or the psychometric model of intelligence (Flanagan, Genshaft, & Harrison, 1997), both of which encompass multiple levels of broader and narrower constructs. Depending on the level of the hierarchy under consideration, one might find broad constructs that have moderate correlations to a wide array of outcomes, or narrower constructs that have higher correlations with a relatively specific set of outcomes. In the assessment of health, for example, this is why some studies assessing health-related quality of life use both generic measures such as the Medical Outcomes Study Short Form (MOS SF-36) and more focused, disease-specific measures (e.g., Clark et al., 2005; Stewart & Ware, 1992).

Acceptance of the multidimensional and hierarchical nature of health has certain consequences, foremost among them, the need for a measure to conform to its theoretical basis. Building on the WHO definition of health as comprising three domains, for example, the RAND Health Insurance Experiment and later, the MOS constructed hierarchical multidimensional measures (e.g., SF-36; Stewart & Ware, 1992) to assess the physical, mental, and social domains of health, rather than relying on the oft-used single item "How would you rate your health?" to assess global health. If a psychologist were to attempt to measure personality or cognition through the use of a similar single-item measure (e.g., "How would you rate your personality?"), we would surely question his or her intentions. However, it should be recognized that global assessments of health are predictive of mortality (Idler & Benyamimi, 1997), and may in certain circumstances be quite useful. However, if our goal is to understand health in its many facets, and changes therein, such a global approach is inappropriate.

These and similar measures of health can be characterized as subjective, in the sense that the person is reporting more or less accurately on his or her own perceptions and states. Health can also be measured more objectively, using a variety of methods (e.g., Elinson, 1988). For example, instead of asking respondents how they would rate their health, one can inquire whether a doctor or health professional has ever given them a diagnosis (e.g., "Has a doctor ever told you that you have diabetes?"). Such questions are, however, subject to reporting error, due to memory or to respondents' reluctance to identify themselves as "sick." Alternatively, one can seek laboratory or diagnostic data from administrative records (e.g., whether a patient in a health care system had a diagnosis of diabetes, or a fasting blood sugar above a critical threshold, or was being treated with insulin). However, all of these sources of information have an associated error; whereas they may vary in degree of objectivity, they also vary in reliability. As in the case of any other construct, the bottom line is that measurement is a challenge, and there is no true "gold standard"; multiple measures should be used. Thus, rather than validating a self-report of disease against an abstracted chart diagnosis, one should think rather of corroborating one type of report against another, and evaluating their sensitivity and specificity (Miller, Rogers, Spiro, & Kazis, 2003). Such a perspective is relatively common with respect to mental disorders, because there are few if any "objective" indicators, and diagnosis generally relies on signs and symptoms as reported by the patient.

The WHO definition, whatever quibbles one might have with the domains identified, defines health explicitly as multidimensional. However, as is the case with intelligence or other multidimensional psychological constructs, having a lot of it in one domain does not necessarily generalize to other domains. We have all known people with a good bit of professional intelligence who are rather retarded with respect to some aspect of practical intelligence. Likewise, someone can have good health in some domains, yet poor health in others.

Continuing the pluralistic focus of a lifespan developmental approach, health is subject to many causal influences; indeed, one could argue that a cottage industry exists simply to enumerate them and develop models of their influence on health (e.g., Evans & Stoddart, 2003). Also with respect to pluralism, health, in at least some of its multiple dimensions, is always changing, declining, and improving from birth until death. Given its multi dimensional and multidirectional nature, we should view health as something positive to be maximized over time, like wealth, and not to be squandered. We should also recognize that there are many aspects of health in which to invest over time, and that these investments may grow or decline at different rates due to a variety of external influences. Like wealth, or financial capital, we should attempt (as the economists would have it) to maximize our health capital (Grossman, 2000), or to preserve rather than expend health, recognizing that it is a lifetime investment. Much like financial investments, the earlier we begin investing in health capital, the greater the rewards in later life.

The third proposition implies that health is best studied and understood *in context*, whether that context is evolutionary, sociohistorical, or ontogenetic. As psychologists, we tend to focus primarily on the latter, but we should encourage and work to understand the former. For example, we should consider Omran's (1971/2005) account of the impact of historical changes on health; or recent work on the evolutionary origins of health and disease, emphasizing the role of maternal health on subsequent development (Gluckman & Hanson, 2004); or the impact of socioeconomic status on health (Marmot, 2004). In our quest to understand health and its developmental changes over the lifespan, we should incorporate all relevant approaches into our models.

The fourth lifespan proposition, that *development is variable* across persons, times, and domains, clearly applies to health. This variability also exists within persons, and this within-person variability should be the focus of developmental approaches to health as well as other developmental constructs (Molenaar, 2004). Irrespective of the domains of health under consideration, a lifespan perspective recognizes that each domain can develop and change at different rates for different persons, as well as vary within the same person over their life. While one person may progress rapidly through the phases of a disease such as lung cancer, another may progress more slowly.

Whether within-person variability in a given domain is meaningful or error variance is a debate largely settled in favor of the former (e.g., Nesselroade, 1991); a more controversial question is whether or not such variability indicates dysfunction, with some (e.g., Lipsitz & Goldberger, 1992) arguing from complexity or chaos theory that within-person variability is good, and its loss is bad, whereas others suggest that greater within-person variability may be predictive of negative outcomes, such as psychopathology (Mroczek et al., 2003) or cognitive decline (MacDonald, Hultsch, & Dixon, 2003).

Given the focus of a lifespan approach on variability within, as well as between persons, what does this suggest about health? For one, we should recognize the heterogeneity of treatment effects among persons. Because most treatments are evaluated based on average effects, which ignore heterogeneity among people (e.g., in disease risk, response to treatment, side effect profiles), we should recognize that not all patients will benefit in the same way from the same treatment (Kravitz, Duan, & Braslow, 2004). The study of patient-by-treatment interactions is an important aspect of a lifespan approach. This is yet another example of the general problem, that a population can actually be a composed of distinct subpopulations (Vaupel & Yashin, 1985). Thus, a modest overall treatment effect may result from a mixture of those who respond substantially, those who benefit somewhat, and those who suffer harm.

## METHODOLOGICAL IMPLICATIONS

### General Methodological Concerns

First, and perhaps most critical, is the recognition that longitudinal data are necessary in developmental studies. In this context, longitudinal studies include both prospective studies (e.g., where risk factors are measured once, and outcomes observed later, as in survival studies), and repeated measures studies (where outcomes are measured multiple times). Longitudinal studies include both long-term studies (over years or decades) and short-term studies (over days or weeks). Second, the methods we adopt should, whenever possible and theoretically justified, allow consideration of differences between persons in aspects of change; that is, we should examine not only average change of a sample in aspects of health over time but also differences among persons in these aspects. As Molenaar (2004) and others have suggested, we should adopt a more idiographic approach methodologically, because our theories are largely idiographic, concerned with change in a person rather than in a population. Third, if we seek to study aging separately from the effects of health or disease, we need to screen and select our samples quite carefully (Fozard et al., 1990). Elimination of participants with prevalent or subclinical disease may render a sample unrepresentative of the general population, but some such selection may be necessary to distinguish the effects of aging from those of disease.

## Use of Theory

We should use theory to guide the design and analysis of studies. If theory suggests that a variable is a potential mediator of the effects of a risk factor on an outcome, use of ordinary regression analysis is a less effective means for testing that theory than is path analysis. The life course approach to epidemiology has made clear the limitations of regression in such a context (Kuh & Ben-Shlomo, 2004; Kuh & Hardy, 2002). If theory specifies a causal chain, then simultaneous entry of the variables in this chain will likely result in the more proximal variables having a significant effect and overlook the effects of the more distal influences (Weitkunat & Wildner, 2002). The use of simultaneous rather than sequential methods of data analysis may account for failures to find a greater role for psychosocial variables in predicting health, relative to biomedical or physiological predictors. This is because psychosocial variables affect health in large part via their effects on physiological processes, and once the latter are included in a simultaneous model, the effects of the former are largely removed. It would be a shame if we continued to use methods that put at a disadvantage our concepts and weaken tests of our theories, especially when alternative methods are available that would permit such tests.

## Choice of Temporal Metameters

In the analysis of longitudinal data, there are a number of options for defining the temporal metameter, or the axis along which data are collected. First, there is the question of scale, perhaps most clearly illustrated when time serves as the axis. Depending on the variable in question, data can be collected over intervals of seconds (e.g., heart rate variability), hours or days (e.g., blood pressure, mood), or months and years (e.g., for personality traits). Second, time can be defined in various ways. Age, measured as time since birth, seems most appropriate for use in developmental studies, but other options include time since an event (e.g., randomization in a clinical trial, first heart attack), or time until an event (e.g., death or first stroke). There are important implications in selecting a temporal metameter for both repeated measures and prospective studies. In repeated measures studies, centering time at the person rather than at the sample mean can result in incorrect estimates, as can use of occasion as the temporal metameter (Mehta & West, 2000).

In survival analysis, use of time on study rather than age as the metameter can likewise result in mistaken inferences (Lamarca, Alonso, Gomez, & Munoz, 1998; Thiebaut & Benichou, 2004). By using age as the temporal metameter in survival analysis, the hazard function is the age-specific incidence of the outcome. In observational studies, in which participants are enrolled based on the time of their assessment, and may or may not have the outcome in question, age would be the preferred metameter. In clinical studies, in which participants who are enrolled are screened and do not have (or have not yet experienced) the outcome, then time since enrollment is a sensible metameter. Under certain conditions, results based on time versus age as the temporal axis will agree, but the results can diverge even when age is used as a stratification variable in models with time on study (Thiebaut & Benichou, 2004). The moral here is that the definition of time used in longitudinal studies can make a meaningful difference in the results.

## Recommended Methods for Longitudinal Studies

Some methods seem especially appropriate for studying health from a life-span perspective. These methods combine theory and data in ways that provide optimal tests of models concerning growth and change, subgroups within change, and consideration of the causes and contexts of change. Foremost among these are growth curve (i.e., multilevel, random effects, or hierarchical) models (Singer & Willett, 2003). These models take into consideration the hierarchical structure of data, such as the nesting of multiple testing occasions within persons, or the nesting of persons within geographic areas (e.g., neighborhoods) or social structures (e.g., marital dyads). Applied to longitudinal data, such models can be used to assess whether there are individual differences in change.

My colleagues and I have used growth curves to examine change in various aspects of personality, and the influence of various social and demographic characteristics on individual differences in change. For the personality traits of neuroticism and extraversion, we found different overall trajectories of change (Mroczek & Spiro, 2003). Positive and negative affect also exhibited different trajectories over time (Griffin, Mroczek, & Spiro, 2006). For both affect and traits, we found predictors of individual differences. For affect, personality traits predicted individual differences in change over time, as did self-rated health and work status. Trajectories varied among birth cohorts, and memory complaints were associated with level, but not change, in both traits. We have also used growth curves to examine changes in health at a daily level in married couples, finding that wives report higher negative affect and lower positive affect on days their husbands report higher symptom levels (Yorgason, Almeida, Neupert, Hoffman, & Spiro, in press).

Growth curves can also be used in situations where the temporal process under investigation has multiple phases or components. For example, Llabre, Spitzer, Saab, and Schneiderman (2001) used piecewise growth curves to model simultaneously two phases of a stress response, reactivity and recovery, in a laboratory challenge task. Multiple measures of blood pressure were taken over a 10-minute span, before and after a cold pressor test. The investigators were able to simultaneously model the two phases of the process, and to consider both predictors and consequences of the two phases. In this example, the two phases were contiguous rather than discrete, but in other applications (e.g., interrupted time-series designs, or studies with multiple assessments both before and after an intervention), piecewise growth curves could also be useful.

A second recent development in growth curves involves multivariate applications, or examining correlated (or coupled) change in outcomes. Sliwinski et al. (2003) examined multiple cognitive abilities over time in an aging sample, some of whom had preclinical dementia. Using age as the temporal metameter, correlations among change in the cognitive dimensions were moderate in the overall sample; however, when the sample was stratified into cases and noncases, the correlations among ability declines were stronger in the cases. When time until disease onset was used as the temporal metameter for the cases, the extent of decline was much greater than in the age-based model, but the correlations among change in abilities were lower than those in the overall sample, although higher than those among the noncases. Other approaches to correlated versus coupled change include the use of structural equation modeling. McArdle et al. (2004), who used structural equation models to test coupled relations between brain size and memory over time, found that an increase in lateral ventricular size was a predictor of decline in memory, but not the reverse.

The final set of methods, known as latent class or growth mixture models, has as its objective the identification of subgroups within the population studied. A common element among these methods is the recognition that the sample under study may be heterogeneous, comprised of subgroups with different patterns or correlates of change. In essence, this approach attempts to fulfill Kluckhohn and Murray's (1948) dictum by identifying the subgroups (see also Vaupel & Yashin, 1985). Alternative approaches have been proposed by Muthén (2001) and Nagin (1999), but the intent in both cases is to identify latent classes that have different patterns of change. A related approach has been used by Aldwin, Spiro, Levenson, and Cupertino (2001), who used growth curves to identify individual trajectories of self-reported health, and then cluster analysis to identify groups of persons with similar health trajectories. The resulting groups differed in demographics, antecedent health behaviors, and personality traits, as well as in their subsequent mortality.

Helgeson, Snyder, and Seltman (2004) used Nagin's (1999) approach to identify distinct trajectories of change in self-assessed physical and mental health among breast cancer patients who were assessed seven times over 4 years with the SF-36 health status measure (Stewart & Ware, 1992). Four groups were found for both mental and physical health trajectories; the groups differed in demographics, psychosocial characteristics, and disease-related variables. Legler, Davis, Potosky, and Hoffman (2004) used Muthén's (2001) approach to examine recovery of sexual function following prostate surgery. Four groups were found with distinct patterns of recovery, and these differed in demographics and in treatment-related variables. McDonough, Sacker, and Wiggins (2005) also used Muthén's (2001) approach to analyze the effects of different poverty groups on trajectories of self-rated health. Four such groups were found, differing in gender, race, and education; these groups had different effects on health trajectories and interacted with age, race, and gender to affect initial health.

## SUMMARY

As discussed here, a lifespan developmental perspective consists of four propositions. These propositions have both theoretical and methodological implications for the study of health. They suggest that we consider health over time, in context, from multiple points of view, and with a recognition of its variability both within and among persons. A lifespan approach advocates a focus on both protective and risk factors, on health and disease. Several governmental organizations have advocated a lifespan approach to health (NPHP, 2001; OBSSR, 2005; WHO, 2000), and a growing body of evidence supports its utility (Kuh & Ben-Shlomo, 2004; Kuh & Hardy, 2002; Lynch & Davey Smith, 2005). Although a lifespan perspective has developed primarily in psychology, there are growing interests from other social and biomedical sciences. Furthermore, a number of methodologists and statisticians have adopted a lifespan view, and more and more methods are being developed to test developmental hypotheses.

A lifespan perspective can be taken on various phenomena related to health. One example is on the development of a disease through its various stages (e.g., Lynch & Davey Smith, 2005); another is the development of disability (Verbrugge & Jette, 1984). At a different level of analysis, a lifespan perspective has implications for the study of health care systems, and for the development and implementation of both prevention and intervention programs (Halfon & Hochstein, 2002; NPHP, 2001). If the trajectory of health can be altered early in life by prevention, then perhaps the onset of disease can be prevented; if the trajectory is altered later in life by intervention, perhaps comorbidity can be compressed and health care use reduced (Fries, 2003).

My goal has been to outline one view of a lifespan perspective of health, and to consider some of its methodological implications. If this chapter motivates others to adopt such an approach to theory or methodology, I believe it will enhance the study of the interplay between health and aging, and lead to better foundation for theory, research, and policy.

## ACKNOWLEDGMENTS

I gratefully acknowledge the support provided by the U.S. Department of Veterans Affairs Merit Review program, and by the Massachusetts Veterans Epidemiology Research and Information Center (MAVERIC) and the Normative Aging Study, funded by the Cooperative Studies Program of the U.S. Department of Veterans Affairs. In addition, support was also provided by Grant Nos. AG18436 (Daniel Mroczek, Principal Investigator) and AG14345 (Martin Albert, Principal Investigator) from the National Institutes of Health. This chapter is dedicated to John R. Nesselroade and Paul B. Baltes, in thanks for their roles in setting me along my developmental trajectory.

## REFERENCES

Aldwin, C. M., Spiro, A., III, Levenson, M. R., & Cupertino, A. P. (2001). Longitudinal findings from the Normative Aging Study: III. Personality, health trajectories, and mortality. *Psychology and Aging, 16*(3), 450–465.

Aldwin, C. M., Spiro, A., III, & Park, C. L. (2006). Health, behavior, and optimal aging: A life span developmental perspective. In J. E. Birren & K. W. Schaie (Eds.), *Handbook of the psychology of aging* (6th ed., pp. 85–104). Burlington, MA: Elsevier.

Baltes, P. B. (1987). Theoretical propositions of life-span developmental psychology: On the dynamics between growth and decline. *Developmental Psychology, 23,* 611–626.

Baltes, P. B., Staudinger, U. M., & Lindenberger, U. (1999). Lifespan psychology: Theory and application to intellectual functioning. *Annual Review of Psychology, 50,* 471–507.

Boorse, C. (1997). A rebuttal on health. In J. Humber & R. Almeder (Eds.), *What is disease?* (pp. 1–134). Totowa, NJ: Humana Press.

Brady, C. B., Spiro, A., III, McGlinchey-Berroth, R., Milberg, W., & Gaziano, J. M. (2001). Stroke risk predicts verbal fluency decline in healthy older men: evidence from the Normative Aging Study. *Journals of Gerontology: Psychological Sciences and Social Sciences, Series B, 56*(6), P340–P346.

Clark, J., Spiro, A., III, Miller, D. R., Fincke, B. G., Skinner, K. M., & Kazis, L. E.

(2005). Patient-based measures of illness severity in the Veterans Health Study. *Journal of Ambulatory Care Management, 28*(3), 264–275.

Elinson, J. (1988). Defining and measuring health and illness. In K. W. Schaie, R. T. Campbell, W. Meredith, & S. C. Rawlings (Eds.), *Methodological issues in aging research* (pp. 231–248). New York: Springer.

Evans, R. G., Stoddart, G. L. (2003). Consuming research, producing policy? *American Journal of Public Health, 93*(3), 371–379.

Finch, C. E., & Crimmins, E. M. (2004). Inflammatory exposure and historical changes in human life-spans. *Science, 305*(5691), 1736–1739.

Flanagan, D. P., Genshaft, J. L., & Harrison, P. L. (Eds.). (1997). *Contemporary intellectual assessment: Theories, tests, and issues.* New York: Guilford Press.

Fogel, R. W. (2003). Secular trends in physiological capital: Implications for equity in health care. *Perspectives in Biology and Medicine, 46*(3, Suppl.), S24–S38.

Fozard, J. L., Metter, E. J., & Brant, L. J. (1990). Next steps in describing aging and disease in longitudinal studies. *Journal of Gerontology, 45*(4), P116–P127.

Fries, J. F. (2003). Measuring and monitoring success in compressing morbidity. *Annals of Internal Medicine, 139*(5, Pt. 2), 455–459.

George, L. K. (2003). What life course perspectives offer the study of aging and health. In R. Settersten (Ed.), *Invitation to the life course* (pp. 161–188). Amityville, NY: Baywood.

Gluckman, P. D., & Hanson, M. A. (2004). Living with the past: evolution, development, and patterns of disease. *Science, 305*(5691), 1733–1736.

Griffin, P. W., Mroczek, D. K., & Spiro, A., III. (2006). Variability in affective change among aging men: Findings from the VA Normative Aging Study. *Journal of Research in Personality.*

Grimley Evans, J. (1988). Ageing and disease. In D. Evered & J. Whelan (Eds.), *Research and the ageing population* (pp. 38–57). Chichester, UK: Wiley.

Grossman, M. (2000). The human capital model. In A. J. Culyer & J. P. Newhouse (Eds.), *Handbook of health economics* (Vol. 1A, pp. 347–408). Amsterdam: Elsevier/North-Holland.

Halfon, N., & Hochstein, M. (2002). Life course health development: An integrated framework for developing health, policy, and research. *Milbank Quarterly, 80*(3), 433–479.

Harris, C. W. (Ed.). (1963). *Problems in measuring change.* Madison: University of Wisconsin Press.

Helgeson, V. S., Snyder., P., & Seltman, H. (2004). Psychological and physical adjustment to breast cancer over 4 years: Identifying distinct trajectories of change. *Health Psychology, 23*(1), 3–15.

Hofer, S. M., & Sliwinski, M. J. (2001). Understanding ageing: An evaluation of research designs for assessing the interdependence of ageing-related changes. *Gerontology, 47*(6), 341–352.

Idler, E., & Benyamini, Y. (1997). Self-rated health and mortality: A review of 27 community studies. *Journal of Health and Social Behavior, 38*, 21–37.

Kluckhohn, C., & Murray, H. A. (1948). Personality formation: The determinants. In C. Kluckhohn & H. A. Murray (Eds.), *Personality: Its nature, society, and culture* (pp. 35–52). New York: Knopf.

Kraemer, H. C., Yesavage, J. A., Taylor, J. L., & Kupfer, D. (2000). How can we learn about developmental processes from cross-sectional studies, or can we? *American Journal of Psychiatry, 157*(2), 163–171.

Kravitz, R. L., Duan, N., & Braslow, J. (2004). Evidence-based medicine, heterogeneity of treatment effects, and the trouble with averages. *Milbank Quarterly, 82*(4), 661–687.

Kuh, D., & Ben-Shlomo, Y. (Eds.). (2004). *A life course approach to chronic disease epidemiology* (2nd ed.). New York: Oxford University Press.

Kuh, D., & Hardy, R. (Eds.). (2002). *A life course approach to women's health.* Oxford, UK: Oxford University Press.

Lamarca, R., Alonso, J., Gomez, G., & Munoz, A. (1998). Left-truncated data with age as time scale: An alternative for survival analysis in the elderly population. *Journals of Gerontology: Biological Sciences and Medical Sciences, Series A, 53*(5), M337–M343.

Legler, J. M., Davis, W. W., Potosky, A. L., & Hoffman, R. M. (2004). Latent variable modelling of recovery trajectories: Sexual function following radical prostatectomy. *Statistics in Medicine, 23*(18), 2875–2893.

Lipsitz, L. A., & Goldberger, A. L. (1992). Loss of complexity and aging: Potential applications of fractals and chaos theory to senescence. *Journal of the American Medical Association, 267*, 1806–1809.

Llabre, M. M., Spitzer, S. B., Saab, P. G., & Schneiderman, N. (2001). Piecewise latent growth curve modeling of systolic blood pressure reactivity and recovery from the cold pressor test. *Psychophysiology, 38*(6), 951–960.

Lynch, J., & Davey Smith, G. (2005). A life course approach to chronic disease epidemiology. *Annual Review of Public Health, 26*, 1–35.

MacDonald, S. W., Hultsch, D. F., & Dixon, R. A. (2003). Performance variability is related to change in cognition: Evidence from the Victoria Longitudinal Study. *Psychology and Aging, 18*(3), 510–523.

Marmot, M. (2004). *The status syndrome: How social standing affects our health and longevity.* New York: Holt.

McArdle, J. J., Hamagama, F., Jones, K., Jolesz, F., Kikinis, R., Spiro, A., III, et al. (2004). Structural modeling of dynamic changes in memory and brain structure using longitudinal data from the Normative Aging Study. *Journals of Gerontology: Psychological Sciences and Social Sciences, Series B, 59*, P294–P304.

McCrae, R. R., & Costa, P. T. (2003). *Personality in adulthood: A five-factor theory perspective.* New York: Guilford Press.

McDonough, P., Sacker, A., & Wiggins, R. D. (2005). Time on my side?: Life course trajectories of poverty and health. *Social Science and Medicine, 61*(8), 1795–1808.

Mehta, P. D., & West, S. G. (2000). Putting the individual back into individual growth curves. *Psychological Methods, 5*(1), 23–43.

Miller, D. R., Rogers, W. H., Spiro, A., III, & Kazis, L. E. (2003, December). *Evaluation of disease status based on patient self-report in the Medicare Health Outcomes Survey: Using linked survey data and computerized medical data from the Veterans Health Administration.* Report to the National Committee for Quality Assurance. Health Outcomes Technologies Program, Boston University School of Public Health and the Institute for Health Outcomes and Policy, Center for Health Quality, Outcomes, and Economic Research, VA Medical Center, Bedford, MA. Available online at www.hosonline.org/surveys/hos/download/hos_evaluation_self-report_disease_status.pdf.

Molenaar, P. C. M. (2004). A manifesto on psychology as idiographic science: Bringing the person back into scientific psychology, this time forever (with Discussion). *Measurement, 2*(4), 201–544.

Mroczek, D. K., & Spiro, A., III. (2003). Modeling intraindividual change in personality traits: Findings from the Normative Aging Study. *Journals of Gerontology: Psychological Sciences and Social Sciences, Series B, 58,* P153–P165.

Mroczek, D. K., Spiro, A., III, & Almeida, D. M. (2003). Between- and within-person variation in affect and personality over days and years: How basic and applied approaches can inform one another. *Ageing International, 28,* 260–278.

Murray, C. J. L., Salomon, J. A., Mathers, C. D., & Lopez, A. D. (2002). *Summary measures of population health: Concepts, ethics, measurement and applications.* Geneva: World Health Organization.

Muthén, B. (2001). Second-generation structural equation modeling with a combination of categorical and continuous latent variables: New opportunities for latent class/latent growth modeling. In L. M. Collins & A. Sayer (Eds.), *New methods for the analysis of change* (pp. 291–322). Washington, DC: American Psychological Association.

Nagin, D.S. (1999). Analyzing developmental trajectories: A semi-parametric, group-based approach. *Psychological Methods, 4,* 139–177.

National Public Health Partnership. (2001). *Preventing chronic disease: A strategic framework.* Melbourne, Australia: Author.

Nesselroade, J. R. (1991). The warp and the woof of the developmental fabric. In R. M. Downs, L. S. Liben, & D. S. Palermo (Eds.), *Visions of aesthetics, the environment and development: The legacy of Joachim F. Wohlwill* (pp. 213–240). Hillsdale, NJ: Erlbaum.

Office of Behavioral and Social Sciences Research. (2005). *Behavioral and social sciences research in the 21st century: Summary of recommendations from 6 NAS reports.* Available online at obssr.od.nih.gov/publications/nrc-reports.htm (last updated January 27, 2005).

Omran, A. R. (2005). The epidemiologic transition: A theory of the epidemiology of population change. *Milbank Quarterly, 83*(4), 731–735. (Original work published 1971)

Pepper, S. (1942). *World hypotheses: A study in evidence.* Berkeley: University of California Press.

Peto, R., & Doll, R. (1997). There is no such thing as aging. *British Medical Journal, 315*(7115), 1030–1032.

Raudenbush, S. W. (2001). Comparing personal trajectories and drawing causal inferences from longitudinal data. *Annual Review of Psychology, 52,* 501–525.

Riley, M. W. (1994). Aging and society: Past, present, and future (the 1993 Kent Lecture). *Gerontologist, 34*(4), 436–446.

Rogosa, D. R. (1995). Myths and methods: Myths about longitudinal research, plus supplemental questions. In J. M. Gottman (Ed.), *The analysis of change* (pp. 3–65). Hillsdale, NJ: Erlbaum.

Settersten, R. A. (Ed.) (2003). *Invitation to the life course.* Amityville, NY: Baywood.

Settersten, R. A. (2006). When nations call: How wartime military service matters for the life course and aging. *Research on Aging, 28,* 12–36.

Singer, J. D., & Willett, J. B. (2003). *Applied longitudinal data analysis: Modeling change and event occurrence.* New York: Oxford University Press.

Sliwinski, M. J., Hofer, S. M., & Hall, C. (2003). Correlated and coupled cognitive change in older adults with and without preclinical dementia. *Psychology and Aging, 18,* 672–683.

Smith, R. (2002). In search of "non-disease." *British Medical Journal, 324,* 883–885.

Smith, T. W., & Spiro, A., III. (2002). Personality, health, and aging: Prolegomenon for the next generation. *Journal of Research in Personality, 36,* 363–394 (Erratum, p. 661).

Spiro, A., III. (2001). Health in midlife: Toward a lifespan view. In M. E. Lachman (Ed.), *Handbook of midlife development* (pp. 156–187). New York: Wiley.

Spiro, A., III, & Brady, C. B. (in press) Integrating health into cognitive aging research (and theory). In S. M. Hofer & D. F. Alwin (Eds.), *The handbook of cognitive aging: Interdisciplinary perspectives.* Thousand Oaks, CA: Sage.

Spiro, A., III, Schnurr, P. P., & Aldwin, C. M. (1997). A life-span perspective on the effects of military service. *Journal of Geriatric Psychiatry, 30,* 91–128.

Stewart, A. L., & Ware, J. E. (1992). *Measuring functioning and well-being: The Medical Outcomes Study approach.* Durham, NC: Duke University Press.

Thiebaut, A. C., & Benichou, J. (2004). Choice of time-scale in Cox's model analysis of epidemiologic cohort data: A simulation study. *Statistics in Medicine, 23*(24), 3803–3820.

Vaupel, J. W., & Yashin, A. I. (1985). Heterogeneity's ruses: Some surprising effects of selection on population dynamics. *American Statistician, 39*(3), 176–185.

Verbrugge, L. M., & Jette, A. M. (1984). The disablement process. *Social Science and Medicine, 38*(1), 1–14.

Weitkunat, R., & Wildner, M. (2002). Exploratory causal modeling in epidemiology: Are all factors created equal? *Journal of Clinical Epidemiology, 55*(5), 436–444.

Wohlwill, J. F. (1973). *The study of behavioral development.* New York: Academic Press.

World Health Organization. (1946). The constitution of the World Health Organization. *WHO Chronicle, 1,* 21.

World Health Organization. (2000). *The implications for training of embracing a life course approach to health.* Available online at www.who.int/ageing/publications/lifecourse/alc_lifecourse_training_en.pdf.

Yorgason, J. B., Almeida, D., Neupert, S., Hoffman, L., & Spiro, A., III (in press). A dyadic examination of daily health symptoms and emotional well-being in later life couples. *Family Relations.*

# PART II

# BIOLOGICAL ISSUES

# CHAPTER 6

# Psychoneuroimmunological Processes in Aging and Health

TARA L. GRUENEWALD *and* MARGARET E. KEMENY

Although we are all susceptible to the increased experience of disease and death associated with aging, progression to these inevitable outcomes is thought to be moderated by individual social, psychological, and behavioral factors. In recent decades, this assertion has been bolstered by research that has identified some of the biological pathways through which psychosocial factors might modulate cognitive and physical declines in health. A greater understanding of the ways the social and psychological characteristics of individuals interact with the functioning of their internal biological regulatory systems may aid in efforts to promote health-conferring environments and lifestyles. The field of psychoneuroimmunology (PNI), which concentrates on linkages between psychosocial factors and nervous, neuroendocrine, and immune processes, may provide useful templates for elucidating the pathways that hasten or slow the progression to poor health outcomes among those of increasing age.

An armory of PNI research has demonstrated that social, psychological, and behavioral factors can modulate immunological processes, with the nervous and endocrine systems acting as primary mediators of this modulation (for reviews, see Ader, 2000; Kemeny & Gruenewald, 2000; Kiecolt-Glaser, McGuire, Robles, & Glaser, 2002; Lutgendorf & Costanzo, 2003). Although PNI processes have the potential to affect disease processes at any age, these linkages may be most critical for health status in the early and later years of life, when the immune system is experiencing maturation or senescence, respectively (Coe & Lubach, 2003). Thus, attention to the contribution of PNI relationships in understanding risk factors for

morbidity and mortality in the young and in the old may prove more fruitful in terms of directing health promotion intervention efforts where they
are most useful.

The importance of understanding the role of PNI processes in health
and well-being in older adults is underscored by the fact that the proportion of aged adults in our population will continue to increase substantially
in coming decades. There were an estimated 35 million Americans age 65
and older in the year 2000, and this number is expected almost to double to
over 70 million by 2030, when one out of every five Americans is expected
to be 65 or older (Federal Interagency Forum on Aging-Related Statistics,
2004). Among older adults, the experience of multiple diseases is common
(MacKnight & Rockwood, 2001). Older adults are also more prone to
contract infections and to experience more severe and longer lasting infectious episodes than younger adults (see Castle, 2000; Plackett, Boehmer,
Faunce, & Kovacs, 2004). This greater vulnerability of older adults is
thought to result from changes in immune functioning and other bodily
systems that occur with aging, rendering older adults less able to resist
pathogens and mutagens. Efforts to identify further psychosocial and other
factors that may act to exacerbate or ameliorate this biological vulnerability may prove fruitful in combating increased infection and disease in older
adults. Such efforts will be important to limit the years that individuals live
with disease and disability, ensuring that individuals live both better and
longer lives.

## BIOLOGICAL AGING

Alterations in the functioning of biological regulatory systems are known
to occur throughout an organism's developmental history, but the nature of
such changes in older adults may lead to increased risk for disease and disability. Increasing age is associated with significant alterations in the primary biological mediators and functioning of many physiological systems,
including neuroendocrine and immune systems. Not only are these systems
important for normal physiological functioning, but they also play a central
role in adaptation to life's challenges, including psychosocial and physiological stressors.

### Neuroendocrine Alterations

Neuroendocrine systems in the body are responsible for the performance of
many bodily processes essential to normal functioning, including metabolic,
cardiovascular, digestive, and reproductive functioning. Thus, changes in
the level or activity of hormones that support such functions may have important implications for functioning and disease. The level and activity of

hormones in a number of neuroendocrine pathways appear to show substantial change during older age (see Epel, Burke, & Wolkowitz, Chapter 7, this volume). Aging is associated with significant alterations in *adrenal* (decreased levels of dehydroepiandrosterone [DHEA], DHEA sulfate [DHEAS], androstenedione, and progesterone; higher DHEA-to-cortisol ratio), *gonadal* (decreased testosterone and estrogen), *growth* (decreased growth hormone [GH], insulin-like growth factor-1 [IGF-1], and *calcium* (decreased calcitonin and vitamin D; increased parathyroid hormone) hormone systems (see Straub, Miller, Scholmerich, & Zietz, 2000). Older adults have also been found to have higher basal levels of hypothalamic–pituitary–adrenal (HPA) hormones in some studies (adrenocorticotropic hormone [ACTH] and cortisol; e.g., Van Cauter, Leproult, & Kupfer, 1996; Ferrari et al., 2000; Luz et al., 2003), as well as impaired diurnal cycles of cortisol (e.g., flattened rhythm, higher evening levels; Ferrari et al., 2000) in comparison to younger adults.

## Immune Alterations

The immune system provides bodily protection against infection and disease, and is the primary defender against external (e.g., viruses, bacteria) and internal (e.g., abnormal cell growth) agents of ill health. Immune system functions can broadly be divided into adaptive and innate processes. Adaptive immunity is characterized by antigen-specific immune functions, including the production of antibodies by β lymphocytes (β-cells; humoral immunity) and cell-mediated functions orchestrated by T lymphocytes (T-cells). Innate immunity refers to disease resistance that is not antigen specific and includes nonspecific cytotoxic and phagocytic processes (e.g., killing of virally infected cells by natural killer (NK) cells and "ingestion" of foreign particles by macrophages), and inflammation. Mediators of both arms of the immune system appear to change with increasing age (for reviews, see Butcher & Lord, 2004; Straub et al., 2000), and age-related alterations in immunity are thought to contribute to the increased rate of morbidity and mortality witnessed in older adults (Castle, 2000; Schroder & Rink, 2003).

Lymphocytes and antigen-presenting cells (APCs) are the primary agents in adaptive immune responses. The two major populations of lymphocytes are β-cells and T-cells. β-cells mature within the bone marrow, where they become antibody-producing cells that express unique antigen-binding receptors on their membranes. Upon first contact with an antigen for which a β-cell is specific, a naive β-cell will differentiate into memory β-cells and plasma cells. Memory cells provide protection in the case of future contact with a specific antigen, and plasma cells provide the backbone of the immediate antibody response by secreting high levels of antibodies within a short period of time.

T-cells also originate in the bone marrow but mature in the thymus gland. Commonly studied T-cells include cytotoxic (CD8+) and helper (CD4+) T-cells. Cytotoxic T-cells recognize specific antigens when presented on the surface of an infected bodily cell and initiate mechanisms to kill the infected cell. Helper T-cells play a central role in the activation of both humoral (antibody-mediated) and cell-to-cell (cell-mediated) immune functions. These functions include the activation and proliferation of β- and T-cells, monocytes, NK cells, and other immune cells. This assistance is carried out by chemical messenger proteins released from activated T-cells, commonly referred to as cytokines (e.g., interleukins [ILs]-2, 3, 4, 5, 6, and 10). The activation of helper T-cells, in turn, is dependent on recognition of specific antigens presented by APCs, such as macrophages, β-cells, and dendritic cells, which is also supported by a variety of cytokines released from APCs.

The majority of research conducted on immune alterations with aging has focused on changes in adaptive immune functioning. Alterations in T-cell number and function with age have been documented in many studies. In terms of T-cell number, there appears to be a decrease in the number of naive CD4 and CD8 T-cells, but an expansion in the number of memory cells in those of older age (for reviews, see Castle, 2000; Globerson & Effros, 2000). The expansion of memory cells is thought to result from chronic antigen exposure (e.g., altered self-antigens, viral infections) over the life course. Decreased T-cell proliferation in response to antigenic stimulation has been observed in many, but not all, studies examining age-associated changes in immune function (Chakravarti & Abraham, 1999).

Reductions in the activation and proliferation of β-cells have also been observed in older adults, as well as lower production of specific antibody and a lower production per cell (Castle, 2000). Vaccination-induced antibody responses have been shown to be impaired in older adults (Bernstein et al., 1999), with impairments more likely to occur when helper T-cell involvement is needed to facilitate the antibody response. Impairments in immune responses to vaccination may partially account for the finding that approximately 90% of deaths to influenza in the United States occur in adults age 65 and older (Castle, 2000).

Age-related changes in innate immunity have been less studied, but there is evidence for reduced function of several innate immune cell lines. Neutrophils play a central role in immune responses to bacterial and fungal infections; these cells are first responders to sites of infected tissue, where neutrophils phagocytize ("ingest") and kill foreign invaders (Schroder & Rink, 2003). Although it appears that neutrophil number is similar in the old and the young, there is evidence of a reduction in the phagocytic (ingestion) capacity of neutrophils in older adults (Butcher et al., 2001; Wenisch, Patrulta, Daxbock, Krause, & Horl, 2000), and in the generation of reactive oxygen species involved in the intracellular killing of pathogens (Braga et al., 1998; Biasi et al., 1996); however, age-associated reductions in the production of oxygen species are not always found (e.g., Butcher et al.,

2001). The significance of potential age-related reductions in the phagocytic and killing capabilities of neutrophils is highlighted by the fact that morbidity and mortality from bacterial and fungal infections are prominent in older adults (Schneider, 1983).

NK cells also play a critical role in innate immunity by targeting and killing virus-infected and mutated (cancerous) cells. Compared to young adults, NK cells represent a higher percent of white blood cells in older adults, with this increased percentage a result of decreased T-cell number and increased NK cell number (Plackett et al., 2004). Reviews of NK activity suggest that killing activity is impaired in older adults; however, the clinical significance of this impairment may be offset by the increased number of circulating NK cells in older adults (Castle, 2000).

Macrophages (also called monocytes) perform a variety of important innate immune functions, such as phagocytosis, killing, and upregulation of other innate effector cells through production of cytokines. Macrophage-produced cytokines also play a central role in the activation or inhibition of adaptive immune functions. Research indicates that the phagocytic activity of macrophages of older adults appears to be intact, but that killing of tumor cells is impaired (Castle, 2004; McLachlan, Serkin, Morrey-Clark, & Bakouche, 1995). Monocytes from older adults have been found to produce less IL-1, a cytokine involved in the regulation of both adaptive and innate immune functions, as well as less reactive oxygen and nitrogen species (McLachlan et al., 1995), which play a key role in killing of tumor cells and intracellular killing of microorganisms.

In contrast to the general reductions in some components of adaptive and innate immune cell function, accumulating evidence documents age-related *increases* in proinflammatory cytokines, the chemical mediators that act to upregulate inflammatory processes. Much of this research has focused on increases in the proinflammatory cytokine IL-6 (Ershler & Keller, 2000). This cytokine orchestrates a number of inflammatory immune processes including attracting immune cells to sites of inflammation, activating lymphocytes, and inducing production of acute-phase proteins, e.g., fibrinogen, C-reactive protein (CRP), in the liver. IL-6 is normally expressed at low levels in the serum unless there is an infection, trauma, or other stressor (Ershler & Keller, 2000). However, a growing body of evidence suggests that among apparently healthy adults, those of older age have higher plasma levels of IL-6 (for review, see Ershler & Keller, 2000), or produce greater levels of IL-6 under conditions of antigenic/mitogenic stimulation (Fagiolo et al., 1993; Roubenoff et al., 1998). Age-related increases in circulating levels or stimulated production of IL-6 are not always found, however (Beharka et al., 2001; Peterson et al., 1994). Evidence is also mixed for age-related increases in levels and production of the proinflammatory cytokine tumor necrosis factor–α (TNF-α; Bruunsgaard et al., 1999; Fagiolo et al., 1993; Peterson et al., 1994; Roubenoff et al., 1998).

It is important to recognize that whereas many of these studies have compared older to younger adults, controlling for a number of potential confounding factors (e.g., disease status), unmeasured factors that coincide with aging (e.g., reductions in level of physical activity, changes in diet, or exposure to stressors that are more frequent with age, such as bereavement), may not have been assessed in every investigation and may provide alternative explanations for age-related alterations in immune parameters. Animal studies have confirmed some of the age-associated immune alterations reviewed earlier, providing support for the notion that such changes are a function of the aging process.

## BIOLOGICAL AGING AND DISEASE

The neuroendocrine and immune alterations associated with aging reviewed here may play an important role in older adults' resistance to declines in cognitive and physical functioning, and disease development. As briefly reviewed below, biological mediators of these physiological systems have been implicated in functional impairments and diseases common in older adults.

### Cognitive Impairment

Cognitive impairments, including memory problems and deterioration in intellectual abilities, are common in older adults. These impairments are characterized as dementia when they are of sufficient degree to interfere with social or occupational function. The prevalence of Alzheimer's disease (AD) and dementia doubles every five years in adults over age 65, with AD prevalence rates ranging from 25 to 50% in those over age 85 (Godbout & Johnson, 2004; Larson, Kukull, & Katzman, 1992). A number of biological variables known to change with increasing age have been implicated in the development or severity of cognitive impairments, including high levels of IL-6 (Godbout & Johnson, 2004; Weaver et al., 2002; Yaffe et al., 2003), low levels of DHEA, high levels of cortisol, impaired glucocorticoid feedback regulation, and a high cortisol-to-DHEA ratio (e.g., Ferrari et al., 2000; Pedersen, Wan, & Mattson, 2001; Polleri, Gianelli, & Murialdo, 2002). These biological states characteristic of older age may work together to provide a neurotoxic milieu, leading to neurodegeneration and plaque formation in the brain.

### Physical Impairment/Frailty

Declines in physical functioning and the development of frailty are also more likely with increasing age. Typical measures of older adults' physical functioning include self-reported ability to perform activities of daily living (e.g., bathing, dressing, walking) and performance-based measures of physical function (e.g., gait speed, grip strength, ability to rise from a seated position). Estimates of the percentage of older adults (age 65 years or older) reporting difficulty in performing activities of daily living range from 6 to 18%, depending on the study (Freedman, Martin, & Schoeni, 2002). No established criteria exist to determine whether individuals' possess impairments in performance-based measures of physical function; however, declines in these functional indicators have been shown to occur with increasing age (e.g., over 20% of a sample of older adults ages 70–79 showed declines in performance-based measures over a 3-year period; Seeman et al., 1994). Frailty has been described as a "wasting syndrome of advanced age" (Walston & Fried, 1999, p. 1173), and is often assessed with combined indicators of unintentional weight loss, weakness, exhaustion, slow gait, and low physical activity level (Fried et al., 2001).

Declines in physical functioning and the development of frailty may also be affected by neuroendocrine and immune changes associated with aging. Inflammatory biomarkers, such as IL-6 and CRP, are associated with levels of physical functioning and disability in older adults (Ferrucci et al., 1999; Taaffe, Harris, Ferrucci, Rowe, & Seeman, 2000). Frail older adults have also been shown to have higher levels of inflammatory biomarkers, such as CRP, compared to their nonfrail counterparts (Walston et al., 2002). Hypothesized routes that may underlie associations between cytokines and physical functioning include direct catabolic processes (e.g., breakdown of muscle mass) and negative effects on bone remodeling processes, as well as indirect processes, such as induced anorexia (i.e., reduced dietary intake) and reductions in the anabolic hormones GH and IGF-1 (Ershler & Keller, 2000; Roubenoff, 2003). Low levels of testosterone and DHEA have been found to be associated with lower levels of muscle mass and strength in men (Valenti et al., 2004) but not women, wheras frail elders of both sexes have been shown to have higher cortisol-to-DHEA ratios and impaired glucocorticoid feedback sensitivity (Carvalhaes-Neto, Huayllas, Ramos, Cendoroglo, & Kater, 2003). More research is needed to determine the role of age-associated immune and neuroendocrine changes in the development of frailty.

## Cardiovascular Disease

Cardiovascular disease (CVD) is the number one cause of death in both males and females in the United States, with over 80% of CVD-related deaths occurring in those age 65 and over (American Heart Association, 2005). Indicators of chronic subclinical inflammation, including high circulating levels of proinflammatory cytokines and mediators, such as IL-6, CRP and fibrinogen, are now recognized as important prognostic indicators of CVD health events and CVD-related mortality (Danesh, Collins, Appleby, & Peto, 1998; Pai et al., 2004). It appears that inflammatory processes play a role in both the initial development of CVD conditions and the progression of the disease (see Cooper, Katzel, & Waldstein, Chapter 8, this volume; Tracy, 2003). Inflammatory processes within the vascular system, including inflammation in response to arterial lipid deposition, as well as those that may take place within or outside the vascular system, such as inflammation in response to acute or persistent infection or autoimmune processes, may contribute to CVD development and progression (Black, 2003). Older adults may be more susceptible to the adverse effects of inflammation on the cardiovascular system as a result of increased lifetime exposure to vascular damage and infection that induces inflammation, compromised ability to mount an efficient immune response to infection, as well as decreased regulatory control of proinflammatory cytokines, resulting in persistent elevations in circulating cytokine levels. As we discuss below, psychosocial factors associated with elevations in proinflammatory cytokines may also play a contributing role in inflammation-associated CVD risk.

## Mortality

Given the prominent role of inflammatory processes in cognitive impairment, physical disability and physical disease, it is not surprising that a growing number of studies provide evidence that elevations in proinflammatory cytokines also prospectively predict mortality in older adults. Circulating levels of proinflammatory cytokines and mediators, including IL-6, TNF-$\alpha$, and CRP, have been found to predict both cardiovascular mortality (Volpato et al., 2001) and all-cause mortality (e.g., Bruunsgaard et al., 2003; Harris et al., 1999; Reuben et al., 2002). More research is needed to determine the various pathways through which elevations in proinflammatory cytokines lead to increased mortality risk; the functioning and disease states associated with inflammation we have reviewed here likely play important roles, although associations between elevated cytokine levels and mortality remain, albeit often somewhat reduced, when accounting for these factors.

## PSYCHOSOCIAL FACTORS, BIOLOGICAL AGING, AND HEALTH

The biological changes associated with aging, and the subsequent increased risks for changes in functioning and disease status that may result from these changes, occur within the context of individuals' psychological, social, and physical environments. Psychosocial and physical variables may act as further risk factors, increasing older adults' vulnerability to adverse mental and physical health states, or they may act as protective factors that may help to soften the blow of biological aging on functioning and health outcomes. Below, we highlight briefly key psychosocial risk or protective factors that may have an impact on health outcomes in older adults, and review, when available evidence permits, biological pathways that may play a role in associations with functioning and health.

## Chronic Stressors

Certain traumatic or chronic stressors are more likely to occur in older adults, including the death of friends and family members, the loss of friends due to disability or relocation (of the friend or the self), caregiving for an ill or disabled spouse, and disability and serious health threats, both those faced by the self and others (e.g., Glass, Kasl, & Berkman, 1997). Much of the research on the physiological and health consequences of chronic stress experience in older adults has examined caregiver models of chronic stress (see Fortinsky, Tennen, Frank, & Affleck, Chapter 12, this volume). It is estimated that approximately 15% of the U.S. adult population cares for a seriously ill or disabled family member, with one-third of caregivers being older adults themselves (American Society on Aging, 2001). Although caregiving may provide positive psychological benefits, it is also characterized by psychological, social, physical, and monetary demands that can be exhausting and stressful (Pinquart & Sorensen, 2003; Schulz & Martire, 2004). Adverse effects of caregiving on psychological states, such as depression and self-efficacy, have been shown to occur in both young and old adult caregivers, although these effects have been shown to be more pronounced in older adult caregivers (Pinquart & Sorensen).

A significant body of research indicates that the chronic stress of long-term caregiving is associated with impairments in immune and neuroendocrine functioning. Compared to noncaregiver older adults, older caregivers have been found to have higher antibody titers for latent viruses (indicating poor immune control over latent viral infections; Glaser & Kiecolt-Glaser, 1997), reduced responsiveness of NK cells to cytokine signals (Esterling, Kiecolt-Glaser, & Glaser, 1996), slower healing of wounds (Kiecolt-Glaser, Marucha, Malarkey, Mercado, & Glaser, 1995), poorer antibody responses to vaccination (Kiecolt-Glaser, Glaser, Gravenstein, Malarkey, & Sheridan, 1996), higher levels of basal cortisol (Vedhara et al., 1999), and indicators of poor metabolic functioning (e.g., high levels of triglycerides and fasting insulin, low levels of high-density lipoprotein [HDL] cholesterol; see Vitaliano, Zhang, & Scanlan, 2003). Consistent with the notion that stressor exposure may interact with age to have more deleterious effects on physiology, caregiving-associated decrements in immune responses to vaccination have been shown to be greater in older compared to younger care-givers (Kiecolt-Glaser et al., 1996). However, immunological and neuro-endocrine differences between caregivers and age-matched controls are not always found, nor is age always found to moderate associations between caregiving status and physiological measures (Vitaliano, Zhang, & Scanlan, 2003), although this may be due in part to the tendency to include age as a covariate rather than a moderator in analyses, and the older and restricted age range of the majority of caregivers studied. The immunological and neuroendocrine alterations associated with caregiving burden that have been observed in many studies, however, may have important functioning and health consequences. Caregiving has been found to be associated with poor cognitive functioning (Lee, Kawachi, & Grodstein, 2004), greater risk for the experience of infectious illness (Kiecolt-Glaser, Dura, Speicher, & Trask, 1991), hypertensive changes in blood pressure (Shaw et al., 1999), and mortality (Schulz & Beach, 1999) in older adults. Future research is needed to determine whether the neuroendocrine and immune alterations observed in caregivers mediate these effects.

## Social Stressors and Resources

Social factors (e.g., social isolation) can affect the health and well-being of both young and old, but older adults may be more likely to experience certain negative social stressors, and may be more vulnerable to their effects on physiology and health (see Rook, Mavandadi, Sorkin, & Zettel, Chapter 14, this volume). Social isolation and low levels of social integration (e.g., small number of social ties) have been found prospectively to predict disability, disease development, and mortality in a number of studies (for review, see Seeman, 2000). Older adults are more likely to experience reductions in social network size due to loss of friends and family members from illness, disability, mortality, and reductions in social and occupational activities (Herzog & House, 1991; Rook et al., Chapter 14, this volume); thus, increasing age and reduced social resources may combine to impact health and longevity in aging adults. Some studies have also found that associations between social integration level and mortality are moderated by age with stronger associations in older adults (e.g., Seeman, Kaplan, Knudsen, Cohen, & Guralnik, 1987; Tucker, Schwartz, Clark, & Friedman, 1999; Yasuda et al., 1997). Although research on the biological pathways that may underlie these effects is limited, low levels of social integration have been found to be associated with elevated levels of inflammatory markers (e.g., fibrinogen, CRP, IL-6) in elderly men (Loucks, Berkman, Gruenewald & Seeman, 2005, 2006), and high levels of allostatic load in both men and women (an index of dysregulation in multiple biological regulatory systems, e.g., cardiovascular, metabolic, immune; Seeman et al., 2004).

Older adults, like their younger counterparts, also appear to derive psychological, physiological, and health benefits from qualitative aspects of their social relationships, including perceived availability of social support from network members (Seeman, 2000). For example, greater perceived availability of emotional support has been found to predict lower levels of cognitive decline in older adults (Seeman, Lusignolo, Albert, & Berkman, 2001) and lower mortality following myocardial infarction (Berkman, Leo-Summers, & Horwitz, 1992). Social support has also been shown to be associated with physiological states that may account for some of these associations; greater levels of actual or perceived support have been found to be associated with more positive indicators of cardiovascular, neuroendocrine, and immune functioning (Uchino, Cacioppo, & Kiecolt-Glaser, 1996). Social support has also been found to moderate physiological responses to acute stressor experience in the laboratory. To date, however, there is little information on whether the physiological benefits of social support vary across the lifespan.

Greater engagement in social activity is also an important predictor of decreased risk for declines in cognitive and physical functioning (Bassuk, Glass, & Berkman, 1999; Unger, Johnson, & Marks, 1997) and mortality (Glass, Mendes de Leon, Marottoli, & Berkman, 1999), even in studies controlling for baseline health status (because health problems might impede individuals' ability to engage in social activity). One social activity/resource in which older adults appear to engage or draw upon more than younger adults is involvement and attendance in religious activities and services (Park, Chapter 16, this volume). Fellowship with other church members can provide both a source of social activity and social support. Attendance at church services has been found to be negatively associated with risk of disability onset (Idler & Kasl, 1997) and mortality (Koenig et al., 1999; Lutgendorf, Russell, Ullrich, Harris, & Wallace, 2004). More frequent church attendance has also been found to be associated with lower levels of the proinflammatory cytokine IL-6 (Koenig et al., 1997; Lutgendorf et al., 2004), and IL-6 levels mediated the association between church attendance and mortality in the investigation by Lutgendorf and associates. Other physiological pathways that may be involved in health benefits of church attendance and engagement in other social activities should be an aim of future research.

## Mood State (Depression, Anxiety, and Positive Mood)

Although older adults appear to be less likely to suffer from major depressive disorders compared to younger adults, minor depressive disorders and depressive symptomatology are more common in older adults, with prevalence estimates of 6–23% (typical prevalence rate is ~15%) in community-dwelling older adults (Gallo & Lebowitz, 1997). Less research on anxiety has been conducted in older adult populations, but the prevalence of anxious symptomatology in community samples is also substantial (e.g., 15%; Mehta et al., 2003).

The relatively high rates of depressive and anxious symptomatology may be due to the high rates of physical disease comorbidity and disability in older adults, but these mood states have also been shown prospectively to predict disability, morbidity, and mortality outcomes, independent of baseline disease and functioning status. Depression and depressed mood has been found to predict declines in physical functioning in a number of studies of older adults (for review, see Stuck et al., 1999). Clinical and subclinical levels of depression and anxiety are consistent and strong predictors of morbidity and mortality. A recent review of large-scale ($N > 500$), prospective cohort studies with initially healthy participants indicated that in all 11 studies, depression and/or anxiety were significant predictors of the development of CHD (Hemingway & Marmot, 1999). Depression or depressed mood has been shown to predict CHD, cancer, and all-cause mortality in samples with disease or those that were initially healthy at the time of baseline evaluation of depression (Brown, Levy, Rosberger, & Edgar, 2003; Burg, Benedetto, & Soufer, 2003; Hemingway & Marmot, 1999).

A number of biological alterations found in individuals with depression may account for the poor functioning and health outcomes associated with depression. Depressed individuals have been found to have increased levels of inflammatory biomarkers, including circulating levels of CRP and fibrinogen, and circulating and mitogen-stimulated levels of IL-6, TNF-$\alpha$, and IL-1$\beta$ (e.g., Penninx et al., 2003; Suarez, Krishnan, & Lewis, 2003; von Kanel, Mills, Fainman, & Dimsdale, 2001). Whether enhanced proinflammatory activity is a cause or consequence of depressive states remains unclear, but there is evidence to support a bidirectional association with cytokines inducing negative mood states (Licinio, Kling, & Hauser, 1998; Valentine, Meyers, Kling, Richelson, & Hauser, 1998), and negative mood induction associated with increased cytokine activity (Mittwoch-Jaffe, Shalit, Srendi, & Yehuda, 1995). Irrespective of the direction of this association, increased inflammatory immune activity appears to be characteristic of depressive states in a number of studies. High levels of cortisol are also well-documented in depression studies, including studies of older adults (e.g., Luz et al., 2003; Trzonknowski et al., 2004), and enhanced inflammatory activity may contribute to this state, because inflammatory cytokines, particularly IL-6, are potent stimulators of the HPA axis (Path, Scherbaum, & Bornstein, 2000). It has been hypothesized that age and associated alterations in neuroendocrine and immune functioning may render older adults more vulnerable to biological impairments associated with depression (Kiecolt-Glaser et al., 2002), although little empirical evidence has directly tested this hypothesis to date.

A growing number of studies have evaluated the ability of positive affective states and subjective well-being to predict disease outcomes, including mortality, in older individuals. These positive psychological states have been measured with the positive affect items found on depression and other mood scales, as well as with measures of happiness, life satisfaction, and subjective well-being. Across a number of studies, a relatively consistent predictive association has been observed between positive affect/well-being and reduced mortality in elderly individuals living in the community (Pressman & Cohen, 2005). A few studies also suggest that positive psychological states predict a lower likelihood of the onset of certain diseases, such as stroke (Ostir, Markides, Peek, & Goodwin, 2001). In a review of this literature, Pressman and Cohen (2005) argue that issues, such as the difficulty in obtaining a "healthy" baseline assessment in these longitudinal studies, as well as other methodological problems, compromise the validity of some of these studies. Whereas positive affect has been associated with changes in the neuroendocrine and immune system, few of these studies have been conducted in older individuals. Therefore, the physiological mediators of the positive affect and health relationships in older adults remain unclear.

## Cognitive Factors

Cognitive factors, such as perceptions of mastery and efficacy, as well as older adults' perceptions regarding aging, may also play an important role in functioning and health outcomes in older adults. Self-efficacy, control, and personal mastery beliefs have been found to predict lower likelihood of declines in cognitive and physical functioning over time in older adults (Femia, Zarit, & Johansson, 1997; Mendes de Leon, Seeman, Baker, Richardson, & Tinetti, 1996; Seeman, McAvay, Merrill, Albert, & Rodin, 1996; Skaff, Chapter 10, this volume). Their perceptions about aging may also play a role in disability development and health outcomes as they age. Older adults with more positive perceptions of aging, including the belief that older adults remain useful and happy, showed less decline in physical functioning over an 18-year period (Levy, Slade, & Kasl, 2002) and lived longer over a 20-year follow-up (Levy, Slade, Kunkel, & Kasl, 2002) than those with less positive perceptions of aging. Perceptions of the self in relation to others have also been found to predict disability and mortality outcomes in older adults. For example, older adults who feel more useful to others and society have been shown to have decreased likelihood of experiencing declines in physical functioning and mortality in a number of investigations (Grand, Grosclaude, Bocquet, Pous, & Albarede, 1988; Gruenewald, Karlamangla, Greendale, Singer, & Seeman, in press; Okamoto & Tanaka, 2004; Pitkala, Laakkonen, Strandberg, & Tilvis, 2004). The physiological pathways that play a role in associations between cognitive perceptions and health outcomes in older adults remain to be elucidated, but such efforts represent an interesting area of new research.

## Psychological Interventions

Although a number of intervention studies have involved psychological approaches with the aim of improving health or modifying neuroendocrine and immune outcomes, few have been conducted with samples of older adults (Miller & Cohen, 2001). In one study of adults over age 60, participants enrolled in a 15-week meditation-based movement training program exhibited an increase in varicella-zoster virus–specific cell-mediated immunity compared to wait-list control participants (Irwin, Pike, Cole, & Oxman, 2003). Varicella-zoster virus causes shingles, a painful condition that increases in incidence and severity with age. In another study, a relaxation program provided individually three times a week for a month improved a variety of immune functions, including NK cell activity, in geriatric residents of independent living facilities, when compared to a social contact intervention or no intervention (Kiecolt-Glaser et al., 1985). More research is needed to determine carefully the physiological and health benefits of such interventions in older adults, as well as the conditions under which they are most effective (e.g., in those with a chronic illness or undergoing chronic stress).

## CONCLUSIONS AND FUTURE DIRECTIONS

Declines in cognitive and physical functioning and the development of disease are common characteristics of older age. Age-associated changes in major biological regulatory systems, including neuroendocrine and immune systems, may play a role in the functioning and disease outcomes we have highlighted in this overview. Alterations in these systems may render older adults more vulnerable to the experience of adverse health outcomes. However, age-associated biological vulnerabilities occur within the context of individuals' psychosocial, behavioral, and physical environments. In this overview, we have highlighted social and psychological factors that are shaped by age, that have been shown to be associated with biomarkers of the neuroendocrine and immune systems, and that may operate synergistically with age-associated alterations in biology to confer either increased or decreased risk for poor functioning and health outcomes in older adults.

As reviewed, there is growing evidence that the chronic stressor of caregiving, social isolation, and depressed and anxious mood are significant predictors of greater disability, disease, and mortality. At the same time, social support, positive mood states, and cognitive appraisals of mastery, efficacy, and usefulness have predicted lower rates of these outcomes.

Neuroendocrine and immune changes are associated with these psychological and social factors, but an understanding of the biological mediators of these relationships remains to be fully elucidated.

Although our primary interest is identifying psychosocial risk and protective factors that may affect the health and well-being of older adults, our ability to identify these factors and critically evaluate their role in functioning and disease outcomes is hindered by several gaps in the research literature. One important gap is the relative dearth of research studies investigating the potential moderating role of age in associations among psychosocial factors, biology, and health outcomes. These associations are often studied in specific age groups (e.g., young or old adults), or age is used as a control variable (covariate) in analyses. Investigations examining age as a moderator of associations between psychosocial factors and biological and functioning/health outcomes would allow for the identification of psychological and social factors most strongly linked to these outcomes in older adults. As with research in those of all ages, more investigations of the mediating role of neuroendocrine and immune factors in associations between psychosocial factors and health are needed. These links may be easiest to study in older adult populations, because the prevalence of poor functioning, morbidity, and mortality outcomes is higher in older compared to younger adult samples. It will also be necessary to characterize more carefully social and psychological factors that are impacted by age and may affect biological functioning and health. The scientific literature on age-associated alterations in biology currently dwarfs the analogous literature on age-related changes in psychosocial variables. Sophisticated assessments of variables at each step in the chain from psychosocial factors to biology to health outcomes are needed to clarify our understanding of relationships among these factors and help us design effective health-promotion interventions.

## REFERENCES

Ader, R. (2000). On the development of psychoneuroimmunology. *European Journal of Pharmacology, 405*(1–3), 167–176.

American Heart Association. (2005). *Heart disease and stroke statistics—2005 update.* Dallas, TX: Author.

American Society on Aging. (2001). *Facts on aging: Profile of informal and family caregivers.* San Francisco: Author.

Bassuk, S. S., Glass, T. A., & Berkman, L. F. (1999). Social disengagement and incident cognitive decline in community-dwelling elderly persons. *Annals of Internal Medicine, 131*(3), 165–173.

Beharka, A. A., Meydani, M., Wu, D., Leka, L. S., Meydani, A., & Meydani, S. N. (2001). Interleukin-6 production does not increase with age. *Journals of Gerontology, Biological Sciences and Medical Sciences, Series A, 56*(2), B81–B88.

Berkman, L. F., Leo-Summers, L., & Horwitz, R. I. (1992). Emotional support and survival after myocardial infarction: A prospective, population-based study of the elderly. *Annals of Internal Medicine, 117*(12), 1003–1009.

Bernstein, E., Kaye, D., Abrutyn, E., Gross, P., Dorfman, M., & Murasko, D. M. (1999). Immune response to influenza vaccination in a large healthy elderly population. *Vaccine, 17*(1), 82–94.

Biasi, D., Carletto, A., Dell'Agnola, C., Caramaschi, P., Montesanti, F., Zavateri, G. et al. (1996). Neutrophil migration, oxidative metabolism, and adhesion in elderly and young subjects. *Inflammation, 20*(6), 673–681.

Black, P. H. (2003). The inflammatory response is an integral part of the stress response: Implications for atherosclerosis, insulin resistance, Type II diabetes and metabolic syndrome X. *Brain, Behavior, and Immunity, 17*(5), 350–364.

Braga, P. C., Sala, M. T., Dal Sasso, M., Mancini, L., Sandrini, M. C., & Annoni, G. (1998). Influence of age on oxidative bursts (chemiluminescence) of polymorphonuclear neutrophil leukocytes. *Gerontology, 44*(4), 192–197.

Brown, K. W., Levy, A. R., Rosberger, Z., & Edgar, L. (2003). Psychological distress and cancer survival: A follow-up 10 years after diagnosis. *Psychosomatic Medicine, 65*(4), 636–643.

Bruunsgaard, H., Andersen-Ranberg, K., Jeune, B., Pedersen, A. N., Skinhoj, P., & Pedersen, B. K. (1999). A high plasma concentration of TNF-alpha is associated with dementia in centenarians. *Journals of Gerontology: Biological Sciences and Medical Sciences, Series A, 54*(7), M357–M364.

Bruunsgaard, H., Ladelund, S., Pedersen, A. N., Schroll, M., Jorgensen, T., & Pedersen, B. K. (2003). Predicting death from tumour necrosis factor-alpha and interleukin-6 in 80-year-old people. *Clinical and Experimental Immunology, 132*(1), 24–31.

Burg, M. M., Benedetto, M. C., & Soufer, R. (2003). Depressive symptoms and mortality two years after coronary artery bypass graft surgery (CABG) in men. *Psychosomatic Medicine, 65*(4), 508–510.

Butcher, S. K., Chahal, H., Nayak, L., Sinclair, A., Henriquez, N. V., Sapey, E., et al. (2001). Senescence in innate immune responses: Reduced neutrophil phagocytic capacity and CD16 expression in elderly humans. *Journal of Leukocyte Biology, 70*(6), 881–886.

Butcher, S. K., & Lord, J. M. (2004). Stress responses and innate immunity: Aging as a contributory factor. *Aging Cell, 3*(4), 151–160.

Carvalhaes-Neto, N., Huayllas, M. K., Ramos, L. R., Cendoroglo, M. S., & Kater, C. E. (2003). Cortisol, DHEAS and aging: Resistance to cortisol suppression in frail institutionalized elderly. *Journal of Endocrinological Investigations, 26*(1), 17–22.

Castle, S. C. (2000). Clinical relevance of age-related immune dysfunction. *Clinical Infectious Diseases, 31*(2), 578–585.

Chakravarti, B., & Abraham, G. N. (1999). Aging and T-cell-mediated immunity. *Mechanisms of Ageing and Development, 108*(3), 183–206.

Coe, C. L., & Lubach, G. R. (2003). Critical periods of special health relevance for psychoneuroimmunology. *Brain, Behavior, and Immunity, 17*(1), 3–12.

Danesh, J., Collins, R., Appleby, P., & Peto, R. (1998). Association of fibrinogen, C-reactive protein, albumin, or leukocyte count with coronary heart disease: Meta-analyses of prospective studies. *Journal of the American Medical Association, 279*(18), 1477–1482.

Ershler, W. B., & Keller, E. T. (2000). Age-associated increased interleukin-6 gene expression, late-life diseases, and frailty. *Annual Review of Medicine, 51,* 245–270.

Esterling, B. A., Kiecolt-Glaser, J. K., & Glaser, R. (1996). Psychosocial modulation of cytokine-induced natural killer cell activity in older adults. *Psychosomatic Medicine, 58*(3), 264–272.

Fagiolo, U., Cossarizza, A., Scala, E., Fanales-Belasio, E., Ortolani, C., Cozzi, E., et al. (1993). Increased cytokine production in mononuclear cells of healthy elderly people. *European Journal of Immunology, 23*(9), 2375–2378.

Federal Interagency Forum on Aging-Related Statistics. (2004). *Older Americans 2004: Key indicators of well-being.* Washington, DC: U.S. Government Printing Office.

Femia, E. E., Zarit, S. H., & Johansson, B. (1997). Predicting change in activities of daily living: A longitudinal study of the oldest old in Sweden. *Journals of Gerontology: Psychological Sciences and Social Sciences, Series B, 52*(6), 294–302.

Ferrari, E., Arcaini, A., Gornati, R., Pelanconi, L., Cravello, L., Fioravanti, M., et al. (2000). Pineal and pituitary–adrenocortical function in physiological aging and in senile dementia. *Experimental Gerontology, 35*(9–10), 1239–1250.

Ferrucci, L., Harris, T. B., Guralnik, J. M., Tracy, R. P., Corti, M. C., Cohen, H. J., et al. (1999). Serum IL-6 level and the development of disability in older persons. *Journal of the American Geriatrics Society, 47*(6), 639–646.

Freedman, V. A., Martin, L. G., & Schoeni, R. F. (2002). Recent trends in disability and functioning among older adults in the United States: A systematic review. *Journal of the American Medical Association, 288*(24), 3137–3146.

Fried, L. P., Tangen, C. M., Walston, J., Newman, A. B., Hirsch, C., Gottdiener, J., et al. (2001). Frailty in older adults: evidence for a phenotype. *Journals of Gerontology: Biological Sciences and Medical Sciences, Series A, 56*(3), 146–156.

Gallo, J. J., & Lebowitz, B. D. (1999). The epidemiology of common late-life mental disorders in the community: Themes for the new century. *Psychiatric Services, 50*(9), 1158–1166.

Glaser, R., & Kiecolt-Glaser, J. K. (1997). Chronic stress modulates the virus-specific immune response to latent herpes simplex virus type 1. *Annals of Behavioral Medicine, 19*(2), 78–82.

Glass, T. A., Mendes de Leon, C., Marottoli, R. A., & Berkman, L. F. (1999). Population based study of social and productive activities as predictors of survival among elderly Americans. *British Medical Journal, 319,* 478–483.

Glass, T. A., Kasl, S. V., & Berkman, L. F. (1997). Stressful life events and depressive symptoms among the elderly: Evidence from a prospective community study. *Journal of Aging and Health, 9*(1), 70–89.

Globerson, A., & Effros, R. B. (2000). Ageing of lymphocytes and lymphocytes in the aged. *Immunology Today, 21*(10), 515–521.

Godbout, J. P., & Johnson, R. W. (2004). Interleukin-6 in the aging brain. *Journal of Neuroimmunology, 147*(1–2), 141–144.

Grand, A., Grosclaude, P., Bocquet, H., Pous, J., & Albarede, J. L. (1988). Predictive value of life events, psychosocial factors and self-rated health on disability in an elderly rural French population. *Social Science and Medicine, 27*(12), 1337–1342.

Gruenewald, T. L., Karlamangla, A. S., Greendale, G. A., Singer, B. H., & Seeman, T. E. (in press). Feeling of usefulness to others, disability and mortality in older adults: The MacArthur Study of Successful Aging. *Journal of Gerontology: Psychological Sciences and Social Sciences.*

Harris, T. B., Ferrucci, L., Tracy, R. P., Corti, M. C., Wacholder, S., Ettinger, W. H., et al. (1999). Associations of elevated interleukin-6 and C-reactive protein levels with mortality in the elderly. *American Journal of Medicine, 106*(5), 506–512.

Hemingway, H., & Marmot, M. (1999). Evidence based cardiology: Psychosocial factors in the aetiology and prognosis of coronary heart disease: Systematic review of prospective cohort studies. *British Medical Journal, 318*(7196), 1460–1467.

Herzog, A. R., & House, J. S. (1991). Productive activities and aging well. *Generations: Journal of the American Society on Aging, 15*(1), 49–54.

Idler, E. L., & Kasl, S. V. (1997). Religion among disabled and nondisabled persons II: Attendance at religious services as a predictor of the course of disability. *Journals of Gerontology: Psychological Sciences and Social Sciences, Series B, 52*(6), 306–316.

Irwin, M. R., Pike, J. L., Cole, J. C., & Oxman, M. N. (2003). Effects of a behavioral intervention, Tai Chi Chih, on varicella-zoster virus specific immunity and health functioning in older adults. *Psychosomatic Medicine, 65*(5), 824–830.

Kemeny, M. E., & Gruenewald, T. L. (2000). Affect, cognition, the immune system and health. *Progress in Brain Research, 122,* 291–308.

Kiecolt-Glaser, J. K., Dura, J. R., Speicher, C. E., & Trask, O. J. (1991). Spousal caregivers of dementia victims: Longitudinal changes in immunity and health. *Psychosomatic Medicine, 53*(4), 345–362.

Kiecolt-Glaser, J. K., Glaser, R., Gravenstein, S., Malarkey, W. B., & Sheridan, J. (1996). Chronic stress alters the immune response to influenza virus vaccine in older adults. *Proceedings of the National Academy of Sciences of the United States of America, 93*(7), 3043–3047.

Kiecolt-Glaser, J. K., Glaser, R., Willinger, D., Stout, J., Messick, G., Sheppard, S., Ricker, D., et al. (1985). Psychosocial enhancement of immunocompetence in a geriatric population. *Health Psychology, 4*(1), 25–41.

Kiecolt-Glaser, J. K., Marucha, P. T., Malarkey, W. B., Mercado, A. M., & Glaser, R. (1995). Slowing of wound healing by psychological stress. *Lancet, 346*(8984), 1194–1196.

Kiecolt-Glaser, J. K., McGuire, L., Robles, T. F., & Glaser, R. (2002). Psychoneuroimmunology and psychosomatic medicine: Back to the future. *Psychosomatic Medicine, 64*(1), 15–28.

Koenig, H. G., Cohen, H. J., George, L. K., Hays, J. C., Larson, D. B., & Blazer, D. G. (1997). Attendance at religious services, interleukin-6, and other biological parameters of immune function in older adults. *International Journal of Psychiatry in Medicine, 27*(3), 233–250.

Koenig, H. G., Hays, J. C., Larson, D. B., George, L. K., Cohen, H. J., et al. (1999). Does religious attendance prolong survival?: A six-year follow-up study of 3,968 older adults. *Journals of Gerontology: Biological Sciences and Medical Sciences, Series A, 54*(7), 370–376.

Larson, E. B., Kukull, W. A., & Katzman, R. L. (1992). Cognitive impairment: Dementia and Alzheimer's disease. *Annual Reviews in Public Health, 13,* 431–449.

Lee, S., Kawachi, I., & Grodstein, F. (2004). Does caregiving stress affect cognitive function in older women? *Journal of Nervous and Mental Disease, 192*(1), 51–57.

Levy, B. R., Slade, M. D., & Kasl, S. V. (2002). Longitudinal benefit of positive self-perceptions of aging on functional health. *Journals of Gerontology: Psychological Sciences and Social Sciences, Series B, 57*(5), 409–417.

Levy, B. R., Slade, M. D., Kunkel, S. R., & Kasl, S. V. (2002). Longevity increased by positive self-perceptions of aging. *Journal of Personality and Social Psychology, 83*(2), 261–270.

Licinio, J., Kling, M. A., & Hauser, P. (1998). Cytokines and brain function: Relevance to interferon-alpha-induced mood and cognitive changes. *Seminars in Oncology, 25*(Suppl. 1), 30–38.

Loucks, E. B., Berkman, L. F., Gruenewald, T. L., & Seeman, T. E. (2005). Social integration is associated with fibrinogen concentration in elderly men. *Psychosomatic Medicine, 67*(3), 353–358.

Loucks, E. B., Berkman, L. F., Gruenewald, T. L., & Seeman, T. E. (2006). Relation of social integration to inflammatory marker concentrations in men and women 70–79 years. *American Journal of Cardiology, 97*, 1010–1016.

Lutgendorf, S. K., & Costanzo, E. S. (2003). Psychoneuroimmunology and health psychology: An integrative model. *Brain, Behavior, and Immunity, 17*(4), 225–232.

Lutgendorf, S. K., Russell, D., Ullrich, P., Harris, T. B., & Wallace, R. (2004). Religious participation, interleukin-6, and mortality in older adults. *Health Psychology, 23*(5), 465–475.

Luz, C., Dornelles, F., Preissler, T., Collaziol, D., da Cruz, I. M., & Bauer, M. E. (2003). Impact of psychological and endocrine factors on cytokine production of healthy elderly people. *Mechanisms of Ageing and Development, 124*(8–9), 887–895.

MacKnight, C., & Rockwood, K. (2001). Use of the chronic disease score to measure comorbidity in the Canadian Study of Health and Aging. *International Psychogeriatrics, 13*(Suppl.), 137–142.

McLachlan, J. A., Serkin, C. D., Morrey-Clark, K. M., & Bakouche, O. (1995). Immunological functions of aged human monocytes. *Pathobiology, 63*(3), 148–159.

Mehta, K. M., Simonsick, E. M., Penninx, B. W., Schulz, R., Rubin, S. M., & Satterfield, S. (2003). Prevalence and correlates of anxiety symptoms in well-functioning older adults: Findings from the Health Aging and Body Composition Study. *Journal of the American Geriatrics Society, 51*(4), 499–504.

Mendes de Leon, C. F., Seeman, T. E., Baker, D. I., Richardson, E. D., & Tinetti, M. E. (1996). Self-efficacy, physical decline, and change in functioning in community-living elders: A prospective study. *Journals of Gerontology: Psychological Sciences and Social Sciences, Series B, 51*(4), 183–190.

Miller, G. E., & Cohen, S. (2001). Psychological interventions and the immune system: A meta-analytic review and critique. *Health Psychology, 20*, 47–63.

Mittwoch-Jaffe, T., Shalit, F., Srendi, B., & Yehuda, S. (1995). Modification of cytokine secretion following mild emotional stimuli. *Neuroreport, 6*(5), 789–792.

Okamoto, K., & Tanaka, Y. (2004). Subjective usefulness and 6-year mortality risks among elderly persons in Japan. *Journals of Gerontology: Psychological Sciences and Social Sciences, Series B, 59*(5), 246–249.

Ostir, G. V., Markides, K. S., Peek, M. K., & Goodwin, J. S. (2001). The association between emotional well-being and the incidence of stroke in older adults. *Psychosomatic Medicine, 63*(2), 210–215.

Pai, J. K., Pischon, T., Ma, J., Manson, J. E., Hankinson, S. E., Joshipura, K., et al. (2004). Inflammatory markers and the risk of coronary heart disease in men and women. *New England Journal of Medicine, 51*(25), 2599–2610.

Path, G., Scherbaum, W. A., & Bornstein, S. R. (2000). The role of interleukin-6 in the human adrenal gland. *European Journal of Clinical Investigation, 30*, 91–95.

Pedersen, W. A., Wan, R., & Mattson, M. P. (2001). Impact of aging on stress-responsive neuroendocrine systems. *Mechanisms of Ageing and Development, 122*(9), 963–983.

Penninx, B. W., Kritchevsky, S. B., Yaffe, K., Newman, A. B., Simonsick, E. M., Rubin, S., et al. (2003). Inflammatory markers and depressed mood in older persons: Results from the Health, Aging and Body Composition Study. *Biological Psychiatry, 54*(5), 566–572.

Peterson, P. K., Chao, C. C., Carson, P., Hu, S., Nichol, K., & Janoff, E. N. (1994). Levels of tumor necrosis factor alpha, interleukin 6, interleukin 10, and transforming growth factor beta are normal in the serum of the healthy elderly. *Clinical Infectious Diseases, 19*(6), 1158–1159.

Pinquart, M., & Sorensen, S. (2003). Differences between caregivers and noncaregivers in psychological health and physical health: A meta-analysis. *Psychology and Aging, 18*(2), 250–267.

Pitkala, K. H., Laakkonen, M. L., Strandberg, T. E., & Tilvis, R. S. (2004). Positive life orientation as a predictor of 10-year outcome in an aged population. *Journal of Clinical Epidemiology, 57*(4), 409–414.

Plackett, T. P., Boehmer, E. D., Faunce, D. E., & Kovacs, E. J. (2004). Aging and innate immune cells. *Journal of Leukocyte Biology, 76*(2), 291–299.

Polleri, A., Gianelli, M. V., & Murialdo, G. (2002). Dementia: A neuroendocrine perspective. *Journal of Endocrinological Investigation, 25*(1), 73–83.

Pressman, S. D., & Cohen, S. (2005). Does positive affect influence health? *Psychological Bulletin, 131*, 925–971.

Reuben, D. B., Cheh, A. I., Harris, T. B., Ferrucci, L., Rowe, J. W., Tracy, R. P., et al. (2002). Peripheral blood markers of inflammation predict mortality and functional decline in high-functioning community-dwelling older persons. *Journal of the American Geratrics Society, 50*(4), 638–644.

Roubenoff, R. (2003). Catabolism of aging: Is it an inflammatory process? *Current Opinion in Clinical Nutrition and Metabolic Care, 6*(3), 295–299.

Roubenoff, R., Harris, T. B., Abad, L. W., Wilson, P. W., Dallal, G. E., & Dinarello, C. A. (1998). Monocyte cytokine production in an elderly population: Effect of age and inflammation. *Journals of Gerontology: Biological Sciences and Medical Sciences, Series A, 53*(1), 20–26.

Schneider, E. L. (1983). Infectious diseases in the elderly. *Annals of Internal Medicine, 98*(3), 395–400.

Schroder, A. K., & Rink, L. (2003). Neutrophil immunity of the elderly. *Mechanism of Ageing and Development, 24*(4), 419–425.

Schulz, R., & Beach, S. R. (1999). Caregiving as a risk factor for mortality: The Caregiver Health Effects Study. *Journal of the American Medical Association, 282*(23), 2215–2219.

Schulz, R., & Martire, L. M. (2004). Family caregiving of persons with dementia:

Prevalence, health effects, and support strategies. *American Journal of Geriatric Psychiatry, 12*(3), 240–249.

Seeman, T., Glei, D., Goldman, N., Weinstein, M., Singer, B., & Lin, Y. (2004). Social relationships and allostatic load in Taiwanese elderly and near elderly. *Social Science and Medicine, 59*(11), 2245–2257.

Seeman, T., McAvay, G., Merrill, S., Albert, M., & Rodin, J. (1996). Self-efficacy beliefs and change in cognitive performance: MacArthur Studies of Successful Aging. *Psychology and Aging, 11*(3), 538–551.

Seeman, T. E. (2000). Health promoting effects of friends and family on health outcomes in older adults. *American Journal of Health Promotion, 14*(6), 362–370.

Seeman, T. E., Charpentier, P. A., Berkman, L. F., Tinetti, M. E., Guralnik, J. M., Albert, M., et al. (1994). Predicting changes in physical performance in a high-functioning elderly cohort: MacArthur Studies of Successful Aging. *Journals of Gerontology: Biological Sciences and Medical Sciences, Series A, 49*(3), 97–108.

Seeman, T. E., Kaplan, G. A., Knudsen, L., Cohen, R., & Guralnik, J. (1987). Social network ties and mortality among the elderly in the Alameda County Study. *American Journal of Epidemiology, 126*(4), 714–723.

Seeman, T. E., Lusignolo, T. M., Albert, M., & Berkman, L. (2001). Social relationships, social support, and patterns of cognitive aging in healthy, high-functioning older adults: MacArthur Studies of Successful Aging. *Health Psychology, 20*(4), 243–255.

Shaw, W. S., Patterson, T. L., Ziegler, M. G., Dimsdale, J. E., Semple, S. J., & Grant, I. (1999). Accelerated risk of hypertensive blood pressure recordings among Alzheimer caregivers. *Journal of Psychosomatic Research, 46*(3), 215–227.

Straub, R. H., Miller, L. E., Scholmerich, J., & Zietz, B. (2000). Cytokines and hormones as possible links between endocrinosenescence and immunosenescence. *Journal of Neuroimmunology, 109*(1), 10–15.

Stuck, A. E., Walthert, J. M., Nikolaus, T., Bula, C. J., Hohmann, C., & Beck, J. C. (1999). Risk factors for functional status decline in community-living elderly people: A systematic literature review. *Social Science and Medicine, 48*(4), 445–469.

Suarez, E. C., Krishnan, R. R., & Lewis, J.G. (2003). The relation of severity of depressive symptoms to monocyte-associated proinflammatory cytokines and chemokines in apparently healthy men. *Psychosomatic Medicine, 65*, 362–368.

Taaffe, D. R., Harris, T. B., Ferrucci, L., Rowe, J., & Seeman, T. E. (2000). Cross-sectional and prospective relationships of interleukin-6 and C-reactive protein with physical performance in elderly persons: MacArthur Studies of Successful Aging. *Journals of Gerontology: Biological Sciences and Medical Sciences, Series A, 55*(12), 709–715.

Tracy, R. P. (2003). Thrombin, inflammation, and cardiovascular disease: an epidemiologic perspective. *Chest, 124*(Suppl. 3), 49–57.

Trzonkowski, P., Mysliwska, J., Godlewska, B., Szmit, E., Lukaszuk, K., Wieckiewicz, J., et al. (2004). Immune consequences of the spontaneous pro-inflammatory status in depressed elderly patients. *Brain, Behavior, and Immunity, 18*(2), 135–148.

Tucker, J. S., Schwartz, J. E., Clark, K. M., & Friedman, H. S. (1999). Age-related changes in the associations of social network ties with mortality risk. *Psychology and Aging, 14*(4), 564–571.

Uchino, B. N., Cacioppo, J. T., & Kiecolt-Glaser, J. K. (1996). The relationship between social support and physiological processes: A review with emphasis on underlying mechanisms and implications for health. *Psychological Bulletin, 119*(3), 488–531.

Unger, J. B., Johnson, C. A., & Marks, G. (1997). Functional decline in the elderly: Evidence for direct and stress-buffering protective effects of social interactions and physical activity. *Annals of Behavioral Medicine, 19*(2), 152–160.

Valenti, G., Denti, L., Maggio, M., Ceda, G., Volpato, S., Bandinelli, S., et al. (2004). Effect of DHEAS on skeletal muscle over the life span: The InCHIANTI study. *Journals of Gerontology: Biological Sciences and Medical Sciences, Series A, 59*(5), 466–472.

Valentine, A. D., Meyers, C. A., Kling, M. A., Richelson, E., & Hauser, P. (1998). Mood and cognitive side effects of interferon-alpha therapy. *Seminars in Oncology, 25*, 39–47.

Van Cauter, E., Leproult, R., & Kupfer, D. J. (1996). Effects of gender and age on the levels and circadian rhythmicity of plasma cortisol. *Journal of Clinical Endocrinology and Metabolism, 81*(7), 2468–2473.

Vedhara, K., Cox, N. K., Wilcock, G. K., Perks, P., Hunt, M., Anderson, S., et al. (1999). Chronic stress in elderly carers of dementia patients and antibody response to influenza vaccination. *Lancet, 353*(9153), 627–631.

Vitaliano, P. P., Zhang, J., & Scanlan, J. M. (2003). Is caregiving hazardous to one's physical health?: A meta-analysis. *Psychological Bulletin, 129*(6), 946–972.

Volpato, S., Guralnik, J. M., Ferrucci, L., Balfour, J., Chaves, P., Fried, L. P., et al. (2001). Cardiovascular disease, interleukin-6, and risk of mortality in older women: The Women's Health and Aging Study. *Circulation, 103*(7), 947–953.

von Kanel, R., Mills, P. J., Fainman, C., & Dimsdale, J. E. (2001). Effects of psychological stress and psychiatric disorders on blood coagulation and fibrinolysis: A biobehavioral pathway to coronary artery disease? *Psychosomatic Medicine, 63*(4), 531–544.

Walston, J., & Fried, L. P. (1999). Frailty and the older man. *Medical Clinics of North America, 83*(5), 1173–1194.

Walston, J., McBurnie, M. A., Newman, A., Tracy, R. P., Kop, W. J., Hirsch, C. H., et al. (2002). Frailty and activation of the inflammation and coagulation systems with and without clinical comorbidities: Results from the Cardiovascular Health Study. *Archives of Internal Medicine, 162*(20), 2333–2341.

Weaver, J. D., Huang, M. H., Albert, M., Harris, T., Rowe, J. W., & Seeman, T. E. (2002). Interleukin-6 and risk of cognitive decline: MacArthur Studies of Successful Aging. *Neurology, 59*(3), 371–378.

Wenisch, C., Patruta, S., Daxbock, F., Krause, R., & Horl, W. (2000). Effect of age on human neutrophil function. *Journal of Leukocyte Biology, 67*(1), 40–45.

Yaffe, K., Lindquist, K., Penninx, B. W., Simonsick, E. M., Pahor, M., Kritchevsky, S., et al. (2003). Inflammatory markers and cognition in well-functioning African-American and white elders. *Neurology, 61*(1), 76–80.

Yasuda, N., Zimmerman, S. I., Hawkes, W., Fredman, L., Hebel, J. R., & Magaziner, J. (1997). Relation of social network characteristics to 5-year mortality among young-old versus old-old white women in an urban community. *American Journal of Epidemiology, 145*(6), 516–523.

# CHAPTER 7

# The Psychoneuroendocrinology of Aging

## Anabolic and Catabolic Hormones

ELISSA S. EPEL, HEATHER M. BURKE,
*and* OWEN M. WOLKOWITZ

As the American population ages, the number of Americans with some form of age-related disease (e.g., heart disease, diabetes, cancer, Alzheimer's disease) will reach epidemic proportions. "Biological age"—based on physiological markers of aging in the absence of disease—may be more predictive of age-related disease than chronological age—based on years of living. Unfortunately, there are few accepted markers of biological age. The neuroendocrine system offers some insight as to one's biological age, and phenotyping neuroendocrine profiles may help to explain variance in longevity.

"Psychoneuroendocrinology" is the study of interactions between mind, brain, and hormonal function. A glance at the neuroanatomy of the endocrine system reveals the intimate connections between the brain and the periphery. Hormones not only regulate peripheral physiology and homeostasis but also act on brain sites to actively affect brain function and neuronal longevity (Sapolsky, Krey, & McEwen, 1986). Subtle yet chronic changes in hormonal patterns can exert pathological effects on health over time. Besides sex, one of the biggest factors shaping the neuroendocrine milieu is aging. Aging causes subtle and blatant changes; initially, blood hormone levels may not be noticeably different, but the amplitude and frequency of hormone pulses are altered, usually decreased (Wise, 1999). Later, in older age, certain hormone deficiencies become more common and on a spectrum with clinical endocrine disorders. This chapter primarily focuses on the hypothalamic–pituitary–adrenal (HPA) axis, because we know the most about this axis.

The pure effects of chronological aging on neuroendocrine function, which we refer to as "primary aging," are difficult to study without taking into account effects of life stress and lifestyle factors, which together promote secondary aging. Despite the sometimes large effects of primary aging on hormones, there is nevertheless great variability between elderly individuals' hormonal profiles. In this chapter, we delineate some of the modifiable behavioral factors that help explain this interindividual variability in hormonal profiles. We propose that many of the effects of primary aging on hormones (e.g., decreases in growth hormone [GH], insulin-like growth factor–1 [IGF-1], and thyroid; increases in cortisol) are not inevitable and are exacerbated by chronic stress and lifestyle factors.

At the micro or cellular level, telomere length of leukocytes may serve as another marker of biological age, in that it serves as an index of cell longevity, and possibly human longevity (Cawthon, Smith, O'Brien, Sivatchenko, & Kerber, 2003), and is also associated with duration of stressful life experiences and impaired allostasis (Epel et al., 2004; Epel, Lin, et al., 2006). Furthermore, it is plausible that neuroendocrine aging promotes cellular aging, based on *in vitro* studies reviewed.

## THE COMMON NEUROENDOCRINE AGING PROFILE: ANABOLIC–CATABOLIC IMBALANCE

Rather than reviewing the changes of single hormones separately, it is helpful to take a systems-level view of the changes. Readers are referred elsewhere for in-depth background on individual hormones (Morrison, 1996; Wolkowitz & Rothschild, 2003). At a most basic (and perhaps overly reductionistic) level, hormonal activity can be classified as having anabolic and catabolic functions. Anabolic functions promote salutary tissue growth (e.g., lean mass, bone, and in some cases, immune cells), whereas catabolic functions catabolize or break down bone or lean tissue for fuel. Hormones have different roles depending on timing of release, amount, and whether they stimulate effectors. Furthermore, it may be the relative balance of these classes of hormones that determines the extent to which there is an overall net catabolic process, especially when considering chronic or long-term changes, which argues for a systems approach. Based on effects of long-term exposure of each hormone on lean mass or bone, we classify cortisol and catecholamines as catabolic, and testosterone, estrogen, dehydroepiandrosterone (DHEA), and IGF-1 as anabolic (Bjorntorp, 1995; Herndon & Tompkins, 2004; Togari, 2002).

In some individuals, aging is associated with a syndromal shift in hormonal milieu from hormones with anabolic functions to those with more catabolic functions. This anabolic–catabolic hormone imbalance ("A/C imbalance") may serve as an index of biological age and thus disease risk. When cortisol is chronically elevated, it reduces lean mass, bone density, shifts fat stores to more atherogenic visceral fat distribution patterns (Dallman, Pecoraro, & la Fleur, 2005), and leads to atrophy of hippocampal cells (Sapolsky et al., 1986). Changes in anabolic and catabolic hormones are significant in that in many cases, hormone levels precede onset of age-related diseases such as osteoporosis, visceral adiposity, and other aspects of the metabolic syndrome, Alzheimer's disease, and major depression, (Bjorntorp, 1995; Goodyer, Herbert, & Altham, 1998; Harris et al., 2000; Otte et al., 2005).

## Catabolic Hormones: The HPA Axis, Focusing on Cortisol

### Basal Diurnal Cortisol

Many studies have examined multiple measures of daily cortisol and whether they vary by age. There is mixed evidence for a relationship between basal HPA axis activity and aging. Basal cortisol and adrenocorticotropic hormone (ACTH) levels tend to be higher in older men and women (Deuschle, Gotthardt, et al., 1997; Ferrari et al., 1995; Van Cauter, Leproult, & Kupfer, 1996), although other studies have not found differences in basal cortisol levels (Kudielka, Schmidt-Reinwald, Hellhammer, & Kirschbaum, 1999; Seeman & Robbins, 1994), especially those using a single time point before administering a stressor or challenge. As might be expected, cortisol tends to be elevated in elderly adults with psychiatric and medical comorbidities (Otte et al., 2005).

The pattern of age-related changes in cortisol in healthy people varies considerably between individuals. Rather than consistent "main effects" of aging across studies, it is more likely that those most vulnerable, presumably due to greater life stress, lifestyle factors, or genetic vulnerabilities, will be those who show increased basal cortisol with age. In a longitudinal study, Lupien et al. (2005), following 51 older individuals over time, demonstrated basal cortisol variability with aging, and potential clinical significance of these individual differences. They found no relation between age and cortisol level or increase in cortisol over a 5-year period. However, they found subgroups with distinct cortisol dynamics: those that had increasing cortisol levels over time, with currently high levels (12); those that had increasing levels over time, with only moderate current levels (29); and those that had *decreasing* levels over time, with current moderate levels (10). These differences were pathophysiologically relevant. The group with increasing cortisol levels and with high initial levels had greater memory impairments, increases in trigylcerides, and showed 14% atrophy of hippocampal volume on a magnetic resonance imaging (MRI) scan compared to the group with decreasing cortisol secretion over the 5 years. This latter group had memory performance equivalent to that of young samples, suggesting that increases in cortisol with age are certainly not inevitable.

Studies also suggest that the correlation between cortisol and age is stronger among those high in distress. In one study of 47- to 78-year-olds with ongoing stressors (bereavement or hospitalization of spouse within the last 2 months), 24-hour urinary cortisol was progressively elevated with age, but only in those with depressive symptoms (Jacobs, Mason, Kosten, Brown, & Ostfeld, 1984). Another study found a correlation between 24-hour plasma cortisol and age in people with current depression, which disappeared when the participants recovered from depression (Asnis et al., 1981). *Thus, there appears to be an interaction between age and depression in terms of effects on the HPA axis, with basal cortisol output increasing with age in some individuals, particularly those who are depressed.*

## Stress Reactivity

Aging may also alter responsivity to environmental demands. Allostasis describes the fluctuations in regulatory systems needed to maintain homeostasis (McEwen, 1998). Many hormonal systems show large fluctuations throughout the day, depending on level of arousal or activity (e.g., eating, exercise, rest). Aging may lead to a breakdown in ability to respond to stressors. This appears to be true with the HPA axis, which has been tested most in response to challenges. Otte et al. (2005) performed a meta-analysis of 45 studies comparing cortisol responses to challenge in young versus older healthy samples, controlling for confounds of smoking, medication use, and health problems. Of these studies, six examined psychosocial stressors and the remainder examined responses to pharmacological challenge. In both types of studies, age was related to greater cortisol responses. Impaired allostasis in the form of cortisol reactivity may extend to middle-aged adults as well (Steptoe, Kunz-Ebrecht, Wright, & Feldman, 2005).

The relationship between cortisol reactivity and aging is three times stronger for women than for men (Otte et al., 2005). It is unclear why gender appears to interact with age in predicting increased reactivity. Estrogen can reduce activity, so this finding may be related to the dramatic decrease in estrogen exposure among aged women (Young, Altemus, Parkison, & Shastry, 2001), greater cumulative burden of life stress or depression in women, or that types of stressors to which older adults are exposed tend to be more interpersonal in nature (Aldwin, Sutton, Chiara, & Spiro, 1996), to which women tend to respond with greater cortisol reactivity than do men (Stroud, Salovey, & Epel, 2002).

## HPA Axis Negative Feedback Sensitivity (Tested by Pharmacological Stimulation)

Another way to test allostasis of the HPA axis is to examine the integrity of the negative feedback loop. According to the glucocorticoid cascade hypothesis, which is based on rat studies, cortisol overexposure damages sites of negative feedback, particularly in the hippocampus (Sapolsky, 1989). Because the hippocampus is an important mediator of negative feedback onto the HPA axis, hippocampal damage further impairs the shutoff response of the HPA axis, leading to progressively higher cortisol levels and further hippocampal destruction.

The Dexamethasone Suppression Test (DST) provides a way to test negative feedback sensitivity, particularly of glucocorticoid receptors in the pituitary. In healthy, nondepressed individuals, administration of dexamethasone lowers endogenous cortisol production, but 30–50% of people with major depression exhibit greater endogenous cortisol responses to the DST, most likely due to corticotripin-releasing hormone (CRH) overdrive, or downregulated or subsensitive cortisol receptors. DST studies comparing older and younger samples find greater post-DST cortisol responses with aging, particularly in women (Otte et al., 2005). Wilkinson et al. (2005), by blocking cortisol synthesis and then infusing hydrocortisone, have repeatedly found deficits in negative feedback suppression of ACTH in aging, and have shown that the age-related deficit in feedback inhibition is linked to altered mineralocorticoid receptor function. In summary, there appear to be losses of and/or reduced sensitivity in glucocorticoid and mineralocorticoid receptors due to primary aging, resulting in more impaired negative feedback, and subsequently slightly higher basal cortisol levels in older individuals than in their younger counterparts.

## The Sympathetic–Adrenomedullary Axis

The sympathetic–adrenomedullary (SAM) axis is part of the sympathetic nervous system and is partially responsible for initiating the "fight-or-flight" response. In the SAM axis, stress stimulates nerves that directly innervate the adrenal medulla, which in turn releases norepinephrine (NE) and epinephrine (EPI) into the bloodstream. Stress may also activate NE's release as a neurotransmitter from the locus coeruleus (LC) in the brain. This has widespread effects, including direct interactions with CRH in the central nucleus of the amygdala. Data suggest that in people with depression or chronic stress, there is a "coactivation" or a mutually reinforcing link between activation of the LC and this CRH pathway, with each being driven and sustained by high levels of cortisol (Wong et al., 2000).

Because nerve impulses directly stimulate the adrenal medulla, the SAM axis has faster and more immediate effects than the slower-acting HPA axis.

Basic effects of SAM hormones (NE and EPI) include increased heart rate, blood pressure, metabolic rate, and alertness. There is some evidence for heightened sympathetic tone with aging, described below. However, very few aging studies have been done on NE and EPI, likely due in part to the difficulty of collecting repeated blood measures (since snapshot measures are usually not informative and may reflect stress from venipuncture). In several studies of men, older men had higher levels of basal NE than their younger counterparts (Barnes, Raskind, Gumbrecht, & Halter, 1982; Esler et al., 1995; Kudielka, Schmidt-Reinwald, Hellhammer, Schurmeyer, & Kirschbaum, 2000). These age differences may be clinically significant, in that older adults with higher EPI and NE have earlier mortality and greater degrees of functional decline (Reuben, Talvi, Rowe, & Seeman, 2000).

Though based on a small number of studies, older adults also tend to show greater SAM stress reactivity. Both older men and women have higher NE responses to cold pressor (Palmer, Ziegler, & Lake, 1978) and, in one study, to psychosocial stressors (Aslan, Nelson, Carruthers, & Lader, 1981), although other studies have not found age differences (Blandini et al., 1992; Ng, Callister, Johnson, & Seals, 1994).

## Anabolic Hormones

### Dehydroepiandrosterone

DHEA, a mild anabolic–androgenic hormone in its own right, serves as the major precursor for the sex steroids testosterone and estrogen. In addition to being synthesized in the adrenal gland and the gonads, DHEA is synthesized in the brain, where it is called a "neurosteroid" and has direct neural effects (Baulieu, 1997). The past two decades have witnessed tremendous interest in DHEA as a possible "antiaging" hormone (Wolkowitz & Reus, 2000). Although empirical studies are putting these expectations into better perspective (Wolf & Kirschbaum, 1998), several compelling lines of evidence have fueled this interest. First, circulating levels of DHEA and its sulfate [DHEAS; together referred to as "DHEA(S)"] progressively decline from young adulthood through the end of the lifespan, making them one of the most reliable biomarkers of age; DHEA(S) levels reach their peak in the mid-20s and approach a nadir (~20% of peak levels) at approximately 65–70 years, the age at which the incidence of many age-related illnesses steeply increases (Regelson, Loria, & Kalimi, 1994).

Second, preclinical studies suggest that DHEA(S) protects against neurodegeneration (Kimonides, Spillantini, Sofroniew, Fawcett, & Herbert, 1999) and various pathological processes seen in illness and aging (Svec & Porter, 1998), although the relevance of many animal studies is questionable given that rodents secrete little DHEA compared to humans. Third, some epidemiological studies suggest that relatively higher DHEA(S) levels are associated with enhanced physical and mental well-being (Wolkowitz & Reus, 2000), whereas lower levels of DHEA(S) are associated with hippocampal atrophy (Magri et al., 2000), depression (Wolkowitz & Reus, 2000), and cardiovascular disease (CVD; Hechter, Grossman, & Chatterton, 1997), although many of the studies on cardiovascular disease may be flawed (Tchernof & Labrie, 2004).

Because cortisol levels typically either rise or do not change with age, there is a highly significant decrease in plasma ratios of DHEA(S)-to-cortisol with age (Hechter, Grossman, & Chatterton, 1997). Several authors have suggested that these ratios are more meaningful than are levels of DHEA(S) or cortisol alone (Hechter et al., 1997; Wolkowitz & Reus, 2000). One study comparing cortisol and DHEA in serum and cerebrospinal fluid (CSF) found low DHEA-to-cortisol ratios with age, mainly due to lower DHEA in people over 60 years old (Guazzo, Kirkpatrick, Goodyer, Shiers, & Herbert, 1996). It was also notable that a cortisol–age relationship was found in CSF but not in serum, suggesting that central age-related changes in HPA axis activity may not be apparent by examining circulating blood cortisol levels. These findings of DHEA-to-cortisol ratio changes with age are consistent with the notion proposed here that "A/C imbalance" plays a role in aging.

## The Somatotropic Axis (Growth Hormone and IGF-1)

Growth hormone (GH) is an important age-related hormone. The hypothalamus secretes growth hormone-releasing hormone (GHRH), which stimulates, and somatostatin, which suppresses the anterior pituitary release of GH. GH then stimulates the liver to synthesize insulin-like growth factors, most notably IGF-1, the major anabolic effector of GH.

Adults vary greatly in their ability to secrete GH. Starting as early as age 25, GH levels begin to decline, and it is estimated that one-third of elderly adults reach a "somatopause," or functional cessation of GH secretion (Martin, Yeo, & Sonksen, 1997; Van Cauter, Leproult, & Plat, 2000). GH deficiency due to aging is associated with the same symptoms as clinical GH deficiency secretion (Martin et al., 1997), including excessive fat mass and hyperlipidemia; reduced muscle mass, strength, and bone density; and greater risk of death from CVD, as well as higher levels of psychological distress and major depression in both genders (Lynch et al., 1994; Vance & Mauras, 1999).

These effects of GH deficiency are largely due to insufficient IGF. Some of GH's direct effects are catabolic, similar to cortisol, such as inducing insulin resistance (by blocking insulin signaling in liver, primarily, and in muscle, and possibly by reducing insulin-sensitizing adipocytokines, e.g., adiponectin; Dominici et al., 2005). Conversely, IGF-1 enhances insulin action, leading to insulin sensitivity, and is critical to skeletal and cardiovascular muscle strength. The effect of IGF-1 then typically overrides the catabolic effects of GH. IGF-1 also exerts negative feedback on the pituitary to shut off GH secretion, and insufficient synthesis of IGF-1 can lead to excessive GH and GH-induced insulin resistance (Yakar, Pennisi, Wu, Zhao, & LeRoith, 2005). In men, despite known declines in GH with aging, aging is related to a lower IGF-1-to-GH ratio, suggesting that relative levels of each hormone—high IGF in relation to GH—are important to healthy aging (Morley et al., 1997). The interrelationships among IGF, GH, and IGF-binding proteins may also change with age (Wise, 1999), so it is helpful to measure each of these three factors when possible.

Although many animal studies find that IGF-1 signaling promotes aging and earlier mortality (Tatar, Bartke, & Antebi, 2003), this may be due in part to the fact that lower species have a shared IGF–insulin receptor, whereas humans have a specific receptor for IGF (Rincon, Rudin, & Barzilai, 2005). This is significant in that insulin exposure, in contrast to IGF-1 effects, promotes abdominal adiposity and the metabolic syndrome, whereas insulin sensitivity is linked to longevity, at least as demonstrated by centenarians (Paolisso et al., 1999). This difference in receptor specificity may explain why IGF-1 promotes aging in lower species but appears to have salutary effects in humans.

### The Hypothalamic–Pituitary–Gonadal Axis

In women, the dramatic fluctuations and then loss of estrogen and progesterone during perimenopause lead to loss of menses and compensatory increases in follicle-stimulating hormone, luteinizing hormone, and mood symptoms (Rehman & Masson, 2005). Men experience more subtle hormonal changes with aging. Testosterone declines with age in males (Morley et al., 1997) and around 2.4 million men have androgen deficiency, with associated symptoms of low libido, erectile dysfunction, and depressive symptoms (Trubo, 2005). Testosterone has anabolic effects in terms of stimulating lean mass, and estrogen and testosterone both promote bone mass. The decline in reproductive hormones is linked to the phenotypic changes with age, including loss of bone mass and redistribution of fat stores toward the abdominal/visceral area. In the Morley et al. (1997) study of healthy men, decreases in testosterone showed the strongest correlation with age, and with cognitive and physical changes.

### Summary: Is There Empirical Support for an A/C Imbalance with Aging?

As described earlier, chronological aging is clearly linked to decreases in anabolic hormones, mainly DHEA, sex hormones such as testosterone and estrogen, GH, and IGF-1. Conversely, cortisol and catecholamines, which tend to have more catabolic effects (in terms of breaking down energy stores) do not tend to decrease with age, and if they do change, they tend to increase basally. Further, the magnitude of the acute stress response of cortisol and catecholamines also tends to increase with aging. Functionally, the HPA axis and the somatrotropic and gonadal axes are coregulated, in that they have antagonistic effects on each other. Thus, increases in activity in an anabolic axis might suppress activity of the HPA axis (and vice versa). For these reasons, with aging and the typical decreases in anabolic hormones, the anabolic-to-catabolic balance is decreased, leading to what we have called "A/C imbalance." These decreases appear to be normative, although they are probably on a spectrum with diagnosable idiopathic endocrine deficiency disorders that appear with age and that are treatable with hormone replacement (e.g., testosterone deficiency, GH deficiency). Furthermore, there is considerable interindividual variability, with some showing little change with aging.

If A/C balance is indeed tied to aging and good health, we should observe a salutary A/C balance in healthy centenarians, especially in those who have avoided major diseases (around 30% of those who live to 100). When compared to a control sample of healthy older adults (less than 100 years old), healthy centenarians tend to show lower fasting insulin and glucose (Paolisso et al., 2001), higher or similar thyroid hormones (Baldelli, Zucchi, Pradelli, Montanini, & DeSantis, 1996; Magri et al., 2002), and similar cortisol and GH levels (Baldelli et al., 1996). These results tend to be based on snapshot blood sampling, which should be interpreted cautiously but nonetheless support the idea that A/C balance does not inevitably deteriorate in older age and is important to good health.

Last, A/C imbalance is merely the most common pattern of hormonal changes with aging; thus, there are many exceptions to this pattern. DHEA tends to decrease less in women than in men, and around 15% of women (vs. 5% of men) show *increases* in DHEA in older age (Tannenbaum, Barrett-Connor, Laughlin, & Platt, 2004). Elevated DHEA(S) has been related to factors such as the metabolic syndrome in women (Barrett-Connor & Ferrara, 1996), and elevated growth factors such as IGF-1 are related to breast cancer. Thus such elevations in anabolic hormones are not always a sign of good neuroendocrine health.

## STRESS AND LIFESTYLE MODERATORS

### Chronic Stress and Distress

Primary aging effects (promoting A/C imbalance) are intertwined with secondary effects from chronic stress, because aging increases exposure to certain chronic stressors. Older adults are vulnerable to negative effects of stress due to both increased exposure to chronic stress and decreased physiological resiliency, most apparent in impaired allostasis when responding to acute stressors. Old age is a time associated with numerous chronic psychosocial stressors, such as social isolation, financial stress, bereavement, and caregiving (Aldwin et al., 1996). Not only are older adults often exposed to more chronic stressors than their younger counterparts, but there is also accumulating evidence that older individuals are less able to recover from the physiological consequences of such stressors, at least in terms of cortisol and catecholamines. The impaired negative feedback of the HPA axis and the A/C imbalance may underlie this vulnerability. With a low reserve of restorative capacity, stress exacerbates an already catabolic milieu, leading to breakdown of bodily resources, without the subsequent repair mechanisms. Thus, stress may accelerate the profile of neuroendocrine changes that comes with aging.

There is empirical support for this, although few studies examine both anabolic and catabolic hormones simultaneously. Traumatic physiological stressors such as burns or other injuries dramatically reduce A/C balance, and psychological stressors may have a more subtle impact. Chronic stress, such as caregiving or work strain, can elevate cortisol (Steptoe, Cropley, Griffith, & Kirschbaum, 2000; Vedhara et al., 1999).

Chronic stress or anxiety have been associated with low levels of DHEA (Wolkowitz & Reus, 2000), and testosterone (Morgan et al., 2000). Low IGF-1 has been linked to subordinate social status in baboons, and to low social status and depression in humans (Epel, Burke, et al., 2005). One prototypical stress-related psychiatric condition, major depression, is often associated with changes in A/C balance. Depressive symptoms are associated with low DHEA (Wolkowitz, 1999), although some contradictory reports exist (see Wolkowitz, Epel, & Reus, 2001), lower or altered GH (Linkowski, 2003), and possibly low testosterone in men (Seidman et al., 2002).

Unlike primary aging, which tends to be associated with normal or low anabolic hormones, chronic distress is also related to reports of higher levels of anabolic hormones. For example, testosterone can also increase in women due to an ongoing stressor (a recent or impending divorce; Powell et al., 2002), and IGF-1 has been reported to be higher in major depression (Deuschle, Blum, et al., 1997). Chronic stress can also lead to alternative or additional deficits in HPA axis function, such as blunted diurnal rhythm (low morning levels and/or elevated evening levels) or hypocortisolemia, a recently recognized profile that may be equally common as elevated cortisol in certain states of chronic stress (Fries, Hesse, Hellhammer, & Hellhammer, 2005). Thus, chronic distress leads to multiple phenotypes of endocrine dysregulation, a common one being A/C imbalance. In this way, there may be synergistic effects of aging and chronic stress, leading to premature neuroendocrine aging that results in an A/C imbalance.

Pruessner et al. (2005) found that age is related to lower hippocampal volume, but mainly for those in the low self-esteem/control group, explaining up to 55% of the variance in the low self-esteem/control group and only 5% of variance in the high self-esteem group. Furthermore, only those in the low self-esteem/control group showed reduced cortisol diurnal rhythm (due to low morning cortisol). Thus, stable self-schemas may have long-term effects on both HPA axis dysregulation and hippocampal volume, possibly through modulating stress appraisal and reactivity, as discussed by Pruessner and colleagues. This serves as an example of how aging may lead to dysregulation, but primarily in the face of ongoing challenge.

## Activity/Fitness

Moderate exercise (vs. overtraining or being sedentary) is likely one of the most potent promoters of a salutary A/C balance. Exercise increases IGF-1–mediated neurogenesis, leading to new hippocampal cells in the adult rat brain (Trejo, Carro, & Torres-Aleman, 2001). In humans, physical fitness is associated with greater GH and IGF-1 levels, higher DHEAS (Abassi et al., 1998), and higher testosterone (Ari et al., 2004). However, many studies find that fitness does not change basal hormones, suggesting that the acute increases in anabolic hormones during exercise may be responsible for salutary effects on body composition (Kraemer & Ratamess, 2005). Fit women tend to secrete more testosterone during exercise compared to unfit women (Keizer et al., 1987). In one study comparing older, fit women with older and younger unfit women, all older women had higher ACTH basally and in response to psychosocial stressors and a cold pressor test. However, older, fit women had cortisol responses similar to those of young, unfit women. Fitness may prevent age-related changes in cortisol reactivity (Traustadóttir, Bosch, & Matt, 2005). Thus, chronic stress and physical fitness may temper in opposite directions the neuroendocrine changes that occur with aging.

## Sleep and Diurnal Rhythms

Aging can lead to circadian shifts that may alter the A/C balance. Diurnal rhythms are regulated in part by the suprachiasmatic nucleus. With age, there tends to be a flattening of diurnal rhythms due to dysregulated signals from the central nervous system, leading to earlier timing and blunted amplitude of most rhythms (Wise, 1999). Melatonin, which regulates several diurnal rhythms, such as cortisol and sleep–wake cycles, tends to decrease with age, potentially contributing to dysregulation of other rhythms (Ferrari et al., 1995).

Sleep plays an important role in maintaining rhythmicity of A/C hormones. The first half of the night's sleep, a highly restorative period, is characterized by elevated GH and low cortisol. However, with aging, sleep architecture changes, leading to decreases in slow wave sleep and rapid eye movement (REM), contributing to blunted GH peaks, as well as less decline in cortisol during sleep. In this way, the typical sleep of older adults and disrupted sleep of younger adults may induce an A/C imbalance (Van Cauter, Plat, Leproult, & Copinschi, 1998).

## HEALTH-RELEVANT OUTCOMES

### Insulin Resistance

We conceptualize insulin resistance as one of the most sensitive and proximal health consequences of A/C imbalance. Elevated cortisol can induce insulin resistance, as demonstrated by Cushing's syndrome, and insulin resistance is responsible for many chronic disease processes (Reaven, 1994). Insulin resistance, adiposity, and hormonal regulation are highly interdependent. A/C imbalance promotes loss of muscle and increases in adiposity. For example, cortisol can break down lean tissue, but in the presence of insulin, it stimulates fat storage, preferentially depositing visceral fat. Furthermore, decreases in GH and sex hormones lead to less lipolysis and increases in visceral adiposity (Bjorntorp, 1996). In turn, increases in relative adiposity promote insulin resistance. Visceral adiposity increases with age and may explain the increase in insulin resistance more so than does chronological aging (Cefalu et al., 1995). Last, visceral adiposity can also influence A/C balance. For example, visceral adiposity and age both suppress the somatotropic axis, leading to lower GH, although they act via different central mechanisms (Veldhuis et al., 2005). Further complicating the picture, visceral fat cells may contain higher cortisol via intracellular production, and this may impact central HPA axis function, leading to lower levels of circulating cortisol (Seckl, 2004). Thus, part of neuroendocrine aging is due to the age-related relative increases in adiposity, especially visceral adiposity, and subsequent insulin resistance. Hormone studies should always take adiposity into account. Insulin resistance can also cause adiposity (Lustig, 2006; Shoelson, Lee, & Yuan, 2003) although this pathway is less studied.

### Telomere/Telomerase Maintenance System and A/C Imbalance

Because systemic or bodily aging is difficult to measure, it can be helpful to look toward markers of cellular aging. The telomere/telomerase maintenance system is one of the best indices of a mitotic cell's longevity. *In vitro*, telomere length shortening is related to cell senescence and, in people, may predict mortality associated with age-related disease (Cawthon et al.,

2003). Telomeres, the DNA sequences that cap the ends of chromosomes, shorten with chronological age, because telomeric DNA can be lost with each cell division (Blackburn, 2005). However, the biochemical milieu of the cell also determines the rate of shortening with each division. Oxidative stress shortens telomeres, whereas telomerase, a cellular ribonucleoprotein reverse transcriptase enzyme, can rebuild and lengthen telomeres (von Zglinicki & Martin-Ruiz, 2005). Furthermore, various lines of *in vitro* evidence suggests that anabolic hormones, including GH (Kiaris & Schally, 1999), IGF-1 (Torella et al., 2004), and estrogen (Kimura et al., 2004), promote telomerase activity in various cell lines, whereas dexamethasone may reduce telomerase activity, at least in a cancer cell line (Akiyama et al., 2002). A caveat is that, these changes may be tissue/cell specific rather than generalizable to all tissues (Kang et al., 1999).

Consistent with the *in vitro* data, our *in vivo* human data show that higher urinary cortisol is associated with shorter telomeres in leukocytes, and higher urinary EPI is linked to both shorter telomeres and lower telomerase activity (Epel, Lin, et al., 2006). Although the magnitude of these relationships was small, high catabolic hormones may be one factor influencing telomerase activity and subsequent telomere shortening. Lifestyle factors can also affect telomere integrity. Recent data have shown that smoking (Valdes et al., 2005), metabolic syndrome (Epel, Lin, et al., 2005), and increases in adiposity (Gardner et al., 2005) are all associated with telomere shortening or low telomerase.

Cellular aging, as assessed by telomere length, is related to many factors associated with overeating—excess adiposity, insulin resistance, and increased leptin levels (Valdes et al., 2005). Thus, caloric excess may be an early proximal promoter of accelerated aging through its effects at the systems level on body composition and insulin sensitivity, and at the cellular level, possibly through affecting the telomere/telomerase system. Based on the research reviewed, we speculate that chronological aging leads to changes in A/C balance that, when combined with years of chronic stress, can impair the telomere/telomerase maintenance system.

## A POSSIBLE PSYCHOLOGY
## OF HEALTHY NEUROENDOCRINE AGING

So how does one maintain a healthy A/C balance? In terms of psychosocial and behavioral factors that can improve neuroendocrine balance, many answers lie within this volume. Managing stress well in older age involves engaging "secondary control" systems—managing one's internal milieu, including managing expectations, goals, and motivation to meet one's goals rather than trying to control external events directly (see Skaff, Chapter 10, this volume), especially when such events tend to be uncontrollable (e.g., chronic disease and loss).

Although older people are exposed to more chronic stressors, they do not necessarily experience greater daily stress. Aldwin et al. (1996) has shown that older people report fewer daily stressors because of changes in cognitive appraisals of events. Development of adaptive cognitive coping strategies such as positive reappraisals, finding meaning (Bower, Kemeny, Taylor, & Fahey, 1998), and strengthening meaningful social ties (see Rook, Mavandadi, Sorkin, & Zettel, Chapter 14, this volume), can aid coping with chronic stress. Finding meaning (Epel, McEwen, & Ickovics, 1998; Moskowitz & Epel, 2006) has been related to more adaptive profiles of HPA axis function (either diurnal rhythm or reactivity) in healthy young women after facing a major stressor. Spiritual or religious beliefs may ultimately also translate into greater coping (See Park, Chapter 16, this volume), such as acceptance and a decreased need for primary control.

If cognitive coping strategies are effective at managing chronic stress and stress arousal, one would expect centenarians to use these strategies. Although there are no studies using psychometrically valid measures, centenarians have been reported to be highly adaptable people, or "stress resistant" (Perls, Silver, & Lauerman, 1995). Centenarians, compared to younger subjects, report greater use of three coping strategies for health problems— acceptance, not worrying, and taking things one day at a time (Martin, Rott, Poon, Courtenay, & Lehr, 2001). Although these may be cohort effects (rather than age effects), they also tend to be cognitive strategies that capitalize on secondary (vs. primary) control strategies, which should theoretically be related to more stress resistance, and a higher A/C balance.

When older people have not developed these more protective appraisals and flexible coping strategies, they may be more vulnerable to stress. This necessitates the need for both formal and informal interventions. Interventions are needed that increase self-efficacy and autonomy, optimistic appraisals, and growth and adaptability (see Golub & Langer, Chapter 2, this volume). These psychological changes can influence the immediate appraisal processes, promoting perceptions of challenge, selective control, or acceptance rather than threat and striving for control. These factors should lower threat appraisals and increase positive affect. These, in turn, may eventually improve A/C balance, although this needs empirical testing. Both pharmacological interventions and behavioral interventions that appear to increase A/C balance are reviewed elsewhere (Wolkowitz, Epel, & Reus, 2001). However, individual and even group-level interventions are not the answer for a public health solution to the health care crisis—the growing number of elderly with multiple comorbidities, including depression and obesity. Rather, a more effective approach would be to change local, national, and societal structures to integrate older adults into meaningful social roles that promote feelings of mastery and belonging (Schulkin,

2005). Such programs have been successful socially, such as the Experience Corp, in which older adults play a crucial mentoring role for at-risk children in inner-city elementary schools (www.experiencecorps.org/), and may have a large-scale health impact as well.

## CONCLUSIONS AND FUTURE RESEARCH

The literature reviewed suggests that chronological aging leads to a decrease in anabolic hormones, greater cortisol reactivity in response to an acute challenge, and possibly greater basal cortisol levels, with a large degree of interindividual variability. We have suggested that the relative imbalance of "anabolic" (i.e., lean tissue building) to "catabolic" (i.e., tissue destroying) hormone activity is the predominant pattern with aging, and is partly responsible for many of the psychiatric and medical diseases associated with aging.

However, many of the neuroendocrine changes that occur with aging are not inevitable, as demonstrated by healthy centenarians. There are modifiable life-style factors that exacerbate age-related changes in neuroendocrine function. Physical activity and sufficient sleep promote A/C balance, whereas chronic stress, inactivity, and adiposity promote imbalance. Aging itself is related to decreased activity, disrupted sleep, increased chronic stressor exposure, and increases in relative adiposity, making it difficult to parse out how much chronological aging per se causes neuroendocrine shifts versus cumulative effects of stress, psychosocial factors, and lifestyle. In other words, both primary and secondary aging forces promote A/C imbalance and must be taken into account.

In Figure 7.1, we demonstrate the idea that stress interacts with chronological age to promote impaired neuroendocrine allostasis—primarily a shift in basal A/C balance and exaggerated reactivity to acute challenges and slow recovery. In turn, A/C imbalance can contribute to insulin resistance, shifts toward visceral fat distribution, as well as accelerated cellular aging. There are likely relations between metabolic aging and cellular aging that are beyond the scope of this chapter. At this stage, A/C imbalance appears to be the most common profile in aging and may be a valuable marker of biological aging. It will be important to test whether A/C imbalance predicts downstream aging processes, such as metabolic syndrome and markers of cellular aging. Future research should examine A/C balance with both macro- and micro-outcomes, such as psychological well-being, autonomy and control, and possibly markers of cellular aging and damage. By integrating across these levels of analysis, we can learn about the effects of meaning-based constructs on reliable biological outcomes. Aging-related outcomes, such as the DHEA-to-cortisol ratio or telomere length may in turn be helpful metrics to assess effectiveness of interventions on health, or

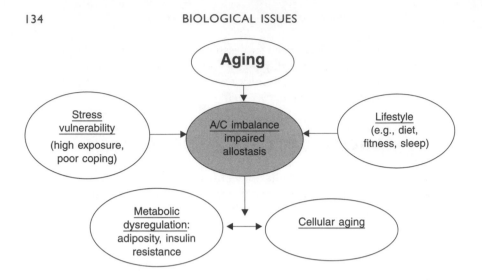

**FIGURE 7.1.** Proposed model of neuroendocrine aging

possibly for understanding mechanisms of change. Further empirical testing of these markers is needed to determine their usefulness.

## ACKNOWLEDGMENTS

This research was supported by grants from the National Institute on Mental Health to Elissa E. Epel (No. K08 MH64110) and Heather M. Burke (No. T32 MH19391). This chapter is dedicated to the memory of Dr. Per Bjorntorp, a broad thinker and empiricist who lucidly described a model of "neuroendocrine aging," long before the data were in. We are still catching up.

## REFERENCES

Abassi, A., Duthie, E., Sheldahl, L., Wilson, C., Sasse, E., Rudman, I., et al. (1998). Association of dehydroepiandrosterone sulfate, body composition, and physical fitness in independent community dwelling older men and women. *Journal of the American Geriatrics Society, 46,* 263–273.

Akiyama, M., Hideshima, T., Hayashi, T., Tai, Y. T., Mitsiades, C. S., Mitsiades, N., et al. (2002). Cytokines modulate telomerase activity in a human multiple myeloma cell line. *Cancer Research, 62*(13), 3876–3882.

Aldwin, C. M., Sutton, K. J., Chiara, G., & Spiro, A., III. (1996). Age differences in stress, coping, and appraisal: Findings from the Normative Aging Study. *Journals of Gerontology: Psychological Sciences and Social Sciences, Series B, 51*(4), P179–P188.

Ari, Z., Kutlu, N., Uyanik, B. S., Taneli, F., Buyukyazi, G., & Tavli, T. (2004). Serum testosterone, growth hormone, and insulin-like growth factor-1 levels, mental reaction time, and maximal aerobic exercise in sedentary and long-term physically trained elderly males. *International Journal of Neuroscience, 114*(5), 623–637.

Aslan, S., Nelson, L., Carruthers, M., & Lader, M. (1981). Stress and age effects on catecholamines in normal subjects. *Journal of Psychosomatic Research, 25*(1), 33–41.

Asnis, G. M., Sachar, E. J., Halbreich, U., Nathan, R. S., Novacenko, H., & Ostrow, L. C. (1981). Cortisol secretion in relation to age in major depression. *Psychosomatic Medicine, 43*(3), 235–242.

Baldelli, M., Zucchi, P., Pradelli, J., Montanini, V., & DeSantis, M. (1996). Hormone levels in centenarians. *Archives of Gerontology and Geriatrics, 5*(Suppl.), 355–362.

Barnes, R. F., Raskind, M., Gumbrecht, G., & Halter, J. B. (1982). The effects of age on the plasma catecholamine response to mental stress in man. *Journal of Clinical Endocrinology and Metabolism, 54*(1), 64–69.

Barrett-Connor, E., & Ferrara, A. (1996). DHEA, DHEAS, obesity, WHR, and NIDDM in postmenopausal women: The Rancho Bernardo Study. *Journal of Clinical Endocrinology and Metabolism, 81,* 5–64.

Baulieu, E. E. (1997). Neurosteroids: A role in aging?: New functions in the central and peripheral nervous systems. *Aging (Milano), 9*(Suppl. 4), 12.

Bjorntorp, P. (1995). Neuroendocrine ageing. *Journal of Internal Medicine, 238,* 401–404.

Bjorntorp, P. (1996). The regulation of adipose tissue distribution. *International Journal of Obesity, 20,* 291–302.

Blackburn, E. H. (2005). Telomeres and telomerase: Their mechanisms of action and the effects of altering their functions. *FEBS Letters, 579*(4), 859–862.

Blandini, F., Martignoni, E., Melzi d'Eril, G. V., Biasio, L., Sances, G., Lucarelli, C., et al. (1992). Free plasma catecholamine levels in healthy subjects: A basal and dynamic study: The influence of age. *Scandinavian Journal of Clinical and Laboratory Investigation, 52*(1), 9–17.

Bower, J., Kemeny, M., Taylor, S., & Fahey, J. (1998). Cognitive processing, discovery of meaning, CD4 decline, and AIDS-related mortality among bereaved HIV-seropostive men. *Journal of Consulting and Clinical Psychology, 66,* 979–986.

Cawthon, R., Smith, K., O'Brien, E., Sivatchenko, A., & Kerber, R. (2003). Association between telomere length in blood and mortality in people aged 60 years or older. *Lancet, 361,* 393–395.

Cefalu, W. T., Wang, Z. Q., Werbel, S., Bell-Farrow, A., Crouse, J. R., III, Hinson, W. H., et al. (1995). Contribution of visceral fat mass to the insulin resistance of aging. *Metabolism, 44*(7), 954–959.

Dallman, M. F., Pecoraro, N. C., & la Fleur, S. E. (2005). Chronic stress and comfort foods: Self-medication and abdominal obesity. *Brain, Behavior, and Immunity, 19*(4), 275–280.

Deuschle, M., Blum, W. F., Strasburger, C. J., Schweiger, U., Weber, B., Korner, A., et al. (1997). Insulin-like growth factor-I (IGF-I) plasma concentrations are increased in depressed patients. *Psychoneuroendocrinology, 22*(7), 493–503.

Deuschle, M., Gotthardt, U., Schweiger, U., Weber, B., Korner, A., Schmider, J., et al. (1997). With aging in humans the activity of the hypothalamus–pituitary–

adrenal system increased and its diurnal amplitude flattens. *Life Sciences, 61,* 2239–2246.

Dominici, F. P., Argentino, D. P., Munoz, M. C., Miquet, J. G., Sotelo, A. I., & Turyn, D. (2005). Influence of the crosstalk between growth hormone and insulin signalling on the modulation of insulin sensitivity. *Growth Hormone and IGF Research, 15*(5), 324–336.

Epel, E., Blackburn, E., Lin, J., Dhabhar, F., Adler, N., Morrow, J. D., et al. (2004). Accelerated telomere shortening in response to exposure to life stress. *Proceedings of the National Academy of Sciences of the United States of America, 101,* 17312–17315.

Epel, E., Burke, H. M., Adler, N., Wolkowitz, O., Sidney, S., & Seeman, T. (2006). *Socio-economic status and the anabolic/catabolic neuroendocrine balance. Annals of Behavioral Medicine, 31,* 50–80.

Epel, E., Lin, J., Wilhelm, F., Mendes, W., Adler, N., Dolbier, C., et al. (2006). Cell aging in relation to stress arousal and cardiovascular disease risk factors. *Psychoneuroendocrinology, 31,* 277–287.

Epel, E., McEwen, B., & Ickovics, J. (1998). Embodying psychological thriving: Physical thriving in response to stress. *Journal of Social Issues, 54,* 301–322.

Esler, M., Kaye, D., Thompson, J., Jennings, G., Cox, H., Turner, A., et al. (1995). Effects of aging on epinephrine secretion and regional release of epinephrine from the human heart. *Journal of Clinical Endocrinology and Metabolism, 80*(2), 435–442.

Ferrari, E., Magri, F., Dori, D., Migliorati, G., Nescis, T., Molla, G., et al. (1995). Neuroendocrine correlates of the aging brain in humans. *Neuroendocrinology, 61*(4), 464–470.

Fries, E., Hesse, J., Hellhammer, J., & Hellhammer, D. H. (2005). A new view on hypocortisolism. *Psychoneuroendocrinology, 30*(10), 1010–1016.

Gardner, J. P., Li, S., Srinivasan, S. R., Chen, W., Kimura, M., Lu, X., et al. (2005). Rise in insulin resistance is associated with escalated telomere attrition. *Circulation, 111*(17), 2171–2177.

Goodyer, I., Herbert, J., & Altham, P. (1998). Adrenal steroid secretion and major depression in 8- to 16-year-olds: III. Influence of cortisol/DHEA ratio at presentation on subsequent rates of disappointing life events and persistent major depression. *Psychological Medicine, 28,* 265–273.

Guazzo, E. P., Kirkpatrick, P. J., Goodyer, I. M., Shiers, H. M., & Herbert, J. (1996). Cortisol, dehydroepiandrosterone (DHEA), and DHEA sulfate in the cerebrospinal fluid of man: Relation to blood levels and the effects of age. *Journal of Clinical Endocrinology and Metabolism, 81*(11), 3951–3960.

Harris, T. O., Borsanyi, S., Messari, S., Stanford, K., Cleary, S. E., Shiers, H. M., et al. (2000). Morning cortisol as a risk factor for subsequent major depressive disorder in adult women. *British Journal of Psychiatry, 177,* 505–510.

Hechter, O., Grossman, A., & Chatterton, R. T., Jr. (1997). Relationship of dehydroepiandrosterone and cortisol in disease. *Medical Hypotheses, 49*(1), 85–91.

Herndon, D. N., & Tompkins, R. G. (2004). Support of the metabolic response to burn injury. *Lancet, 363*(9424), 1895–1902.

Jacobs, S., Mason, J., Kosten, T., Brown, S., & Ostfeld, A. (1984). Urinary-free cortisol excretion in relation to age in acutely stressed persons with depressive symptoms. *Psychosomatic Medicine, 46*(3), 213–221.

Kang, H. K., Kim, M. S., Kim, N. D., Yoo, M. A., Kim, K. W., Kim, J., et al. (1999). Downregulation of telomerase in rat during the aging process. *Molecules and Cells, 9*(3), 286–291.

Keizer, H. A., Beckers, E., de Haan, J., Janssen, G. M., Kuipers, H., van Kranenburg, G., et al. (1987). Exercise-induced changes in the percentage of free testosterone and estradiol in trained and untrained women. *Inernational Journal of Sports Medicine, 8*(Suppl. 3), 151–153.

Kiaris, H., & Schally, A. V. (1999). Decrease in telomerase activity in U-87MG human glioblastomas after treatment with an antagonist of growth hormone-releasing hormone. *Proceedings of the National Academy of Sciences of the United States of America, 96*(1), 226–231.

Kimonides, V. G., Spillantini, M. G., Sofroniew, M. V., Fawcett, J. W., & Herbert, J. (1999). Dehydroepiandrosterone antagonizes the neurotoxic effects of corticosterone and translocation of stress-activated protein kinase 3 in hippocampal primary cultures. *Neuroscience, 89*(2), 429–436.

Kimura, A., Ohmichi, M., Kawagoe, J., Kyo, S., Mabuchi, S., Takahashi, T., et al. (2004). Induction of hTERT expression and phosphorylation by estrogen via Akt cascade in human ovarian cancer cell lines. *Oncogene, 23*(26), 4505–4515.

Kraemer, W. J., & Ratamess, N. A. (2005). Hormonal responses and adaptations to resistance exercise and training. *Sports Medicine, 35*(4), 339–361.

Kudielka, B. M., Schmidt-Reinwald, A. K., Hellhammer, D. H., & Kirschbaum, C. (1999). Psychological and endocrine responses to psychosocial stress and dexamethasone/corticotropin-releasing hormone in healthy postmenopausal women and young controls: The impact of age and a two-week estradiol treatment. *Neuroendocrinology, 70*(6), 422–430.

Kudielka, B. M., Schmidt-Reinwald, A. K., Hellhammer, D. H., Schurmeyer, T., & Kirschbaum, C. (2000). Psychosocial stress and HPA functioning: No evidence for a reduced resilience in healthy elderly men. *Stress, 3*(3), 229–240.

Linkowski, P. (2003). Neuroendocrine profiles in mood disorders. *International Journal of Neuropsychopharmacology, 6*(2), 191–197.

Lupien, S. J., Schwartz, G., Ng, Y. K., Fiocco, A., Wan, N., Pruessner, J. C., et al. (2005). The Douglas Hospital Longitudinal Study of Normal and Pathological Aging: Summary of findings. *Journal of Psychiatry and Neuroscience, 30*(5), 328–334.

Lustig, R. (2006). Childhood obesity: Behavioral aberration or biochemical drive? Reinterpreting the First Law of Thermodynamics. *Nature Clinical Practice, 2*, 447–462.

Lynch, S., Merson, S., Beshyah, S. A., Skinner, E., Sharp, P., Priest, R. G., et al. (1994). Psychiatric morbidity in adults with hypopituitarism. *Journal of the Royal Society of Medicine, 87*, 445–447.

Magri, F., Muzzoni, B., Cravello, L., Fioravanti, M., Busconi, L., Camozzi, D., et al. (2002). Thyroid function in physiological aging and in centenarians: Possible relationships with some nutritional markers. *Metabolism, 51*(1), 105–109.

Magri, F., Terenzi, F., Ricciardi, T., Fioravanti, M., Solerte, S. B., Stabile, M., et al. (2000). Association between changes in adrenal secretion and cerebral morphometric correlates in normal aging and senile dementia. *Dementia and Geriatric Cognitive Disorders, 11*(2), 90–99.

Martin, P., Rott, C., Poon, L., Courtenay, B., & Lehr, U. (2001). A molecular view of coping behavior in older adults. *Journal of Aging and Health, 13*, 72–91.

Martin, F., Yeo, A., & Sonksen, P. (1997). Growth hormone secretion in the elderly: Ageing and the somatopause. *Balliere's Clinical Endocrinology and Metabolism, 11*, 223–249.

McEwen, B. (1998). Protective and damaging effects of stress mediators. *New England Journal of Medicine, 338*, 171–179.

Morgan, C. A., III, Wang, S., Mason, J., Southwick, S. M., Fox, P., Hazlett, G., et al. (2000). Hormone profiles in humans experiencing military survival training. *Biological Psychiatry, 47*(10), 891–901.

Morley, J., Kaiser, F., Raum, W., Perry, H., Flood, J., Jensen, J., et al. (1997). Potentially predictive and manipulable blood serum correlates of aging in the healthy human male: Progressive decreases in bioavailable tesosterone, dehydroepiandrosterone sulfate, and the ratio of insulin-like growth factor 1 to growth hormone. *Proceedings of the National Academy of Sciences of the United States of America, 94*, 7537–7542.

Morrison, M. (Ed.). (1996). *Hormones, gender and the aging brain: The endocrine basis of geriatric psychiatry.* Cambridge University Press, Cambridge, UK.

Moskowitz, J., & Epel, E. (2006). Benefit finding and positive affect: Effects on diurnal cortisol rhythm. *Journal of Positive Psychology, 1*, 83–91.

Ng, A. V., Callister, R., Johnson, D. G., & Seals, D. R. (1994). Sympathetic neural reactivity to stress does not increase with age in healthy humans. *American Journal of Physiology, 267*(1, Pt. 2), H344–H353.

Otte, C., Hart, S., Neylan, T. C., Marmar, C. R., Yaffe, K., & Mohr, D. C. (2005). A meta-analysis of cortisol response to challenge in human aging: Importance of gender. *Psychoneuroendocrinology, 30*(1), 80–91.

Palmer, G. J., Ziegler, M. G., & Lake, C. R. (1978). Response of norepinephrine and blood pressure to stress increases with age. *Journal of Gerontology, 33*(4), 482–487.

Paolisso, G., Barbieri, M., Rizzo, M. R., Carella, C., Rotondi, M., Bonafe, M., et al. (2001). Low insulin resistance and preserved beta-cell function contribute to human longevity but are not associated with TH-INS genes. *Experimental Gerontology, 37*(1), 149–156.

Paolisso, G., Tagliamonte, M. R., Rizzo, M. R., Rotondi, M., Gualdiero, P., Gambardella, A., et al. (1999). Mean arterial blood pressure and serum levels of the molar ratio of insulin-like growth factor-1 to its binding protein-3 in healthy centenarians. *Journal of Hypertension, 17*(1), 67–73.

Perls, T., Silver, M., & Lauerman, J. (1995). *Living to 100: Lessons in living to your maximum potential at any age.* New York: Basic Books.

Powell, L. H., Lovallo, W. L., Matthews, K. A., Meyer, P., Midgley, A. R., Baum, A., et al. (2002). Physiologic markers of chronic stress in middle-aged women. *Psychosomatic Medicine, 64*, 502–509.

Pruessner, J. C., Baldwin, M. W., Dedovic, K., Renwick, R., Mahani, N. K., Lord, C., et al. (2005). Self-esteem, locus of control, hippocampal volume, and cortisol regulation in young and old adulthood. *NeuroImage, 28*, 815–826.

Reaven, G. (1994). Syndrome X: 6 years later. *Journal of Internal Medicine, 236*, 13–22.

Regelson, W., Loria, R., & Kalimi, M. (1994). Dehydroepiandrosterone (DHEA)—the "mother steroid": I. Immunologic action. *Annals of the New York Academy of Sciences, 719*, 553–563.

Rehman, H. U., & Masson, E. A. (2005). Neuroendocrinology of female aging. *Gender Medicine, 2*(1), 41–56.

Reuben, D. B., Talvi, S. L., Rowe, J. W., & Seeman, T. E. (2000). High urinary catecholamine excretion predicts mortality and functional decline in high-functioning, community-dwelling older persons: MacArthur Studies of Successful Aging. *Journals of Gerontology: Biological Sciences and Medical Sciences, Series A, 55*(10), M618–M624.

Rincon, M., Rudin, E., & Barzilai, N. (2005). The insulin/IGF-1 signaling in mammals and its relevance to human longevity. *Experimental Gerontology*.

Sapolsky, R. (1989). Hypercortisolism among socially subordinate wild baboons originates at the CNS level. *Archives of General Psychiatry, 46*, 1047–1051.

Sapolsky, R., Krey, L., & McEwen, B. (1986). The neuroendocrinology of stress and aging: The glucocorticoid cascade hypothesis. *Endocrine Review, 7*, 284–301.

Schulkin, J. (2005). *Allostasis, homeostasis, and the costs of physiological adaptation.* Cambridge, UK: Cambridge University Press.

Seckl, J. R. (2004). 11beta-hydroxysteroid dehydrogenases: Changing glucocorticoid action. *Current Opinion in Pharmacology, 4*(6), 597–602.

Seeman, T., & Robbins, R. (1994). Aging and hypothalamic–pituitary–adrenal response to challenge in humans. *Endocrine Reviews, 15*(2), 233–259.

Seidman, S. N., Araujo, A. B., Roose, S. P., Devanand, D. P., Xie, S., Cooper, T. B., et al. (2002). Low testosterone levels in elderly men with dysthymic disorder. *American Journal of Psychiatry, 159*(3), 456–459.

Shoelson, S. E., Lee, J., & Yuen, M. (2003). Inflammation and the IKK beta/I kappa B/NF-kappa B axis in obesity- and diet-induced insulin resistance. *International Journal of Obesity and Related Metabolic Disorders, 27*(Suppl. 3), S49–S52.

Steptoe, A., Cropley, M., Griffith, J., & Kirschbaum, C. (2000). Job strain and anger expression predict early morning elevations in salivary cortisol. *Psychosomatic Medicine, 62*, 286–292.

Steptoe, A., Kunz-Ebrecht, S. R., Wright, C., & Feldman, P. J. (2005). Socioeconomic position and cardiovascular and neuroendocrine responses following cognitive challenge in old age. *Biological Psychology, 69*(2), 149–166.

Stroud, L., Salovey, P., & Epel, E. (2002). Sex differences in adrenocortical reactivity to achievement versus interpersonal stressors. *Biological Psychiatry, 53*, 318–327.

Svec, F., & Porter, J. R. (1998). The actions of exogenous dehydroepiandrosterone in experimental animals and humans. *Proceedings of the Society of Experimental Biology and Medicine, 218*, 174–191.

Tannenbaum, C., Barrett-Connor, E., Laughlin, G. A., & Platt, R. W. (2004). A longitudinal study of dehydroepiandrosterone sulphate (DHEAS) change in older men and women: The Rancho Bernardo Study. *European Journal of Endocrinology, 151*(6), 717–725.

Tatar, M., Bartke, A., & Antebi, A. (2003). The endocrine regulation of aging by insu-lin-like signals. *Science, 299*(5611), 1346–1351.

Tchernof, A., & Labrie, F. (2004). Dehydroepiandrosterone, obesity and cardiovas-cular disease risk: A review of human studies. *European Journal of Endocrinol-ogy, 151*(1), 1–14.

Togari, A. (2002). Adrenergic regulation of bone metabolism: Possible involvement of sympathetic innervation of osteoblastic and osteoclastic cells. *Microscopy Re-search and Technique, 58*(2), 77–84.

Torella, D., Rota, M., Nurzynska, D., Musso, E., Monsen, A., Shiraishi, I., et al. (2004). Cardiac stem cell and myocyte aging, heart failure, and insulin-like growth factor-1 overexpression. *Circulation Research, 94*(4), 514–524.

Traustadóttir, T., Bosch, P. R., & Matt, K. S. (2005). The HPA axis response to stress in women: Effects of aging and fitness. *Psychoneuroendocrinology, 30*(4), 392–402.

Trejo, J. L., Carro, E., & Torres-Aleman, I. (2001). Circulating insulin-like growth factor I mediates exercise-induced increases in the number of new neurons in the adult hippocampus. *Journal of Neuroscience, 21*(5), 1628–1634.

Trubo, R. (2005). Hormone changes in aging adults probed. *Journal of the American Medical Association, 294*(6), 663–667.

Valdes, A. M., Andrew, T., Gardner, J. P., Kimura, M., Oelsner, E., Cherkas, L. F., et al. (2005). Obesity, cigarette smoking, and telomere length in women. *Lancet, 366*(9486), 662–664.

Van Cauter, E., Leproult, R., & Kupfer, D. (1996). Effects of gender and age on the lev-els and circadian rhythmicity of plasma cortisol. *Journal of Clinical Endocrinol-ogy and Metabolism, 81*, 2468–2473.

Van Cauter, E., Leproult, R., & Plat, L. (2000). Age-related changes in slow wave sleep and REM sleep and relationship with growth hormone and cortisol levels in healthy men. *Journal of the American Medical Association, 284*, 861–868.

Van Cauter, E., Plat, L., Leproult, R., & Copinschi, G. (1998). Alterations of circadian rhythmicity and sleep in aging: Endocrine consequences. *Hormone Research, 49*(3–4), 147–152.

Vance, M., & Mauras, N. (1999). Growth hormone therapy in adults and children. *New England Journal of Medicine, 341*, 1206–1216.

Vedhara, K., Cox, N., Wilcock, G., Perks, P., Hunt, M., Anderson, S., et al. (1999). Chronic stress in elderly carers of dementia patients and antibody response to in-fluenza vaccination. *Lancet, 353*, 627–631.

Veldhuis, J. D., Erickson, D., Mielke, K., Farhy, L. S., Keenan, D. M., & Bowers, C. Y. (2005). Distinctive inhibitory mechanisms of age and relative visceral adiposity on GH secretion in pre- and postmenopausal women studied under a hypogo-nadal clamp. *Journal of Clinical Endocrinology and Metabolism, 90*(11), 6006–6013.

von Zglinicki, T., & Martin-Ruiz, C. M. (2005). Telomeres as biomarkers for ageing and age-related diseases. *Current Molecular Medicine, 5*(2), 197–203.

Wilkinson, C. W., Peskind, E. R., Lash, B., Susan, E., Rieskse, R., Raskind, M., et al. (2005, September). *Aging-related deficits in glucocorticoid feedback inhibition reflect altered mineralocorticoid receptor function.* Paper presented at the Inter-national Society of Psychoneuroendocrinology, Montreal, Canada.

Wise, P. (1999). Neuroendocrine correlates of aging. In P. Conn & M. Freeman (Eds.), *Neuroendocrinology in physiology and medicine*. Totowa, NJ: Humana Press.

Wolf, O., & Kirschbaum, C. (1998). Wishing a dream came true: DHEA as a rejuvenating treatment? *Journal of Endocrinological Investigation, 21*, 133–135.

Wolkowitz, O. (1999). Neuropsychiatric effects of dehydroepiandrosterone (DHEA). In M. Kalimi & W. Regelson (Eds.), *Dehydroepiandrosterone (DHEA)*. Berlin: Walter de Gruyter.

Wolkowitz, O., Epel, E., & Reus, V. (2001). Stress hormone-related psychopathology: Pathophysiological and treatment implications. *World Journal of Biological Psychiatry, 2*, 113–141.

Wolkowitz, O., & Reus, V. (2000). Neuropsychiatric effects of dehydroepiandrosterone (DHEA). In M. Kalimi & W. Regelson (Eds.), *Dehydroepiandrosterone (DHEA): Biochemical, physiological and clinical aspects* (pp. 271–298). Berlin: de Gruyter.

Wolkowitz, O., & Rothschild, A. (Eds.). (2003). *Psychoneuroendocrinology: The scientific basis of clinical practice*. Washington, DC: American Psychiatric Publishing.

Wong, M. L., Kling, M. A., Munson, P. J., Listwak, S., Licinio, J., Prolo, P., et al. (2000). Pronounced and sustained central hypernoradrenergic function in major depression with melancholic features: Relation to hypercortisolism and corticotropin-releasing hormone. *Proceedings of the National Academy of Sciences of the United States of America, 97*(1), 325–330.

Yakar, S., Pennisi, P., Wu, Y., Zhao, H., & LeRoith, D. (2005). Clinical relevance of systemic and local IGF-I. *Endocrine Development, 9*, 11–16.

Young, E. A., Altemus, M., Parkison, V., & Shastry, S. (2001). Effects of estrogen antagonists and agonists on the ACTH response to restraint stress in female rats. *Neuropsychopharmacology, 25*(6), 881–891.

# CHAPTER 8

# Cardiovascular Reactivity in Older Adults

DENISE C. COOPER, LESLIE I. KATZEL,
*and* SHARI R. WALDSTEIN

Cardiovascular disease (CVD) affects over 27 million Americans ages 65 and older. It is the leading cause of death, with about 84% of such deaths occurring among older Americans (American Heart Association, 2005). Traditional risk factors (e.g., high cholesterol, smoking, diabetes, obesity, family history) predict only around half of the variance in new cases of CVD (Treiber et al., 2003). Substantial literature suggests that additional variance in CVD may be predicted by psychosocial factors (e.g., hostility, see Berg, Smith, Henry, & Pearce, Chapter 3, this volume) or psychophysiological factors, such as acute cardiovascular reactions (i.e., reactivity), which occur in response to emotional and environmental situations that evoke stress (Rozanski, Blumenthal, & Kaplan, 1999). Cardiovascular reactivity (CVR), which is also called sympathetic nervous system hyperreactivity, refers to "an individual's propensity to experience cardiovascular reactions of greater or lesser magnitude, in relation to those of other persons, when encountering behavioral stimuli experienced as engaging, challenging, or aversive" (Manuck, 1994, p. 7).

CVR has been conceptualized as a possible mechanism through which stress exerts detrimental effects on health, specifically, the health and function of the cardiovascular system. Initial support of this role for CVR in the development of CVD came most strongly from animal studies of atherosclerosis and hypertension, with converging evidence later provided by human studies on healthy populations and patients with hypertension and other CVDs. The repeated elevations of blood pressure, heart rate, and related parameters in response to stress are hypothesized to promote pathogenic changes in the cardiovascular system that lead to disease. Given that cardiovascular health largely reflects the cumulative effects of decades-long exposures to many factors, including stress, longitudinal studies from younger to older ages would be most informative about the relation of CVR to age-associated increases in CVD.

Although a large literature exploring cardiovascular responses to stress has been developed, there is a dearth of longitudinal data assessing age-related changes in CVR throughout the lifespan. Therefore, this chapter focuses on older adults (ages 65–74: young-old; 75–84: middle-old; 85 and over: old-old; National Center for Health Statistics, 2003) and provides a selective summary of the CVR studies that have included adults ages 65 and over. To provide a foundation for understanding this research, the chapter begins with a description of theories and empirical research linking CVR to CVD. Next, we provide an overview of cardiovascular physiology and the effects of aging on cardiovascular function that are likely to impact cardiovascular response patterns in older adulthood. We then examine a variety of constitutional and psychosocial influences on CVR. The chapter concludes with recommendations for future directions in this area of research.

## LINKS BETWEEN CVR AND CVD

Laboratory assessment of CVR involves measurement of cardiovascular responses while individuals complete one or more experimental tasks designed to induce psychological (e.g., mental arithmetic, public speaking) and/or physical (e.g., cold pressor) stress. The "reactivity hypothesis" suggests that individuals with a dispositional tendency to exhibit larger cardiovascular responses ("hot reactors") may be at higher risk for CVD than those who tend to show smaller responses ("cold reactors"). An underlying assumption of the reactivity hypothesis is that stress responses differ among individuals, and that the tendency to exhibit more or less reactivity to stressful stimuli is a relatively stable individual difference (Manuck, 1994). Furthermore, reactivity assessed in the laboratory is presumed to demonstrate the temporal stability (i.e., similarity of responses to the same type of challenge at different times), intertask consistency (i.e., stability of responses to different challenges), and laboratory-to-field generalization necessary to be considered a proxy for stress-induced responses that repeatedly occur in natural settings and eventually lead to disease. Whereas generalizability has varied, partially due to methodological limitations, CVR has shown temporal stability and intertask consistency among younger and older adults (Burleson et al., 2003; Hawkley et al., 2001; Turner, 1994; Uchino, Holt-Lunstad, Bloor, & Campo, 2005). In addition, individual consistency in response patterns may increase with age (Ditto, Miller, & Maurice, 1987; Garwood, Engel, & Capriotti, 1982).

CVR research focuses on the magnitude of responses to stress. However, the duration of these responses is also of interest, because prolonged cardiovascular arousal might adversely alter regulatory processes involved in blood pressure control. Consequently, some CVR studies include assessments of poststress (or posttask) cardiovascular recovery to measure how long or to what degree cardiovascular parameters remain elevated after stress exposure. Currently, less is known about poststress recovery (e.g., its temporal stability, intertask consistency, and generalizability) than about CVR. However, the duration of stress-induced cardiovascular responses could be quite informative as an index of the adaptive functioning of cardiovascular recovery mechanisms, with sustained arousal reflecting potentially pathogenic processes. Over time, individuals who typically respond to stress with prolonged elevations in blood pressure, heart rate, or other cardiovascular parameters could be at increased risk of CVD.

In fact, CVR has been linked prospectively to hypertension and coronary heart disease, as well as some of their pathogenic precursors, such as elevated blood pressure, increased atherosclerosis, and enlarged left ventricular mass (Manuck, 1994; Treiber et al., 2003). Enhanced blood pressure reactivity also has been associated with greater prevalence of silent cerebrovascular disease (Waldstein et al., 2004), lower levels of cognitive function (Waldstein & Katzel, 2005), and increased risk of incident stroke (Everson et al., 2001). In addition, data suggest that delayed poststress recovery may be related to hypertension (Schuler & O'Brien, 1997; Schwartz et al., 2003; Stewart & France, 2001). Although this body of literature links CVR (and poststress recovery) to CVD, the specific nature of these associations remains uncertain. The role played by exaggerated stress-induced cardiovascular responses could be that of a marker of disease risk or a pathogenic mechanism that promotes CVD.

Hypertension is not only a form of CVD that causes morbidity and mortality, but it is also a risk factor for other types of CVD. Whereas less than 10% of hypertension cases can be traced to a particular source (i.e., secondary hypertension), the cause of most hypertension is uncertain (i.e., essential or primary hypertension). Essential hypertension may be initiated and maintained through several mechanisms, including a shift in the normal dynamic balance between the sympathetic and parasympathetic branches of the autonomic nervous system (Oparil, Zaman, & Calhoun, 2003). This autonomic imbalance usually involves increases in sympathetic excitatory activity (mobilizing energy resources to meet the demands of episodic physical and mental challenges) and decreases in parasympathetic or vagal inhibitory activity (restoring and preserving energy resources to allow the body to "rest and digest").

Autonomic imbalance may develop in part from sympathetic hyperactivity that develops in association with frequent exposures to psychosocial stress and results in physiological ("fight-or-flight") responses of augmented magnitude and/or duration. It is possible that exaggerated cardiovascular responses to stress are only a marker of correlated processes, such as chronic sympathetic activation, which has been posited to lead to hypertension via down-regulation of beta-adrenergic receptors in the heart and peripheral vasculature. However, investigators have more frequently considered pronounced and/or prolonged stress-induced elevations of cardiac and vascular parameters as a possible mechanism that may directly promote CVD. Specifically, repeatedly heightened vasoconstrictive stress responses may lead to structural changes in the peripheral vessels, characterized by vascular hypertrophy (thickening of vessel walls) and alterations in autoregulatory processes. In addition to enhancing vascular reactivity, such adaptations might produce the progressively increased levels of peripheral resistance and blood pressure that result in hypertension (Anderson, McNeilly, & Myers, 1993; Turner, 1994).

Similarly, frequently pronounced cardiovascular responses to stress might contribute to the development of CVD in part by inflicting injury to the inner lining of artery walls, called the endothelium (Manuck, 1994). Such injury promotes inflammation and the adhesion of lipids to the endothelium, which fosters the development of atherosclerosis or buildup of plaque deposits at sites of injury along the endothelium. Most clinical manifestations of CVD (e.g., coronary heart disease) arise from atherosclerosis of the arteries supplying blood to the heart (i.e., coronary artery disease), the brain (i.e., carotid artery disease), and the extremities (i.e., peripheral artery disease). Lipids (fats) and other cellular debris begin accumulating along artery walls during childhood to eventually form fatty streaks, which become more numerous with aging. Progressing asymptomatically over the course of many years, some fatty streaks develop into atherosclerotic plaques, which are raised, cholesterol-laden lesions along the endothelium that narrow the lumen or arterial space through which the blood flows. As the buildup of atherosclerotic plaque continues, blockage of the blood flow in an artery may be caused by a large lesion that either occludes the lumen or restricts passage through the lumen so much that a thrombus (blood clot) can become plugged into the narrowed arterial opening. The particular clinical manifestation (e.g., myocardial infarction, stroke) that emanates from the interrupted blood supply depends on the extent and location of the artery blockage.

Whereas this discussion focuses on cardiovascular responses mediated primarily by the sympathetic nervous system, the concomitant stress-induced activities of other physiological systems (e.g., neuroendocrine response of increased cortisol) that may also play roles in CVD are beyond the scope of this chapter. Nevertheless, the tendency to respond to stress with pronounced and prolonged cardiovascular responses may be related to increased disease risk via pathogenic changes in structure or function that are precursors to many clinical forms of CVD. Although atherosclerosis and blood pressure typically rise with aging, people who characteristically exhibit heightened CVR could have earlier initiation of increases in these precursors and/or faster progression toward clinical disease states. Moreover, patients with CVD who are hyperreactive may be at greater risk for new clinical events (Treiber et al., 2003).

Given that a variety of psychological predispositions and environmental exposures are associated with CVD, CVR is a possible mechanism through which these factors may contribute to poor cardiovascular health over time. Additionally, cardiovascular responses to acute severe psychological stress (e.g., extreme anger) among vulnerable individuals may actually elicit clinical events, such as myocardial infarction or sudden cardiac death, by acutely promoting myocardial ischemia, arrhythmia, plaque rupture, or coronary thrombosis (Kop, 1999; Krantz, Kop, Santiago, & Gottdiener, 1996). With vulnerability conferred by underlying coronary artery disease and risk factors (e.g., hyperlipidemia), the high rates of these conditions among older adults could place them at higher risk for cardiac events induced by acute psychological stress.

CVD has a multifactorial etiology that likely involves complex interactions between physiological processes and an array of psychological, behavioral, environmental, and genetic factors. Consequently, ascertaining the specific nature of relations between CVD and reactivity in the cardiovascular system requires elaborate, decades-long, population-based studies designed to assess interactions among these factors simultaneously. To date, most CVR research has been cross-sectional, and the relatively few longitudinal studies conducted have often been limited by fairly short follow-up intervals and small convenience samples. Thus, despite the considerable literature linking stress-induced cardiovascular responses to preclinical and clinical states of CVD, a definitive role for CVR has not yet been established. Regardless of whether CVR proves to be a mechanism that directly promotes disease or a marker that might identify those at increased disease risk, people who characteristically respond to mental stress with pronounced and/or prolonged elevations in blood pressure, heart rate, and related parameters might have increased vulnerability to CVD. Moreover, such vulnerability may increase with aging.

## AGE-RELATED CARDIOVASCULAR CHANGES AND CVR

The effects of aging on the cardiovascular system have been studied extensively. One of the main challenges in performing this research is to distinguish changes due to primary aging (biological aging) from those due to adverse lifestyle (secondary aging), and changes caused by diseases (tertiary aging) common in older people, such as coronary artery disease. The dramatic, age-related increase in subclinical or occult diseases, such as silent coronary atherosclerosis, further complicates our understanding of the effect of aging on the cardiovascular system. For in-depth reviews of the effects of aging on the cardiovascular system, see Lakatta (2003), and Lakatta and Levy (2003a, 2003b). A brief review of age-related changes in the cardiovascular system that may alter CVR follows.

## Cardiac Function at Rest and during Exercise

Most studies indicate that healthy people exhibit relatively minor effects of aging on cardiac function at rest. Basal resting heart rate does not differ among younger and older individuals. However, heart rate variability (beat-to-beat variability of the heart rhythm), which is regulated by sympathetic and parasympathetic tone, significantly diminishes over the lifespan. Low heart rate variability, reflecting decreased parasympathetic regulation and/or increased sympathetic stimulation of the heart, is related to cardiovascular events and mortality. The major structural change occurring in the heart is age-associated increased stiffness in the left ventricle, which adversely impacts its ability to fill with blood, both at rest and during exercise. Still, aging has only modest effects on cardiac volumes at rest. Commonly observed structural changes in the left ventricle include increased left ventricular wall thickness, decreased numbers of cardiac myocytes, enlargement of the left atrium, and prolonged myocardial contraction. These changes likely occur largely in response to systemic arterial stiffening.

The effects of aging on cardiovascular function during exhaustive exercise are well studied. Maximal heart rate declines by about one beat per minute per year, due to reduced efficacy of beta-adrenergic stimulation. Accordingly, older people show less increase in heart rate than younger people in response to postural changes and orthostatic stress. The ability to perform exhaustive exercise, as indexed by the maximal amount of oxygen consumed during exercise (maximal aerobic capacity), decreases by about 1% per year. This decrease in maximal aerobic capacity is due to a reduction in cardiac reserve, which is largely attributable to declines in maximal heart rate, peripheral skeletal muscle mass, and oxidative enzymes in skeletal muscles, as well as physical deconditioning. However, age-related declines in maximal aerobic capacity may be attenuated in athletes who continue to exercise vigorously.

## Age-Associated Increase in Blood Pressure

Epidemiological studies show that blood pressure, particularly systolic blood pressure, increases with aging (Lenfant, Chobanian, Jones, & Roccella, 2003). Hypertension prevalence may exceed 75% among adults above 80

years of age. Cardiac output (amount of blood ejected by the heart per minute) and peripheral vascular resistance ultimately determine blood pressure,
such that blood pressure is equal to cardiac output multiplied by total
peripheral resistance (total resistance to blood flow in the systemic blood
vessels). Because aging exerts minimal effects on resting cardiac output,
studies have largely focused on factors that impact peripheral resistance.

## Increased Sympathetic Nervous System Activity and Increased Arterial Tone

The autonomic nervous system plays a major role in maintaining blood
pressure, particularly in the regulation of arterial tone. Arterial tone reflects
several factors that stimulate smooth muscle to relax or constrict. Increased
arterial tone may be due to increases in factors that cause constriction and/
or decreases in factors that stimulate relaxation of smooth muscle. Sympathetic activation releases catecholamines (e.g., norepinephrine and epinephrine) that act on receptors to stimulate blood vessels to narrow (vasoconstriction) or widen (vasodilation). Accordingly, enhanced sympathetic activity
and/or dampened parasympathetic activity produce increases in peripheral
vascular resistance, cardiac output, plasma renin, and norepinepherine levels,
as well as an increased pressor response to physical and mental stressors.

Another influence on blood pressure is the renin–angiotensin system.
The enzyme renin converts angiotensinogen to angiotensin I, which is then
converted to angiotensin II, a potent vasoconstrictor. Angiotensin II activates receptors in the heart and in the central and autonomic nervous systems that amplify its vasoconstrictive effects. It also stimulates aldosterone
synthesis to increase sodium retention by the kidney. In the absence of compensatory mechanisms, these metabolic changes, collectively, would produce hypertension.

Aging is associated with increases in sympathetic activity and arterial
tone. Basal levels of the catecholamines (hormones) epinephrine and
norepinephrine are elevated in older people. Age-related changes in receptor and/or postreceptor sensitivity to hormone levels also may impact vascular tone. Whereas the response to vasodilators (beta-adrenergic) appears
to decrease with aging, the vasoconstrictor response to alpha-adrenergic
stimuli remains well preserved with aging. The renin–angiotensin system is
suppressed, resulting in decreased levels of renin and aldosterone among
older people. These changes are probably due to the negative feedback loop
in response to chronically established hypertension.

## Baroreflex Sensitivity

Blood pressure is regulated in part by arterial baroreceptors in the carotid
sinus and in the aortic arch. Normally, when the baroreceptors are acti-

vated by an increase in blood pressure or in central venous pressure, there should be a compensatory decrease in heart rate and blood pressure by vagal stimulation and sympathetic inhibition. However, aging and chronic hypertension may lead to a decrease in the sensitivity of baroreceptors. A reactivity study of healthy middle-aged and older adults suggested that baroreflex sensitivity is inversely correlated with mean arterial blood pressure increases, whereas carotid artery stiffness is positively associated with mean arterial blood pressure and heart rate increases in response to a mental stress task (Lipman, Grossman, Bridges, Hamner, & Taylor, 2002).

## Increased Arterial Stiffness

Numerous changes occur in vascular structure and function with healthy aging. Cross-sectional studies indicate age-associated increases in arterial stiffness, arterial wall thickness, endothelial dysfunction, and arterial pulse pressure (the difference between systolic blood pressure and diastolic blood pressure). This results in increased afterload on the left ventricle, an increase in systolic blood pressure, and left ventricular hypertrophy, as well as other changes in the left ventricular wall that prolong relaxation of the left ventricle in diastole. The increased stiffness of the larger arteries causes an age-associated increase in systolic blood pressure, particularly among people over 60 years of age. Indeed, the increase in the prevalence of hypertension with aging may be due largely to increased vascular resistance. Nevertheless, the magnitude of age-related changes in vascular compliance is potentially modifiable through lifestyle-related factors such as physical activity, dietary composition/salt intake, and weight control.

These age-associated changes in arterial compliance have several physiological consequences. The increased arterial stiffness and decreased systemic compliance results in reduced tolerance for changes in blood and fluid volumes among older adults, which in turn causes them to have greater blood pressure swings than do younger people. In addition, decreased arterial compliance may affect how older people respond to stressors. For example, Huisman et al. (2002) reported that decreased arterial compliance with increasing age is related to response patterns elicited by the cold pressor test being shifted from its usual diastolic blood pressure pattern to a more systolic blood pressure pattern.

## Endothelial Dysfunction

The endothelial cells that line the walls of the arterial system play a major role in the regulation of arterial tone (vasomotor function). Endothelial function progressively declines with aging (Celermajer et al., 1994). Specifically, the vascular endothelium shows a marked decline in the production of nitric oxide (a vasodilator), which is likely due to age-related alterations in the enzyme endothelial nitric oxide synthase (eNOS). The endothelin-1 (a vasoconstrictor) and angiotensin II pathways also may play a role in age-related endothelial dysfunction. Nitric oxide is regarded as a protective factor against atherosclerosis. Thus, the net effect is that the age-related decline in endothelial function increases the risk for atherosclerosis. One potential mechanism whereby psychosocial factors influence cardiovascular risk is through interactions between the autonomic nervous system and the vascular endothelium (Harris & Matthews, 2004). Still, age-related endothelial dysfunction is potentially modifiable by exercise training, vitamin C, and aggressive pharmacological therapy for hypertension and dyslipidemia.

Thus, age-associated changes in the cardiovascular system, especially increases in arterial stiffness, endothelial dysfunction, impaired baroreflexes, and increased sympathetic nervous system activity, may enhance cardiovascular responses among older people. To that end, one might expect dampened heart rate reactivity with increasing age, accompanied by enhanced blood pressure and total peripheral resistance responses. However, surprisingly little is known about age-related differences in the magnitude and patterning of CVR and poststress recovery.

## PREDICTORS OF INDIVIDUAL DIFFERENCES IN CVR

Genetic and physiological variations between persons contribute to individual differences in how they characteristically respond to stress. In addition, the stress-induced cardiovascular responses of groups of individuals have been found to vary in part as a function of several factors that have been linked to CVD. Whereas such research among older adults is rather limited, members of this population have been examined for CVR differences in terms of constitutional (e.g., age, gender, race/ethnicity, health status) and psychosocial (e.g., dispositional, affective, social) characteristics. The following describes research assessing constitutional and psychosocial influences on cardiovascular stress responses.

### Age

To our knowledge, no longitudinal studies have followed people over major portions of the lifespan to document age-related changes in CVR or poststress recovery across young, middle, and older ages. Although people over age 65 have rarely been included in samples, cross-sectional work on predominantly young and middle-aged samples suggests some age differences in CVR. Preliminary data suggest that reactivity of blood pressure, particularly systolic blood pressure, may indeed heighten with aging, in accordance with the aforementioned age-related changes in the cardiovascular system (Steptoe, Moses, & Edwards, 1990). Few investigations of aging and CVR have included assessments of the hemodynamic underpinnings of blood pressure: cardiac output and total peripheral resistance. Results have been mixed for associations between age and cardiac output reactivity, with reports of positive relations (Uchino, Uno, Holt-Lunstad, & Flinders, 1999), negative relations (Boutcher & Stocker, 1996), and some null findings (Jennings et al., 1997; Uchino et al., 2005). Although results are not entirely consistent (Uchino et al., 2005), age has been positively related to reactivity of total peripheral resistance (Boutcher & Stocker, 1996; Jennings et al., 1997; Uchino et al., 1999).

In addition, the relations of age to heart rate reactivity have been examined in several studies, including some that have sampled older people. Although the literature is mixed, older adults often display smaller heart rate increases in response to laboratory stressors than younger adults (Kudielka, Buske-Kirschbaum, Hellhammer, & Kirschbaum, 2004; Labouvie-Vief, Lumley, Jain, & Heinze, 2003). These results are consistent with age-related changes in cardiovascular physiology and have been found using a variety of experimental tasks.

Notwithstanding the age-related dampening of cardiac responses often found in studies utilizing emotion-inducing laboratory stressors, the accompanying affective responses in these investigations tend to contradict notions that emotional capacity widely diminishes with aging. Such research has revealed that older adults generally show comparably high levels of subjective affective responses to emotional inductions, though this has varied somewhat with the use of different experimental methods to induce emotion (Labouvie-Vief et al., 2003; Levenson, Carstensen, Friesen, & Ekman, 1991; Tsai, Levenson, & Cartensen, 2000). With regard to utilizing cognitive tasks as laboratory stressors, such as those measuring memory and intellectual speed, older adults have shown smaller heart rate increases than younger adults, as well as slower poststress recovery for heart rate (Faucheux et al., 1989; Faucheux, Dupuis, Baulon, Lille, & Bourlière, 1983). However, relations between age and cardiovascular responses to cognitive, emotional, and other types of laboratory stressors (e.g., social, physical) may vary in part as a function of several influences. Among these influences are emotional regulation, task engagement, and quality of performance, which could be affected by age-related changes in various cognitive resources. Consequently, older adults may show greater heart rate reactivity to stress than younger adults under certain conditions (Jennings, Nebes, & Brock, 1988).

In summary, relatively little research has directly contrasted older and younger adults for differences in the magnitude of stress-induced cardiovascular responses, and even less data are available regarding the duration of such responses. Moreover, cross-sectional studies of CVR and poststress recovery present a number of interpretive concerns, including age cohort effects and selective survival. Whereas age differences reported in these studies certainly reflect age-related physiological changes, the relative contribution of emotional, cognitive, and other factors (e.g., psychomotor) to such differences cannot be determined from the existing data.

## Gender

In light of men's higher cardiovascular risk before old age, gender differences in physiological stress responses have been explored in many studies of younger people (Stoney, Davis, & Matthews, 1987). Nevertheless, the information regarding gender influences on CVR among older adults is scant and inconsistent. In gender comparisons among healthy and clinical samples of older adults, cardiovascular responses to a variety of cognitive and interpersonal stressors have been higher among healthy men (Traustadóttir, Bosch, & Matt, 2003), higher among socially phobic women (Grossman, Wilhelm, Kawachi, & Sparrow, 2001), or generally comparable between men and women (Kudielka et al., 2004; Labouvie-Vief et al., 2003; Levenson et al., 1991). Although older women sometimes report more intense emotional responses to stressors than do older men, these relatively higher subjective reactions may or may not be accompanied by greater CVR (Grossman et al., 2001; Levenson et al., 1991). The presence of gender differences in poststress recovery is unclear, but some data suggest that healthy older women may exhibit more prolonged heart rate elevation than do older men (Kudielka et al., 2004).

Postmenopausal women have been shown to exhibit greater CVR than premenopausal women or men (Bairey Merz et al., 1998; Owens, Stoney, & Matthews, 1993; Saab, Matthews, Stoney, & McDonald, 1989). Consequently, research has explored the effects of estrogen on stress responses. Compared to their nonuser counterparts, postmenopausal long-term users of estrogen replacement therapy have exhibited higher heart rate reactivity (Burleson et al., 1998) and lower systolic blood pressure reactivity (Matthews, Flory, Owens, Harris, & Berga, 2001). Illustrating the more acute effects of estrogen, blood pressure responses to stress were attenuated among postmenopausal women after receiving transdermal estrogen (Manhem, Brandin, Ghanoum, Rosengren, & Gustafsson, 2003) and among older men receiving estrogen after treatment for prostrate cancer (Komesaroff, Fullerton, Esler, Jennings, & Sudhir, 2002).

All in all, older men and older women often exhibit similar magnitudes of cardiovascular responses to stress, though their subjective responses to particular types of laboratory stressors may vary somewhat by gender. The limited data available suggest that estrogen may be associated with reduced blood pressure responses to stress. Perhaps one mechanism by which estrogen exerts cardioprotective effects is through attenuation of CVR.

## Race/Ethnicity

Cardiovascular morbidity and mortality disproportionately affect some ethnic minorities, especially African Americans compared to European Americans. Accordingly, researchers have compared these groups for possible differences in CVR that might contribute to the disparities in CVD. Albeit not entirely consistent across various types of laboratory stressors, this literature suggests that European American adults frequently exhibit a relatively greater myocardial (or beta-adrenergic) response to stress, with increases of blood pressure, heart rate, cardiac output, and stroke volume (blood volume pumped from the left ventricle in a single heartbeat). By contrast, African American adults, particularly men, often exhibit relatively greater blood pressure reactivity and show more of a vascular (or alpha-adrenergic) response pattern, involving increased blood pressure accompanied by increased total peripheral resistance associated with smooth muscle vasoconstriction (Anderson et al., 1993).

It is unclear whether these differences in hemodynamic patterning are found among older populations. Few studies of CVR have mentioned inclusion of older African Americans, and even fewer have had sufficient power to allow for race-specific analyses. However, in one such study, differences were observed for poststress recovery rather than CVR, with African Americans exhibiting more prolonged elevations of diastolic blood pressure than European Americans (Fredrickson et al., 2000). Ethnic group differences in physiological responses may be influenced by a variety of factors, including cultural differences in perceptual and emotional processes. Preliminary data suggest that African American and European American older adults might use different culturally influenced strategies for coping with chronic stress, such as caregiver stress, which could contribute to racial differences in physiological stress responses (Knight & McCallum, 1998). Whereas cultural norms influence how members of different ethnic groups perceive and respond to stressors, some groups may demonstrate more similarities than differences. For example, older Asian Americans and European Americans have displayed similar behavioral and cardiovascular responses to emotion-inducing laboratory stressors (Tsai et al., 2000). Still, there is a paucity of data regarding CVR among older African Americans and Asian Americans, with even less information available for older Hispanic and Native Americans.

Most of the CVR literature was derived from predominantly European American samples, which makes the generalizability to ethnic minorities uncertain. Research addressing the influence of race/ethnicity on CVR has primarily focused on comparing ethnic minorities to European Americans for detection of between-group differences, with less information available about within-group differences. Given that older members of some minority groups have especially high rates of CVD, further examination of their cardiovascular responses to stressful conditions is warranted to elucidate factors that possibly underlie their increased disease risk.

## Health Status

With advancing age, many medical conditions (e.g., atherosclerosis, diabetes) become more prevalent. Accordingly, disease risk factors (e.g., elevated blood pressure) and medication use (e.g., antihypertensives) tend to be greater with aging. Older individuals with these health issues are frequently excluded from CVR research, because medical illnesses, cardiovascular risk factors, and medications can produce confounding effects on stress responses. Indeed, the extent to which these health status variables influence CVR is uncertain among men and women over the age of 65. In a study of middle-aged men, the small amount of variance in CVR explained by age was found to be similar or slightly greater than the variance accounted for by medication or any single disease (e.g., coronary heart disease, diabetes, respiratory disease), though age, medication, and hypertension were each independent predictors (Jennings et al., 1997). Whereas this study found that disease states contributed rather modest amounts of variance to CVR among middle-aged men, the effects may be larger among older men and women in light of their higher comorbidity and potentially greater levels of disease severity.

CVR has been shown prospectively to predict subclinical and clinical disease states (Treiber et al., 2003), but these conditions are also potential influences on stress responses that must be considered in research designs. Although many CVR studies restrict inclusion to only very healthy people, other work shows the utility of examining patients with medical conditions. For example, in a prospective study of patients ages 37 to 78 with coronary artery disease, subsequent cardiac events (e.g., cardiac death, nonfatal myocardial infarctions) occurred more frequently among those who exhibited mental stress–induced ischemia or tended to show greater diastolic blood pressure responses to laboratory stressors (Krantz et al., 1999).

Elevated resting blood pressure and family history of hypertension are cardiovascular risk factors that have been found to predict CVR, although family history might show fewer relations with stress-induced responses among African Americans than among European Americans (Anderson et al., 1993). Relatively little is known about relations between reactivity and other cardiovascular risk factors, especially among older adults. However, one study of middle-aged to older African Americans revealed that subjects with higher central adiposity (measured by waist circumference) showed greater blood pressure and heart rate reactivity, independent of several other cardiovascular risk factors (Waldstein, Burns, Toth, & Poehlman, 1999).

Overall, age-associated increases in comorbidity, cardiovascular risk factors, and medication use are potential confounders that have contributed to older adults being excluded from many studies of physiological stress responses. Nevertheless, it is important for research to consider these health status issues along with the likely age-associated changes in CVR, because these vulnerabilities may act synergistically in older adults to elevate their risk of cardiovascular morbidity and mortality.

## Psychosocial Factors

The burgeoning body of evidence linking psychosocial factors to the development and course of CVD stimulated a converging literature indicating similar relations between these factors and exaggerated cardiovascular responses to stress. Though the findings on psychosocial factors have not been completely consistent in either the CVD or CVR literatures, the data have largely supported the view of reactivity as a potential pathway through which these factors could lead to increased cardiovascular risk. Older men and women have been included in samples of several such studies that examined relations with psychosocial factors, such as hostility, anxiety, alexithymia, chronic stress, and social support.

As previously noted, stress-induced cardiovascular responses to extreme anger are potential triggers of acute cardiac events, particularly among vulnerable individuals. Earlier interests in relations between anger and CVD were fueled by research that suggested certain characteristics collectively referred to as Type A coronary-prone personality (e.g., angry, impatient, competitive, irritable) predicted coronary heart disease. However, subsequent cardiovascular studies found less support for the overall Type A personality construct. More recent cardiovascular research indicates that a primary toxic element of the Type A construct is dispositional hostility, which involves cognitive (e.g., cynical mistrust), behavioral (e.g., aggression), and emotional (e.g., anger) factors. Prospective and cross-sectional data have established hostility as a predictor of hypertension and coronary heart disease, as well as the severity of coronary artery disease, subclinical atherosclerosis, and myocardial ischemia (Berg et al., Chapter 3, this volume; Rozanski et al., 1999). It has been hypothesized that highly hostile individuals may have more frequent stressful interpersonal experiences and exhibit exaggerated responses to psychosocial stressors than less hostile individuals (Williams, Barefoot, & Shekelle, 1985). Evidence of associations between higher levels of hostility and increased CVR has primarily come from studies of younger samples (Suls & Wan, 1993). However, one study found that hostile middle-aged to older adults, as identified by a structured interview, had more pronounced and prolonged blood pressure responses to anger (Fredrickson et al., 2000).

Another focus of research has been the dispositional tendency frequently and intensely to experience negative affect, such as depression or anxiety. Prospective studies have found evidence that depression (either depressive symptoms or episodic major depression) is predictive of future cardiac events in healthy populations and recurrent cardiac events among patient populations. Similarly, associations between depressive symptoms and pronounced CVR have been noted, perhaps more strongly for heart rate reactivity, though little is known about such relations among older adults (Kibler & Ma, 2004). With regard to anxiety, research suggests that it may be related to increased risk for coronary heart disease and death, particularly sudden cardiac death (Rozanski et al., 1999). The physiological stress responses of adults with phobic anxiety disorders, particularly social phobia, have been of interest, because these individuals tend to report greater emotional and somatic arousal during social stressors than to nonanxious adults. Although CVR studies have examined older adults with social phobia (Grossman et al., 2001), little is known about the stress responses of people over age 65 with other forms of anxiety.

A more recent topic of interest in emotional–cardiovascular research involves individual differences in emotional expression. Alexithymia is a cognitive-affective style in which one has a limited ability to understand, express, or differentiate one's own emotions. Although the underlying mechanism is uncertain, alexithymia has been associated prospectively with all-cause mortality after controlling for traditional cardiovascular risk factors (Kauhanen, Kaplan, Cohen, Julkunen, & Salonen, 1996). CVR may be a mechanism for this relation, as suggested by the preliminary finding of greater blood pressure reactivity among middle-aged to older adults with higher alexithymia (Waldstein, Kauhanen, Neumann, & Katzel, 2002). Further study is needed to discern whether relations between alexithymia and disease outcomes are independent or due primarily to correlations with other factors, such as anxiety, depression, or hostility.

Other major areas of investigation involve examining the cardiovascular effects of factors related to the social environment, such as exposure to chronic stress (e.g., job stress) and supportive resources available from social networks (see Rook, Mavadandi, Sorkin, & Zettel, Chapter 14, this volume). Researchers have found that higher levels of chronic stress and lower levels of social support are associated with increased risk for coronary heart disease (Rozanski et al., 1999; Smith & Ruiz, 2002). Chronic stress and social support have shown similar relations with exaggerated blood pressure reactivity and/or delayed poststress recovery (Gump & Matthews, 1999; Uchino, Cacioppo, & Kiecolt-Glaser, 1996). One source of chronic stress, caregiving for family members with dementia, has been examined for relations with CVR. Limited data on samples involving older adults suggest that older female caregivers might differ little from their noncaregiver counterparts in terms of reactivity, but may show higher resting levels of cardiovascular parameters (Cacioppo et al., 2000). However, if older male and female caregivers are hypertensive, they may show greater stress-induced cardiovascular responses than noncaregivers (Vitaliano, Russo, Bailey, Young, & McCann, 1993). Moreover, lower levels of social support may be associated with heightened CVR among chronically stressed caregivers (Uchino, Kiecolt-Glaser, & Cacioppo, 1992). Though higher levels of social support may buffer against the harmful effects of chronic stress, all social relationships are not necessarily beneficial to health. For example, the number of ambivalent network ties (i.e., individuals who are sources of both positivity and negativity in one's social network) has predicted greater cardiovascular responses to mental stress as a function of age (Uchino, Holt-Lunstad, Uno, & Flinders, 2001).

Whereas psychosocial factors are typically examined separately, they often occur in clusters, which may add to their influence on CVD. This clustering also may increase the variance predicted in CVR and/or post-stress recovery, as suggested by findings among older adult samples (Vitaliano et al., 1993; Vitaliano, Russo, Paulsen, & Bailey, 1995). However, given that psychosocial factors are often intercorrelated and have overlapping constructs, it is uncertain whether relations with cardiovascular conditions are attributable to a single psychosocial factor or to an underlying characteristic shared by several factors. In addition, many of these factors have relations with other pathways to CVD, such as adverse health behaviors (e.g., smoking, poor treatment adherence) and traditional risk factors (e.g., obesity), as well as inflammatory and immunological processes (Suls & Bunde, 2005). Still, psychosocial characteristics influence individuals' concomitant emotional, cognitive, behavioral, and physiological responses to acutely stressful situations, as well as the frequency at which they experience certain stressors. Overall, the literature suggests that several psychosocial factors linked to CVD are also associated with the tendency to respond to stress with enhanced physiological responses. Although the existing studies are not sufficient to provide confirmation, these data generally support CVR as a plausible pathophysiological mechanism linking psychosocial factors and CVD.

## SUMMARY AND CONCLUSIONS

Stress-induced cardiovascular responses of heightened magnitude and/or prolonged duration have been prospectively associated with preclinical forms of CVD (e.g., atherosclerosis, enlarged left ventricular mass), as well as some of its clinical manifestations, such as hypertension, coronary heart disease, and cerebrovascular disease. The precise role of CVR in CVD is uncertain, but it may play a direct role in disease pathogenesis, be a mechanism through which psychosocial factors exert effects, or serve as a disease marker. It also is a potential trigger of pathological states that precede acute cardiac events, particularly among vulnerable older adults. The cardiovascular stress responses of older adults likely become more enhanced and/or prolonged in part because of potentially modifiable (e.g., diet, medication), aging-related changes in the cardiovascular system, such as increased arterial stiffness, endothelial dysfunction, baroreflex impairment, and increased sympathetic nervous system activity, as well as reduced heart rate variability. In addition, several constitutional and psychosocial factors linked to increased cardiovascular risk may contribute to individual differences in CVR and/or poststress recovery.

Although promising, the literature on stress-induced cardiovascular responses among older adults is relatively sparse, with information about a particular topic often limited to a single study. Likewise, the range of potential influences on cardiovascular responses examined in this age group is narrower than the wide array of factors explored in younger age groups. Furthermore, existing data on some topics were derived from relatively small, predominantly European American samples that focused on one gender, which leaves uncertain the generalizability to other groups. Whereas some studies included adults over age 65, few were designed to study aging, and most did not provide age-specific analyses. Information specific to older adults is needed given that hypertension and atherosclerosis may increase their vulnerability to potentially adverse effects of exaggerated cardiovascular responses to mental stress. On the whole, older adults have been underrepresented in CVR research, but the literature to date provides the groundwork for future study of this age group.

## FUTURE DIRECTIONS

CVD incidence and prevalence will likely increase as the expected growth in the older population occurs. The expansion of CVR research among older adults that utilizes larger, diverse samples may shed light on the development and course of the disease. Future research should broaden the examination of constitutional and psychosocial predictors of variability in CVR. For example, more information is needed about how CVR is influenced by cardiovascular risk factors, comorbidity, and medication use, including estrogen. Moreover, research should include greater examination of anxiety and other psychological traits, which might cumulatively influence cardiovascular function over the lifespan. Given the many stressful life changes that may occur with aging (e.g., retirement, increasing medical needs, deaths of loved ones), the relations of reactivity to depression and related factors, such as hopelessness and vital exhaustion (i.e., demoralization, irritability, fatigue), should be explored. Dispositional negative affect could be especially pertinent among older men and women with lower socioeconomic status and/or ethnic/minority status, who face the added demands of coping with a variety of chronic stressors, such as poverty or discrimination. Furthermore, differences in exposure to life stressors and potential interactive effects with genetic risk (e.g., family history of hypertension) or other sources of vulnerability should receive greater consideration in upcoming work (Schwartz et al., 2003).

Whereas research has focused on the magnitude and patterning of cardiovascular responses, the duration of these responses and psychological factors (e.g., rumination) that might prolong them require more attention. In addition, investigations should incorporate strategies to enhance lab-to-life generalizability, such as aggregating across multiple tasks and utilizing socially oriented tasks (e.g., recalled emotional experiences, role-played scenarios) that are representative of real-life stressors among older adults. Future studies should use integrative designs for more comprehensive examinations of physiological stress responses. For example, it may be informative to measure both cardiovascular and neuroendocrine (e.g., cortisol, norepinephrine) reactivity to mental stress, as well as concomitant heart rate variability, to obtain a broader assessment of potential contributors to risk for CVD.

Prior cross-sectional work suggests aging-related changes in cardiovascular responses to stress, but these studies are limited by inferences drawn from data affected by cohort effects and selective survival. Thus, longitudinal studies extending across major portions of the lifespan into old age are sorely needed to determine the true effects of aging on CVR. Through such studies, changes resulting from primary aging (biological aging) might be distinguished from those due to unhealthy lifestyles (secondary aging) and those related to disease (tertiary aging). Moreover, it is difficult to discern from cross-sectional data whether the effects of psychosocial factors on CVR are relatively consistent across the lifespan, or whether they change with aging. Furthermore, longitudinal studies could allow for assessment of the prognostic significance and the specific role played by CVR in various forms of CVD. If its role is pathogenic, reduction of CVR could be a goal of research on pharmacological or behavioral interventions (e.g., exercise, relaxation training), which in turn, might expand the approaches used to reduce CVD.

## REFERENCES

American Heart Association. (2005). *Heart disease and stroke statistics—2005 update*. Dallas, TX: Author.

Anderson, N. B., McNeilly, M., & Myers, H. (1993). A biopsychosocial model of race differences in vascular reactivity. In J. Blascovich & E. S. Katkin (Eds.), *Cardiovascular reactivity to psychological stress and disease* (pp. 83–108). Washington, DC: American Psychological Association.

Bairey Merz, C. N., Kop, W., Krantz, D. S., Helmers, K. F., Berman, D. S., & Rozanski, A. (1998). Cardiovascular stress response and coronary artery disease: Evidence of an adverse postmenopausal effect in women. *American Heart Journal, 135,* 881–887.

Boutcher, S. H., & Stocker, D. (1996). Cardiovascular response of young and older males to mental challenge. *Journals of Gerontology: Psychological Sciences and Social Sciences, Series B, 51,* P261–P267.

Burleson, M. H., Malarkey, W. B., Cacioppo, J. T., Poehlmann, K. M., Kiecolt-Glaser, J. K., Berntson, G. G., et al. (1998). Postmenopausal hormone replacement: Effects on autonomic, neuroendocrine, and immune reactivity to brief psychological stressors. *Psychosomatic Medicine, 60,* 17–25.

Burleson, M. H., Poehlmann, K. M., Hawkley, L. C., Ernst, J. M., Berntson, G. G., Malarkey, W. B., et al. (2003). Neuroendocrine and cardiovascular reactivity to stress in mid-aged and older women: Long-term temporal consistency of individual differences. *Psychophysiology, 40,* 358–369.

Cacioppo, J. T., Burleson, M. H., Poehlmann, K. M., Malarkey, W. B., Kiecolt-Glaser, J. K., Berntson, G. G., et al. (2000). Autonomic and neuroendocrine responses to mild psychological stressors: Effects of chronic stress on older women. *Annals of Behavioral Medicine, 22,* 140–148.

Celermajer, D. S., Sorensen, K. E., Spiegelhalter, D. J., Georgakopoulos, D., Robinson, J., & Deanfield, J. E. (1994). Aging is associated with endothelial dysfunction in healthy men years before the age-related decline in women. *Journal of the American College of Cardiology, 24,* 471–476.

Ditto, B., Miller, S., & Maurice, S. (1987). Age differences in the consistency of cardiovascular response patterns in healthy patterns in healthy women. *Biological Psychology, 25,* 23–31.

Everson, S. A., Lynch, J. W., Kaplan, G. A., Lakka, T. A., Sivenius, J., & Salonen, J. T. (2001). Stress-induced blood pressure reactivity and incident stroke in middle-aged men. *Stroke, 32,* 1263–1270.

Faucheux, B. A., Dupuis, C., Baulon, A., Lille, F., & Bourlière, F. (1983). Heart rate reactivity during minor mental stress in men in their 50s and 70s. *Gerontology, 29,* 149–160.

Faucheux, B. A., Lille, F., Baulon, A., Landau, J., Dupuis, C, & Bourlière, F. (1989). Heart rate and blood pressure reactivity during active coping with a mental task in healthy 18- to 73-year-old subjects. *Gerontology, 35,* 19–30.

Fredrickson, B. L., Maynard, K. E., Helms, M. J., Haney, T. L., Siegler, I. C., & Barefoot, J. C. (2000). Hostility predicts magnitude and duration of blood pressure response to anger. *Journal of Behavioral Medicine, 23,* 229–243.

Garwood, M., Engel, B. T., & Capriotti, R. (1982). Autonomic nervous system function and aging: Response specificity. *Psychophysiology, 19,* 378–385.

Grossman, P., Wilhelm, F. H., Kawachi, I., & Sparrow, D. (2001). Gender differences in psychophysiological responses to speech stress among older social phobics: Congruence and incongruence between self-evaluative and cardiovascular reactions. *Psychosomatic Medicine, 63,* 765–777.

Gump, B. B., & Matthews, K. A. (1999). Do background stressors influence reactivity to and recovery from acute stressors? *Journal of Applied Social Psychology, 29,* 469–494.

Harris, K. F., & Matthews, K. A. (2004). Interactions between autonomic nervous system activity and endothelial function: A model for the development of cardiovascular disease. *Psychosomatic Medicine, 66,* 153–164.

Hawkley, L. C., Burleson, M. H., Poehlmann, K. M., Berntson, G. G., Malarkey, W. B., & Cacioppo, J. T. (2001). Cardiovascular and endocrine reactivity in older females: Intertask consistency. *Psychophysiology, 38,* 863–872.

Huisman, H. W., Van Rooyen, J. M., Malan, N. T., Eloff, F. C., Laubscher, P. J., Steyn, H. S., et al. (2002). Cardiovascular reactivity patterns elicited by the cold pressor test as a function of aging. *Aging Clinical and Experimental Research, 14,* 202–207.

Jennings, J. R., Kamarck, T., Manuck, S., Everson, S. A., Kaplan, G., & Salonen, J. T. (1997). Aging or disease?: Cardiovascular reactivity in Finnish men over the middle years. *Psychology and Aging, 12,* 225–238.

Jennings, J. R., Nebes, R., & Brock, K. (1988). Memory retrieval in noise and psychophysiological response in the young and old. *Psychophysiology, 25,* 633–644.

Kauhanen, J., Kaplan, G. A., Cohen, R. A., Julkunen, J., & Salonen, J. T. (1996). Alexithymia and risk of death in middle-aged men. *Journal of Psychosomatic Research, 41,* 541–549.

Kibler, J. L., & Ma, M. (2004). Depressive symptoms and cardiovascular reactivity to laboratory behavioral stress. *International Journal of Behavioral Medicine, 11,* 81–87.

Knight, B. G., & McCallum, T. J. (1998). Heart rate reactivity and depression in African-American and white dementia caregivers: Reporting bias or positive coping? *Aging and Mental Health, 2,* 212–221.

Komesaroff, P. A., Fullerton, M., Esler, M. D., Jennings, G., & Sudhir, K. (2002). Oestrogen supplementation attenuates responses to psychological stress in elderly men rendered hypogonadal after treatment for prostate cancer. *Clinical Endocrinology, 56,* 745–753.

Kop, W. J. (1999). Chronic and acute psychological risk factors for clinical manifestations of coronary artery disease. *Psychosomatic Medicine, 61,* 476–487.

Krantz, D. S., Kop, W. J., Santiago, H. T., & Gottdiener, J. S. (1996). Mental stress as a trigger of myocardial ischemia and infarction. *Cardiology Clinics, 14,* 271–287.

Krantz, D. S., Santiago, H. T., Kop, W. J., Bairey Merz, C. N., Rozanski, A., & Gottdiener, J. S. (1999). Prognostic value of mental stress testing in coronary artery disease. *American Journal of Cardiology, 84,* 1292–1297.

Kudielka, B. M., Buske-Kirschbaum, A., Hellhammer, D. H., & Kirschbaum, C. (2004). Differential heart rate reactivity and recovery after psychosocial stress (TSST) in healthy children, younger adults, and elderly adults: The impact of age and gender. *International Journal of Behavioral Medicine, 11,* 116–121.

Labouvie-Vief, G., Lumley, M. A., Jain, E., & Heinze, H. (2003). Age and gender differences in cardiac reactivity and subjective emotion responses to emotional autobiographical memories. *Emotion, 3,* 115–126.

Lakatta, E. G. (2003). Arterial and cardiac aging: Major shareholders in cardiovascular disease enterprises—Part III: Cellular and molecular clues to heart and arterial aging. *Circulation, 107,* 490–497.

Lakatta, E. G., & Levy, D. (2003a). Arterial and cardiac aging: Major shareholders in cardiovascular disease enterprises—Part I: Aging arteries: a "set up" for vascular disease. *Circulation, 107,* 139–146.

Lakatta, E. G., & Levy, D. (2003b). Arterial and cardiac aging: Major shareholders in cardiovascular disease enterprises—Part II: The aging heart in health: Links to heart disease. *Circulation, 107,* 346–354.

Lenfant, C., Chobanian, A. V., Jones, D. W., & Roccella, E. J. (2003). Seventh report of the Joint National Committee on the Prevention, Detection, Evaluation, and Treatment of High Blood Pressure (JNC 7): Resetting the hypertension sails. *Hypertension, 41,* 1178–1179.

Levenson, R. W., Carstensen, L. L., Friesen, W. V., & Ekman, P. (1991). Emotion, physiology, and expression in old age. *Psychology and Aging, 6,* 28–35.

Lipman, R. D., Grossman, P., Bridges, S. E., Hamner, J. W., & Taylor, J. A. (2002). Mental stress response, arterial stiffness, and baroreflex sensitivity in healthy aging. *Journal of Gerontology: Biological Sciences, and Medical Sciences, Series A, 57,* B279–B284.

Manhem, K., Brandin, L., Ghanoum, B., Rosengren, A., & Gustafsson, H. (2003). Acute effects of transdermal estrogen on hemodynamic and vascular reactivity in elderly postmenopausal healthy women. *Journal of Hypertension, 21,* 387–394.

Manuck, S. B. (1994). Cardiovascular reactivity in cardiovascular disease: "Once more unto the breach." *International Journal of Behavioral Medicine, 1,* 4–31.

Matthews, K. A., Flory, J. D., Owens, J. F., Harris, K. F., & Berga, S. L. (2001). Influence of estrogen replacement therapy on cardiovascular responses to stress of healthy postmenopausal women. *Psychophysiology, 38,* 391–398.

National Center for Health Statistics. (2003). *Health, United States, 2003.* Hyattsville, MD: Author.

Oparil, S., Zaman, M. A., & Calhoun, D. A. (2003). Pathogenesis of hypertension. *Annals of Internal Medicine, 139,* 761–776.

Owens, J. F., Stoney, C. M., & Matthews, K. A. (1993). Menopausal status influences ambulatory blood pressure levels and blood pressure changes during mental stress. *Circulation, 88,* 2794–2802.

Rozanski, A., Blumenthal, J. A., & Kaplan, J. (1999). Impact of psychological factors on the pathogenesis of cardiovascular disease and implications for therapy. *Circulation, 99,* 2192–2217.

Saab P. G., Matthews, K. A., Stoney, C. M., & McDonald, R. H. (1989). Premenopausal and postmenopausal women differ in their cardiovascular and neuroendocrine responses to behavioral stressors. *Psychophysiology, 26,* 270–280.

Schuler, J. L. H., & O'Brien, W. H. (1997). Cardiovascular recovery from stress and hypertension risk factors: A meta-analytic review. *Psychophysiology, 34,* 649–659.

Schwartz, A. R., Gerin, W., Davidson, K. W., Pickering, T. G., Brosschot, J. F., Thayer, J. F., et al. (2003). Toward a causal model of cardiovascular responses to stress and the development of cardiovascular disease. *Psychosomatic Medicine, 65,* 22–35.

Smith, T. W., & Ruiz, J. M. (2002). Psychosocial influences on the development and course of coronary heart disease: Current status and implications for research and practice. *Journal of Consulting and Clinical Psychology, 70,* 548–568.

Steptoe, A., Moses, J., & Edwards, S. (1990). Age-related differences in cardiovascular reactions to mental stress tests in women. *Health Psychology, 9,* 18–34.

Stewart, J. C., & France, C. R. (2001). Cardiovascular recovery from stress predicts longitudinal changes in blood pressure. *Biological Psychology, 58,* 105–120.

Stoney, C. M., Davis, M. C., & Matthews, K. A. (1987). Sex differences in physiological responses to stress and in coronary heart disease: A causal link? *Psychophysiology, 24,* 127–131.

Suls, J., & Bunde, J. (2005). Anger, anxiety, and depression as risk factors for cardiovascular disease: The problems and implications of overlapping affective dispositions. *Psychological Bulletin, 131,* 260–300.

Suls, J., & Wan, C. K. (1993). The relationship between trait hostility and cardiovascular reactivity: A quantitative review and analysis. *Psychophysiology, 30,* 615–626.

Traustadóttir, T., Bosch, P. R., & Matt, K. S. (2003). Gender differences in cardiovascular and hypothalamic–pituitary–adrenal axis responses to psychological stress in healthy older adult men and women. *Stress, 6,* 133–140.

Treiber, F. A., Kamarck, T., Schneiderman, N., Sheffield, D., Kapuku, G., & Taylor, T. (2003). Cardiovascular reactivity and development of preclinical and clinical disease states. *Psychosomatic Medicine, 65,* 46–62.

Tsai, J. L., Levenson, R. W., & Cartensen, L. L. (2000). Autonomic, subjective, and expressive responses to emotional films in older and younger Chinese Americans and European Americans. *Psychology and Aging, 15,* 684–693.

Turner, J. R. (1994). *Cardiovascular reactivity and stress: Patterns of physiological response.* New York: Plenum.

Uchino, B. N., Cacioppo, J. T., & Kiecolt-Glaser, J. K. (1996). The relationship between social support and physiological processes: A review with emphasis on underlying mechanisms and implications for health. *Psychological Bulletin, 119,* 488–531.

Uchino, B. N., Holt-Lunstad, J., Bloor, L. E., & Campo, R. A. (2005). Aging and cardiovascular reactivity to stress: Longitudinal evidence for changes in stress reactivity. *Psychology and Aging, 20,* 134–143.

Uchino, B. N., Holt-Lunstad, J., Uno, D., & Flinders, J. B. (2001). Heterogeneity in the social networks of young and older adults: Prediction of mental health and cardiovascular reactivity during acute stress. *Journal of Behavioral Medicine, 24,* 361–382.

Uchino, B. N., Kiecolt-Glaser, J. K., & Cacioppo, J. T. (1992). Age-related changes in cardiovascular response as a function of a chronic stressor and social support. *Journal of Personality and Social Psychology, 63,* 839–846.

Uchino, B. N., Uno, D., Holt-Lunstad, J., & Flinders, J. B. (1999). Age-related differences in cardiovascular reactivity during acute psychological stress in men and women. *Journals of Gerontology: Psychological Sciences and Social Sciences, Series B, 54,* P339–P346.

Vitaliano, P. P., Russo, J., Bailey, S. L., Young, H. M., & McCann, B. S. (1993). Psychosocial factors associated with cardiovascular reactivity in older adults. *Psychosomatic Medicine, 55,* 164–177.

Vitaliano, P. P., Russo, J., Paulsen, V. M., & Bailey, S. L. (1995). Cardiovascular recovery from laboratory stress: Biopsychosocial concomitants in older adults. *Journal of Psychosomatic Research, 39,* 361–377.

Waldstein, S. R., Burns, H. O., Toth, M. J., & Poehlman, E. T. (1999). Cardiovascular reactivity and central adiposity in older African Americans. *Health Psychology, 18,* 221–228.

Waldstein, S. R., & Katzel, L. I. (2005). Stress-induced blood pressure reactivity and cognitive function. *Neurology, 64,* 1746–1749.

Waldstein, S. R., Kauhanen, J., Neumann, S. A., & Katzel, L. I. (2002). Alexithymia and cardiovascular risk in older adults: Psychosocial, psychophysiological, and biomedical correlates. *Psychology and Health, 17,* 597–610.

Waldstein, S. R., Siegel, E. L., Lefkowitz, D., Maier, K. J., Pelletier Brown, J. R., Obuchowski, A. M., et al. (2004). Stress-induced blood pressure reactivity and silent cerebrovascular disease. *Stroke, 35,* 1294–1298.

Williams, R. B., Barefoot, J. C., & Shekelle, R. B. (1985). The health consequences of hostility. In M. A. Chesney & R. H. Rosenman (Eds.), *Anger and hostility in cardiovascular and behavioral disorders* (pp. 173–185). Washington, DC: Hemisphere.

# PART III

# PSYCHOSOCIAL ISSUES

# CHAPTER 9

# A Lifespan Approach
# to Personality and Longevity

## The Case of Conscientiousness

HOWARD S. FRIEDMAN *and* LESLIE R. MARTIN

It has long been recognized that individuals vary considerably in their likelihood of illness or premature mortality, but efforts to characterize these individual differences have often proved inconclusive. We intuitively understand and research confirms that a person who is distressed, depressed, hostile, bored, frustrated, isolated, or helpless is more likely to become ill (and die prematurely) than is someone who feels emotionally balanced and efficacious, is in a fulfilling and interesting career, has stable and supportive social relationships, and is well integrated into the community (Booth-Kewley & Friedman, 1987; Cohen & Williamson, 1991; Friedman & Booth-Kewley, 1987; House, Landis, & Umberson, 1988; Kiecolt-Glaser, Glaser, Cacioppo, & Malarkey, 1998; Miller, Smith, Turner, Guijarro, & Hallett, 1996; Repetti, Taylor, & Seeman, 2002; Smith & Gallo, 2001). Efforts to measure, identify, and characterize such people, however, have often led to a morass of weak and hard-to-replicate findings.

Some of the confusion has resulted from differing approaches to individual differences, with some notions deriving from trait research (e.g., hostility, disagreeableness), others arising primarily from psychoanalytic psychosomatic theories (e.g., repressive style, alexithymia), and still others being named as medical syndromes, without any theoretical considerations at all (e.g., Type A behavior). But an emerging consensus about five or so prime personality dimensions of interest (Neuroticism, Extraversion, Openness, Agreeableness, and Conscientiousness) has helped focus research in this area (Marshall et al., 1994; Smith & Gallo, 2001). "Personality," which can be defined as a relatively stable set of cognitive-motivational and socioemotional traits and behavior patterns, has emerged as a valuable construct in understanding individual differences in health.

Personality forms in childhood as temperament encounters socialization; it remains relatively stable thereafter but is by no means immutable. As people mature and encounter different environments and social relations, aspects of their personalities are altered, usually gradually (Costa, Herbst, McCrae, & Siegler, 2000; Twenge, 2000, 2001, 2002). Personality captures a combination of genetic, familial, and sociocultural elements; thus, it is a useful summary construct. As we shall see, one broad trait, conscientiousness, is especially relevant to healthy aging for a variety of reasons.

Another source of past confusion involved the fragmentation of research efforts into a wide variety of disease outcomes, well-being outcomes, and mortality outcomes. Thus, we had some researchers studying hostile struggle and coronary disease, other researchers studying repressed anxiety and asthma, some studying rebelliousness and substance abuse, and still others studying coping processes and longevity. The studies were derived from different models of health, funded by different kinds of agencies, and published in widely disparate sorts of journals.

Rather than studying psychology and healthy aging trait by trait and disease by disease, it is conceptually and heuristically superior to start with a coordinated, unified paradigm. Such an approach maximizes construct validity and helps us avoid doing studies for example, in which cardiovascular mortality is examined but all-cause mortality is ignored. Taking this broader, integrative perspective, the question of "Who gets sick and who stays well?" can be addressed with empirically based concepts that Friedman has termed *disease-prone personalities* and *self-healing personalities* (Friedman 1991/2000b, 1998; Friedman & Booth-Kewley, 1987; Friedman & VandenBos, 1992).

It turns out that there are associations between various psychological disturbances (e.g., chronic anger or anxiety or depression) and multiple diseases, impaired conditions, and risks of premature mortality; that is, there is increasing evidence for a generic disease-prone personality, with the particular negative predictors and outcomes dependent on a host of other biopsychosocial factors. Analogously, this line of thinking is confirmed by growing behavioral and nutritional research, which shows that a cluster of behaviors, such as inactivity and failing to eat an array of fruits and vegetables, is not only associated with poor heart health but also raises risk of cancer, impaired immune response, and so on. As we shall see, there are various complex reasons why a disease-prone personality is at higher risk for sundry adverse outcomes.

In contrast, the "self-healing personality" refers to a healing socioemotional style involving a match between the individual and the environment that maintains a physiological and psychosocial homeostasis, and through which good mental health promotes good physical health (Friedman, 1998). Self-healing, emotionally balanced people may be calm and conscientious, but they are also often responsive, energetic, curious, and constructive; they have better odds of living a longer, healthier life. Importantly, a self-healing style depends on the extant environment and does not involve a lack of challenge; many self-healing individuals enthusiastically embrace challenge. Self-healing personalities often contain elements of the mentally healthy orientations involving efficacy and commitment, described by humanistic and clinical psychologists (Antonovsky, 1979; Bandura, 1997; Csikszentmihalyi, 1991; Maddi & Kobasa, 1984).

Aside from a few insurance company actuaries, the reason we want to understand individual differences in health is to understand the causal pathways to illness; eventually we want to intervene to diminish illness and delay death. For both laypeople and scientists, the first thing one usually thinks about after hearing of an association between an individual characteristic (e.g., hostile struggle, or lack of exercise) and a negative outcome (e.g., coronary heart disease or colon cancer) is the possible causal explanation (e.g., too much psychological/physiological stress). The second thing both laypeople and scientists usually consider is how to prevent the negative outcome in their own cases (e.g., "I am going to play tennis and hang out with friends this weekend"). It is interesting to note how easy it is to slip from hearing about an association to searching for or assuming causal pathways, even though all scientists and many laypersons well appreciate that correlation does not imply causation.

Careful use of longitudinal and quasi-experimental designs can lead to comprehensive causal models of the links between personality and health, despite the fact that we cannot randomly assign people to personality and conduct a randomized trial (Aldwin, Spiro, Levenson, & Cupertino, 2001). However, explanatory models that ignore life trajectories often fail to consider the many different reasons for unhealthy socioemotional and motivational–behavioral patterns. With a lifespan approach, personality can be an important factor for understanding long-term biopsychosocial processes. In particular, it is useful to consider dynamisms, mechanisms, and tropisms (Friedman, 2000a).

## DYNAMISMS, MECHANISMS, TROPISMS

### Dynamisms

Dynamisms are processes responsible for development. These are the reasons different children set off on different health pathways. At a very early age, temperament forms as a function of genetic influences, *in utero* hormonal exposure, perinatal circumstances, and development during a time of rapid nervous system maturing. These personal characteristics then interact with the psychosocial environments created by children's families, their peers, and the broader culture (Caspi, 2000; Kuh & Ben-Shlomo, 1997; Tinsley, 1992). For example, longitudinal studies of children recruited at age 3 have shown that health-relevant factors such as delay of gratification, depression, and drug abuse in the teenage years could be predicted from a knowledge of childhood personality and social pressures, but only if the developmental processes were scrutinized. Certain oversocialized, overcontrolled girls later became depressed, but it was impulsive, undercontrolled boys who were at high risk for depression (Block, Block, & Keyes, 1988; Block, Gjerde, & Block, 1991). This striking gender difference is not a simple function of sex chromosomes; rather, it is a process particular to certain predispositions developing in a particular culture.

Analogously, although longevity tends to run in families, and many diseases have a hereditary component, there is rarely a simple genetic cause of such associations. For example, a comparison of the longevity of thousands of identical and fraternal twins in the Swedish Twin Registry (including twin pairs reared apart) showed the genetic effect to be quite modest; nonshared, individual specific environmental factors accounted for most of the variation (Ljungquist, Berg, Lanke, McClearn, & Pedersen, 1998). It has also been argued that environmental influences during pregnancy and infancy set in motion degenerative processes that appear as chronic diseases decades later (Barker, 1990).

In short, two errors are commonly made when long-term developmental processes are not considered in studies of personality and health. The first error is overlooking those early factors that influence both personality and health, also sometimes termed "underlying third variables." The second mistake is overexplaining a personality-to-disease link in terms of genetic or other relatively stable biological variables.

## Mechanisms

Mechanisms are the mediators between personality and health. Causal mechanisms accounting for associations between individual differences and health outcomes are usually divided into two classes. First, there are the patterns of psychophysiological reactions (including emotional reactions) that affect health-relevant internal processes. Included here are cardiovascular reactivity and immune reactions, both of which are affected by stress. Second, there are the patterns of health behaviors. Important behavioral patterns include tobacco and alcohol use, nutrition (overeating or poor eating), drug abuse, (lack of) exercise, sexual promiscuity, trauma-prone hobbies (e.g., parachuting), or nonadherence to prescribed medical treatments.

This division of mechanisms into two classes is, in some sense, inaccurate, because psychophysiological reactions and health behaviors are intimately related. For example, stress hormones and serum cholesterol have close ties to glucose levels and other elements of metabolism. These are all affected by use of nicotine and alcohol, physical activity, and diet. Similarly, levels of nicotine, glucose, alcohol, and other chemicals in one's body have dramatic effects on health behaviors, and smoking and drug-taking then affect physiology and risk-taking, and so on, in a complicated cycle. Furthermore, an individual's stable biological systems, especially those involving neurotransmitters such as serotonin, affect one's physiology and propensity toward health-relevant behaviors.

Conceptualizing these causal links in a comprehensive manner is important, because it affects selection of variables and which causal models one can and will investigate. Furthermore, without comprehensive causal models, the selection of control variables is often not well conceived. As noted, because we cannot randomly assign people to personality, long-term longitudinal designs are essential.

## Tropisms

Tropisms are the forces that pull phototropic plants toward a source of light, pull some individuals toward more health-promoting spaces, and push other individuals toward darker, health-threatening environments. Some of these forces are partly temperament based, as shown in research indicating a significant role for temperament in the development of alcoholism (Bennett & Miller, 1998). Other tropisms are more heavily environmental (e.g., punishments and rewards that push and pull certain children toward certain life paths). Work with adolescents demonstrates that those who value school, participate in family and religious or community activities, have well-socialized peers as friends, and value health are more likely later to engage in healthy behaviors such as eating a balanced diet, exercising, and using a seat belt (Jessor, Turbin, & Costa, 1998).

It is often assumed, incorrectly, that most life events (stressors) are unpredictable happenings or accidents. An important insight to emerge from modern personality research, however, is that personality can predict life events. For example, neuroticism tends to foretell negative life events; that is, it is often wrong to think of personality, located within the individual, as randomly encountering stressful or unstressful events (Bolger & Zuckerman, 1995; Magnus, Diener, Fujita, & Payot, 1993; McCartney, Harris, & Bernieri, 1990; Scarr & McCartney, 1984; Van Heck, 1997). For example, a longitudinal analysis of personality and work experiences showed that personality at age 18 predicted both objective and subjective work experiences at age 26. Furthermore, the traits that pushed individuals into specific work experiences were the traits that most changed in response to those work environments (Roberts, Caspi, & Moffitt, 2003).

A sensible research approach is therefore to assess the basic dimensions of personality in childhood, track developmental pathways, study health-relevant behaviors and social relations, and examine disease outcomes, including longevity and cause of death. Because this is rarely done, and perhaps because of all the attention to individual characteristics that seem to have a strong emotional component (e.g., attention to the psychophysiological correlates of Type A competition and emotional struggle), it is not surprising that a key personality predictor of health has long been overlooked. "Conscientiousness"—a tendency to be prudent, planful, persistent, and dependable—is not highly related to the personality measures typically used in health psychology research (Booth-Kewley & Vickers, 1994; Friedman, Tucker, & Reise, 1995; Marshall et al., 1994), but it turns out to be highly relevant to pathways to health.

The consideration of dynamisms, mechanisms, and tropisms leads to a complex picture of individual differences and health, and is probably closer to the truth than simple cause–effect models. For example, at certain times or in certain situations in one's life, it may be helpful (healthy) to be worrying (neurotic) or hostile (disagreeable). Similarly, extraversion might be associated with problems (e.g., the sociable drinking buddy) or solutions (e.g., social support in time of need). Conscientiousness, on the other hand, seems likely to be associated with a wide range of healthy processes. It thus proves to be a good illustration of how to move beyond prior difficulties in understanding the relations of personality and health.

## CONSCIENTIOUSNESS

Conscientiousness has a history of decades of scattered study in predicting mental health, although the concept usually has gone by other names. For example, using a sociological perspective, the classic California Psychological Inventory (dating from the 1950s) developed a Socialization scale that was used to classify individuals along a continuum of prosocial, normative behavior (Gough, 1994). This scale differentiates between those who are willing and able to adopt the norms of society, and those who are more deviant or delinquent. Low scorers tend to have trouble imagining and setting long-term goals, and being prudent and moderate in their behavior. They are more likely to end up as substance abusers, have unstable relations, and commit antisocial and illegal acts. Thus, this approach was one of the first to suggest and document that a conscientiousness-relevant dimension is very important to understanding and predicting poor mental health and poor health behaviors. Other commonly used concepts of past decades were impulse control, self-control, disinhibition, and sense of responsibility (Bogg & Roberts, 2004; Clark & Watson, 1999). Yet not until 1993, with publication of new data derived from and collected on the Terman and

Oden (1947) sample, did modern research efforts focus directly on conscientiousness, health, and longevity.

## Conscientiousness in the Terman Data

For the past 15 years, we have been studying personality and longevity in the Terman cohort. The Terman Gifted Children Study (later renamed the Terman Life Cycle Study) began in 1921–1922, when most of the 1,528 participants were in elementary school. Continued until the present, it is the longest study of a single cohort ever conducted, with rich data collected regularly throughout the lifespan (from childhood to late adulthood and death). Along with our colleagues (especially Kathleen Clark, Michael Criqui, Joseph Schwartz, Carol Tomlinson-Keasey, and Joan Tucker), we have made major efforts to follow up on and improve the data set. Data have been collected and refined on subjects' social relations, education, personality, habits, careers, families, mental health, life stress, physical activities, and physical health; most importantly, we have collected death certificates and coded dates and causes of death (Friedman, Tucker, Schwartz, Tomlinson-Keasey, et al., 1995). Until our project began, the study aimed primarily to describe the life course of gifted individuals (Terman & Oden, 1947); that is, the study originally focused on addressing issues such as whether bright children were introverted eggheads (it turned out that they were not). Few predictive studies using the data had been undertaken, with little or no study of health as a function of individual differences. Because of the richness of the psychosocial data across many decades, and because of long-range and valid health outcomes (especially longevity and cause of death), these data provided an excellent opportunity to study personality and longevity.

### The Sample

Terman's aim was to secure a reasonably random sample of bright California children, so Terman searched most public schools in the San Francisco and Los Angeles areas in the early 1920s. Bright children were nominated by their teachers and tested by Terman. The sample was later characterized as a productive, intelligent segment of 20th-century, middle-class American men and women (mostly white) (Sears, 1979, 1984; Subotnik, Karp, & Morgan, 1989). The average birthdate was 1910. Most were preadolescents when first studied. The data were collected prospectively, without any knowledge of the eventual health outcome, thus avoiding several common sources of bias in the data collection phase.

The sample is relatively homogeneous on dimensions of intelligence and social class. A resulting advantage is that these people had the ability to understand medical advice, places to exercise, routine health care, and so on; thus, the sample allows a clearer focus on the effects of psychosocial variables. As with all cohort studies, the results are not directly generalizable to other groups, in other times, in other circumstances, but there is little reason to suspect that the relationships being analyzed will be strongly distorted by the characteristics of this sample; that is, there is no reason to suspect that the relationship between a personality trait like conscientiousness and an outcome such as longevity is different for bright people than it is for people of average intelligence. (The sample is actually much more representative of the population than the various prospective studies that followed samples of physicians or nurses.) The homogeneous nature of the sample might restrict the range on some of the predictor variables; however, our work shows that this is not the case for conscientiousness. Overall, the data are remarkably complete. A low attrition rate of only 6% applies to most longevity analyses. Those lost from the sample do not differ in any known ways on relevant variables.

### Childhood Conscientiousness and Longevity

In statistical survival analyses with 1,178 males and females, we first tested whether variables representing major dimensions of personality could predict longevity across the lifespan (Friedman et al., 1993).

In 1922, one of the participant's parents (usually the mother, or both parents together) and the participant's teacher were asked to rate the participant on 25 trait dimensions (using a 13-point scale) chosen to measure intellectual, volitional, moral, emotional, aesthetic, physical, and social functioning. The scales used are remarkably modern in their appearance, and our measure of Conscientiousness–Social Dependability included four items: prudence, conscientiousness, freedom from vanity/egotism, and truthfulness. This corresponds roughly to the five-factor model (McCrae & John, 1992) dimension of Conscientiousness, and we have documented the correspondence between conscientiousness measured with this scale and the contemporary NEO Personality Inventory—Revised (NEO PI-R) conscientiousness scale (Martin & Friedman, 2000). However, it is not identical to the NEO PI-R measure.

Conscientiousness in childhood was clearly related to survival in middle to old age, establishing that childhood personality is related to survival decades into the future. For example, a person at the 75th percentile on Conscientiousness had only 77% of the risk of a person at the 25th percentile of dying in any given year (Friedman et al., 1993).

In a major follow-up (Friedman, Tucker, Schwartz, Martin, et al., 1995), we examined possible behavioral mechanisms for this robust association by gathering cause-of-death information and considering the possible mediating influences of drinking alcohol, smoking, and overeating. Survival analyses suggested that the protective effect of conscientiousness is not primarily due to accident avoidance. We obtained death certificates for the deceased from state bureaus and professionally coded deaths from injury (accidents and violence, coded 800–999 according to the *International Classification of Diseases*, 9th edition). Only 9% of the low-conscientious quartile and only 5% of the high-conscientious quartile, died as a result of injury; those who died from injury were more likely to be in the low-conscientiousness quartile; but, overall, few people died as the result of injury, so the overall effect of conscientiousness was not simply explained.

Similarly, the protective effect of conscientiousness cannot be mostly explained by abstinence from unhealthy substance intake. Conscientious children were less likely to grow up to be heavy drinkers and smokers, but these health behaviors alone did not explain away the effect. Conscientiousness seems to have more far-reaching and general effects.

### Adult Conscientiousness and Longevity

We next derived (from the archival Terman data) personality measures for adulthood that we likewise validated by showing them to be consistent with the five-factor contemporary conceptions (Martin & Friedman, 2000; Martin, Friedman, & Schwartz, in press). Conscientiousness was "measured" when participants were in their 30s and 40s.

As of the year 2000, 70% of the men and 51% of the women in this sample had verified deaths; median age of death for those who died was 72.7 years for men and 74.0 years for women. We again found conscientiousness (this time measured in adulthood) to be significantly related to mortality risk. Those low on adult conscientiousness died earlier.

Interestingly, we conducted a survival analysis in which both child and adult measures of conscientiousness were entered into the same equation. Each indicator of conscientiousness retained statistical significance, and with equal strength (each interquartile relative hazard = 0.85, $p < .01$). There was no evidence of a gender interaction. This analysis indicates that childhood conscientiousness did *not* predict mortality risk solely through its link with adult conscientiousness. Note that the childhood measure was derived from parent and teacher ratings, and most closely corresponded with the facets of self-discipline and dutifulness, as described by the well-validated NEO PI-R (Costa & McCrae, 1992), whereas the adulthood measure of conscientiousness was based on self-report data and was most closely related to the NEO PI-R facets of achievement striving, self-discipline, and deliberation (Martin & Friedman, 2000). In addition, the substantial time lag from childhood in 1922 to midlife in 1940–1950 likely produced some real change in personality. There is also unreliability of assessment. Nevertheless, these conscientiousness measures complement one another and the overall findings show the importance of this dimension.

## Conscientiousness in Follow-Up Studies by Others

The real test of the relevance of conscientiousness comes from whether these findings can be replicated in other samples by other researchers. Fortunately, the dramatic nature of these findings has inspired many such efforts.

### Longevity

Evidence substantiating our longevity findings is now emerging from replication studies. This is the most striking confirmation of our results. One study examined the relation of personality to mortality in 883 older Catholic clergy members, about two-thirds of whom were female. The NEO Five-Factor Inventory (a short form of the NEO Inventory) was administered at baseline. They were followed for a little more than 5 years, during which time 182 died. Those scoring very high on conscientiousness were about half as likely to die as those with a very low score (Wilson, Mendes de Leon, Bienias, Evans, & Bennett, 2004).

Another key study examined participants in a Medicare demonstration study with over 1,000 participants, ages 65–100 (Weiss & Costa, 2005). Importantly, this prospective study was of people who were older, sicker, and more representative of the elderly population than other such studies to date. Over the 5 years of follow-up, persons higher in conscientiousness were significantly less likely to die.

Some studies of personality have examined and followed patients for whom the issue of adherence to medical treatment (including adherence to special diet) is especially important. For example, in a study of conscientiousness and renal deterioration in patients with diabetes, time to renal failure was longer in those with higher conscientiousness (Brickman, Yount, Blaney, Rothberg, & De-Nour, 1996). In another prospective study of chronic renal insufficiency, patients with low conscientiousness had a substantially increased mortality rate over the 4-year term of the study (Christensen et al., 2002). (Both studies also found effects of neuroticism.)

An interesting study of U.S. presidents looked at personality, health behaviors, and longevity. The personality assessments were done by panels of experts using well-validated measures of the five-factor approach to personality. Here again, conscientiousness emerged as the predictor of longevity, with smoking and drinking explaining some of the association (McCann, 2005).

Since the 1993 study by Friedman et al., there has been remarkable confirmation of the importance of conscientiousness to longevity. Importantly, longevity is a much more reliable and valid outcome than is self-reported health (which often shares method variance with personality assessment). Longevity is not self-reported, and it is generally seen to be an important outcome in analyses of health.

## Dynamisms

Emerging evidence is confirming the importance of conscientiousness to understanding the development and emergence of healthy reaction patterns in children and adolescents (Graziano & Ward, 1992). For example, one study of fifth-grade girls (age 10) showed unconscientious girls to be more susceptible to developing risky behaviors (Markey, Markey, & Tinsley, 2003). Furthermore, as noted earlier, health-relevant factors such as drug abuse, depression, and smoking in the teenage years can be predicted from a knowledge of childhood personality and social pressures, if the developmental processes are carefully analyzed (Flay, 2002; Wills, Resko, Ainette, & Mendoza, 2004); that is, peer groups, commercial advertising, parental behavior, and cultural and subcultural influences are a key part of the emerging health identity in childhood and adolescence (Wakefield, Flay, Nichter, & Giovino, 2003). Precise models of the role of conscientiousness in these early health reaction patterns have not been developed, however.

Evidence for the generality of the conscientiousness effect comes from a study that used the Midlife Development in the United States Survey, a nationally representative sample of 3,032 noninstitutionalized civilian adults (Goodwin & Friedman, in press). This study examined the association between the five-factor traits of personality and common mental and physical disorders. The results showed that conscientiousness (protectively) was reliably associated with reduced risk of illness. On the mental health side, those with major depression, panic attacks, generalized anxiety disorder, and alcohol/substance use disorders had reliably lower levels of conscientiousness compared to those without these disorders. Diagnoses were based on the Composite International Diagnostic Interview (CIDI) scales, a series of diagnostic-specific scales that were developed from item-level analyses of the CIDI questions in the National Comorbidity Survey. In terms of illness traditionally termed "physical health," those with diabetes, hypertension, sciatica, urinary problems, stroke, hernia, tuberculosis, and joint problems likewise had significantly lower levels of conscientiousness compared to those without each physical disorder. Illnesses were assessed by self-report of past 12-month prevalence.

## Mechanisms

There is now emerging evidence for various kinds of mechanisms linking conscientiousness and health. These include both psychophysiological and behavioral mechanisms. For example, in terms of psychophysiological disease mechanisms, one study examined conscientiousness (NEO-PI) and subclinical cardiovascular disease (atherosclerosis) in a healthy community sample of 353 subjects (51% female). This study used sonography to measure intima-media thickness and collected physiological measures, including 24-hour urinary catecholamines. As expected, conscientiousness was associated with less thickening, with urinary norepinephrine emerging as a partial mediator (Witzig, Kamarck, Muldoon, & Sutton-Tyrrell, 2003).

In terms of psychophysiological mechanisms involving underlying factors (third variables), there are some hints that serotonin function may be relevant (Williams et al., 2004). For example, serotonergic functioning influences individual variability on dimensions such as aggression and impulse control, although the degree to which this might be true in the general population versus restricted to particular clinical groups is less clear. Manuck et al. (1998) demonstrated an inverse relationship between serotonergic functioning and both aggression and impulse control in a nonclinical sample. Researchers studying the effects of a mu-opioid receptor mutation found that not only did chemical blocking of opioids result in differential cortisol responses and increases in adrenocorticotropic hormone (ACTH) for those with the variant polymorphism but these individuals also scored significantly lower on NEO PI-R Conscientiousness than did those without it (Wand et al., 2002). These researchers suggest that those with the variant serotonin transporter might have abnormal hypothalamic–pituitary–adrenal (HPA) axis responses to stress and corresponding personality traits that are regulated by mu-opioid receptor activation. These lines of thought are supported by the growing body of evidence that childhood conscientiousness has far-reaching effects in adulthood (as our own studies suggest), so it is likely a fundamental human personality dimension.

In terms of health behaviors, a wide-ranging and comprehensive meta-analysis looked at conscientiousness-related traits (e.g., responsibility, self-discipline, impulsivity, prudence, harm avoidance, and self-control) and their associations with a range of important health behaviors, such as tobacco use, physical activity, alcohol abuse, diet, violence, risky sexual behavior, dangerous driving, suicide, and drug abuse (Bogg & Roberts, 2004) The striking findings revealed that conscientiousness-related traits were negatively associated with all risky health-related behaviors and positively related to all beneficial health-related behaviors. This meta-analysis is an exemplar of how to think about and study behavioral mechanisms—that health behaviors mediate between personality on the one hand, and health and longevity on the other. It uses multiple measures of personality and multiple health behaviors in a clear analytic framework.

## Tropisms

It is well established that married individuals (especially men) live longer than those who are "single," a category that includes those who are divorced or widowed. This phenomenon provides a good example of the limits of traditional approaches to understanding variability in longevity.

Although it is tempting to assume that the marriage itself is health protective (and indeed, pop health advice often recommends "Get married"), such a time-limited conclusion ignores both the precursors of the married state and the sequelae of being married. To look at the full picture across time, we used our expanded information about the Terman cohort to examine this issue (Tucker et al., 1996).

We studied the association between marital history at midlife (in 1950) and mortality (as of 1991) in over 1,000 Terman study participants. It turned out that both precursors and consistency of marriage were relevant. Consistently married individuals lived longer than those who had experienced marital breakup, but this was not necessarily due to the protective effects of marriage itself. In fact, individuals who were currently married but had previously experienced a divorce were at significantly higher mortality risk compared with consistently married individuals. Furthermore, persons who had not married by midlife were not at higher mortality risk compared with those consistently married. Finally, we found evidence for selection into marriage; that is, part of the relationship between marital history and mortality risk seemed to be explained by childhood psychosocial variables that were associated with both future marital history and mortality risk. Notably, consistently married individuals were more conscientious children than were inconsistently married individuals. Overall, there probably were detrimental effects of divorce and underlying personality factors relevant both to who stayed married and who lived long.

Other evidence confirms that there is self-selection into marriage—for example, a heritable influence on propensity to marry (Johnson, McGue, Krueger, & Bouchard, 2004). Furthermore, conscientious college women experience lower rates of divorce (Roberts & Bogg, 2004), and early individual traits affect later marital stability (Larson & Holman, 1994). Thus, divorce, rather than being a random stressor, is somewhat predictable. Add the fact that divorce rates vary dramatically across time and culture, and one can see how simple-minded it is to advise, "Get married to stay healthy."

Similar complex life pathways arise when socioeconomic status (SES) is considered. People with higher SES are more likely to be married, to have access to nutritious food, and to have greater access to a variety of health-protective resources such as expert medical care and safe, unpolluted housing. Furthermore, those who are more controlled, secure, and hardworking by age 18 are headed to better careers within a decade, which in turn can further enhance both their health and subsequent conscientiousness (Hogan & Ones, 1997; Judge & Ilies, 2002; Roberts et al., 2003). Conscientious persons are more likely to follow life pathways to enhanced health. Yet, shockingly, many studies of predictors of health and longevity control (statistically) for SES on the grounds that it is some sort of "noise" factor. By doing so, the researchers may eliminate important predictive factors.

Taken together, and considering full models, the predictive power of conscientiousness is remarkable. Because this dimension has been mostly overlooked in studies of personality and health, and longevity, the confirmation of its relationship to health and recognition of the several ways in which it has key influence suggest numerous possibilities for better understanding the complex interrelationships among personality and psychosocial factors on one hand, and physical health and well-being on the other.

## LESSONS FOR UNDERSTANDING AGING

A conscientious, dependable personality, in appropriate environments, is a key predictor and may be a central underlying causal factor of health and longevity. This is likely not because conscientiousness is isomorphic with a self-healing personality, with simple associations to health. Rather it is mostly because conscientious people generally have a predisposition to salutary reaction patterns; wind up with healthy coping styles, habits, and behaviors; and move toward and create environments beneficial to good health. Environments, in turn, can further influence serotonergic activity, behaviors, and subsequent environments.

Efforts to promote healthy aging are often aimed at adults at a single point in time, with little attention to the lifespan trajectories along which the individuals are already traveling. Such models, which undervalue or ignore life trajectories, fail to consider the many different pathways to healthy or unhealthy patterns. For example, different people are obese, or poorly nourished, or inactive for a variety of reasons in their life histories, and are unlikely to benefit from exactly the same programs of change.

As noted, other personality factors are also relevant to health and indeed may become especially germane to certain situations commonly (but not necessarily) encountered by the aged (Friedman, 2007). Detailed consideration of conscientiousness, however, helps force examination of the multidimensional, interacting processes across time. Interventions to promote healthy aging that do not consider life pathways are inherently weak and incomplete. This is a special problem in a culture where health promotion efforts and the public health system are too often built around a pathology model derived from traditional conceptions of treating acute disease. Healthy aging is a chronic process, indeed, a lifelong passage.

## ACKNOWLEDGMENT

This work was supported by Grant No. AG08825 from the National Institute on Aging (NIA). The views expressed herein are those of the authors and not those of the NIA.

## REFERENCES

Aldwin, C. M., Spiro, A., Levenson, M. R., & Cupertino, A. P. (2001). Longitudinal findings from the normative aging study: III. Personality, individual health trajectories, and mortality. *Psychology and Aging, 16,* 450–465.

Antonovsky, A. (1979). *Health, stress and coping.* San Francisco: Jossey-Bass.

Bandura, A. (1997). *Self-efficacy: The exercise of control.* New York: Freeman.

Barker, D. J. (1990). The fetal and infant origins of adult disease. *British Medical Journal, 301,* 1111.

Bennett, M. E., & Miller, W. R. (1998). Alcohol problems. In H. S. Friedman (Ed.), *Encyclopedia of mental health* (Vol. 1, pp. 53–64). San Diego: Academic Press.

Block, J., Block, J. H., & Keyes, S. (1988). Longitudinally foretelling drug usage in adolescence: Early childhood personality and environmental precursors. *Child Development, 59,* 336–355.

Block, J. H., Gjerde, P. F., & Block, J. H. (1991). Personality antecedents of depressive tendencies in 18-year-olds: A prospective study. *Journal of Personality and Social Psychology, 60,* 726–738.

Bogg, T., & Roberts, B. W. (2004). Conscientiousness and health-related behaviors: A meta-analysis of the leading behavioral contributors to mortality. *Psychological Bulletin, 130*(6), 887–919.

Bolger, N., & Zuckerman, A. (1995). A framework for studying personality in the stress process. *Journal of Personality and Social Psychology, 69,* 890–902.

Booth-Kewley, S., & Friedman, H. S. (1987). Psychological predictors of heart disease: A quantitative review. *Psychological Bulletin, 101,* 343–362.

Booth-Kewley, S., & Vickers, Jr., R. R. (1994). Associations between major domains of personality and health behavior. *Journal of Personality, 62,* 281–298.

Brickman, A. L., Yount, S. E., Blaney, N. T., Rothberg, S. T., & De-Nour, A. K. (1996). Personality traits and long-term health status: The influence of neuroticism and conscientiousness on renal deterioration in Type-1 diabetes. *Psychosomatics, 37*(5), 459–468.

Caspi, A. (2000). The child is father of the man: Personality continuities from childhood to adulthood. *Journal of Personality and Social Psychology, 78,* 158–172.

Christensen, A. J., Ehlers, S. L., Wiebe, J. S., Moran, P. J., Raichle, K., Ferneyhough, K., et al. (2002). Patient personality and mortality: A 4-year prospective examination of chronic renal insufficiency. *Health Psychology, 21,* 315–320.

Clark, L. A., & Watson, D. (1999). Temperament: A new paradigm for trait psychology. In L. Pervin & O. John (Eds.), *Handbook of personality: Theory and research* (2nd ed., pp. 399–423). New York: Guilford Press.

Cohen, S., & Williamson, G. M. (1991). Stress and infectious disease in humans. *Psychological Bulletin, 109,* 5–24.

Costa, P. T., Jr., & McCrae, R. R. (1992). *The Revised NEO Personality Inventory professional manual.* Odessa, FL: Psychological Assessment Resources.

Costa, P. T., Jr., Herbst, J. H., McCrae, R. R., & Siegler, I. C. (2000). Personality at midlife: Stability, intrinsic maturation, and response to life events. *Assessment, 7,* 365–378.

Csikszentmihalyi, M. (1991). *Flow: The psychology of optimal experience*. New York: HarperCollins.

Flay, B. R. (2002). Positive youth development requires comprehensive health promotion programs. *American Journal of Health Behavior, 26,* 407–424.

Friedman, H. S. (Ed.). (1998). Self-healing personalities. In *Encyclopedia of mental health*. (Vol. 3, pp. 453–459). San Diego: Academic Press.

Friedman, H. S. (2000a). Long-term relations of personality and health: Dynamisms, mechanisms, tropisms. *Journal of Personality. 68,* 1089–1108.

Friedman, H. S. (2000b). *Self-healing personality: Why some people achieve health and others succumb to illness*. New York: Republished by: Universe (www.iuniverse.com). (Original work published 1991)

Friedman, H. S. (2007). Personality, disease, and self-healing. In H. S. Friedman & R. C. Silver (Eds.), *Foundations of health psychology*. New York: Oxford University Press.

Friedman, H. S., & Booth-Kewley, S. (1987). The "disease-prone personality": A meta-analytic view of the construct. *American Psychologist, 42,* 539–555.

Friedman, H. S., Tucker, J. S., & Reise, S. (1995). Personality dimensions and measures potentially relevant to health: A focus on hostility. *Annals of Behavioral Medicine, 17,* 245–253.

Friedman, H. S., Tucker, J., Schwartz, J. E., Martin, L. R., Tomlinson-Keasey, C., Wingard, D., et al. (1995). Childhood conscientiousness and longevity: Health behaviors and cause of death. *Journal of Personality and Social Psychology, 68,* 696–703.

Friedman, H. S., Tucker, J. S., Schwartz, J. E., Tomlinson-Keasey, C., Martin, L. R., Wingard, D. L., et al. (1995). Psychosocial and behavioral predictors of longevity: The aging and death of the "Termites." *American Psychologist, 50,* 69–78.

Friedman, H. S., Tucker, J., Tomlinson-Keasey, C., Schwartz, J., Wingard, D., & Criqui, M. H. (1993). Does childhood personality predict longevity? *Journal of Personality and Social Psychology, 65,* 176–185.

Friedman, H. S., & VandenBos, G. (1992). Disease-prone and self-healing personalities. *Hospital and Community Psychiatry, 43,* 1177–1179.

Goodwin, R. G., & Friedman, H. S. (2006). Health status and the five factor personality traits in a nationally representative sample. *Journal of Health Psychology, 11,* 643–654.

Gough, H. G. (1994). Theory, development, and interpretation of the CPI Socialization Scale. *Psychological Reports, 75*(1, Pt. 2), 651–700.

Graziano, W. G., & Ward, D. (1992). Probing the Big Five in adolescence: Personality and adjustment during a developmental transition. *Journal of Personality, 60,* 426–439.

Hogan, J., & Ones, D. S. (1997). Conscientiousness and integrity at work. In R. Hogan, J. A. Johnson, & S. R. Briggs (Eds.), *Handbook of personality psychology* (pp. 849–870). San Diego: Academic Press.

House, J. S., Landis, K. R., & Umberson, D. (1988). Social relationships and health. *Science, 241,* 540–545.

Jessor, R., Turbin, M. S., & Costa, F. M. (1998). Protective factors in adolescent health behavior. *Journal of Personality and Social Psychology, 75,* 788–800.

Johnson, W., McGue, M., Krueger, R. J., & Bouchard, T. J., Jr. (2004). Marriage and personality: A genetic analysis. *Journal of Personality and Social Psychology, 86,* 285–294.

Judge, T. A., & Ilies, R. (2002). Relationship of personality to performance motivation: A meta-analytic review. *Journal of Applied Psychology, 87*(4), 797–807.

Kiecolt-Glaser, J. K., Glaser, R., Cacioppo, J. T., & Malarkey, W. B. (1998). Marital stress: Immunologic, neuroendocrine, and autonomic correlates. *Annals of the New York Academy of Sciences, 840,* 656–663.

Kuh, D., & Ben-Shlomo, Y. (Eds.). (1997). *A life course approach to chronic disease epidemiology.* New York: Oxford University Press.

Larson, J. H., & Holman, T. B. (1994). Premarital predictors of marital quality and stability. *Family Relations, 43,* 228–237.

Ljungquist, B., Berg, S., Lanke, J., McClearn, G. E., & Pedersen N. L. (1998). The effect of genetic factors for longevity: A comparison of identical and fraternal twins in the Swedish Twin Registry. *Journals of Gerontology, Biological Science and Medical Science, Series A, 53*(6), M441–M446.

Maddi, S. R., & Kobasa, S. C. (1984). *The hardy executive: Health under stress.* Homewood, IL: Dow Jones–Irwin.

Magnus, K., Diener, E., Fujita, F., & Payot, W. (1993). Extraversion and neuroticism as predictors of objective life events: A longitudinal analysis. *Journal of Personality and Social Psychology, 65,* 1046–1053.

Manuck, S. B., Flory, J. D., McCaffery, J. M., Matthews, K. A., Mann, J. J., & Muldoon, M. F. (1998). Aggression, impulsivity, and central nervous system serotonergic responsivity in a nonpatient sample. *Neuropsychopharmacology, 19,* 287–299.

Markey, C. N., Markey, P. M., & Tinsley, B. J. (2003). Personality, puberty, and preadolescent girls' risky behaviors: Examining the predictive value of the five-factor model of personality. *Journal of Research in Personality, 37,* 405–419.

Marshall, G. N., Wortman, C. B., Vickers, R. R., Kusulas, J. W., & Hervig, L. K. (1994). The five-factor model of personality as a framework for personality–health research. *Journal of Personality and Social Psychology, 67,* 278–286.

Martin, L. R., & Friedman, H. S. (2000). Comparing personality scales across time: An illustrative study of validity and consistency in life-span archival data. *Journal of Personality, 68,* 85–110.

Martin, L. R., Friedman, H. S., & Schwartz, J. E. (in press). Personality and mortality risk across the lifespan: The importance of conscientiousness as a biopsychosocial attribute. *Health Psychology.*

McCann, S. J. (2005). Longevity, Big Five personality factors, and health behaviors: Presidents from Washington to Nixon. *Journal of Psychology, 139,* 273–286.

McCartney, K., Harris, M. J., & Bernieri, F. (1990). Growing up and growing apart: A developmental meta-analysis of twin studies. *Psychological Bulletin, 107,* 226–237.

McCrae, R. R., & John, O. (1992). An introduction to the five-factor model and its applications. *Journal of Personality, 60,* 175–215.

Miller, T. Q., Smith, T. W., Turner, C. W., Guijarro, M. L., & Hallett, A. J. (1996). A meta-analytic review of research on hostility and physical health. *Psychological Bulletin, 119,* 322–348.

Repetti, R. L., Taylor, S. E., & Seeman, T. E. (2002). Risky families: Family social environments and the mental and physical health of offspring. *Psychological Bulle-tin, 128,* 330–366.

Roberts, B. W., & Bogg, T. (2004). A longitudinal study of the relationships between conscientiousness and the social environmental factors and substance use behaviors that influence health. *Journal of Personality, 72,* 325–353.

Roberts, B. W., Caspi, A., & Moffitt, T. (2003). Work experiences and personality development in young adulthood. *Journal of Personality and Social Psychology, 84,* 582–593.

Scarr, S., & McCartney, K. (1984). How people make their own environments: A theory of genotype–environment effects. *Annual Progress in Child Psychiatry and Child Development,* 98–118.

Sears, P. S. (1979). The Terman studies of genius, 1922–1972. In A. H. Passow (Ed.), *The gifted and talented: Their education and development: The seventy-eighth yearbook of the National Society for the Study of Education* (pp. 75–96) Chicago: University of Chicago Press.

Sears, R. R. (1984). The Terman gifted children study. In S.A. Mednick, M. Harway, & K. M. Finello (Eds.), *Handbook of longitudinal research* (Vol. 1, pp. 398–414). New York: Praeger.

Subotnik, R. F., Karp, D. E., & Morgan, E. R. (1989). High IQ children at midlife: An investigation into the generalizability of Terman's Genetic Studies of Genius. *Roeper Review, 11*(3), 139–145.

Smith, T. W., & Gallo, L. C. (2001). Personality traits as risk factors for physical illness. In A. Baum, T. A. Revenson, & J. E. Singer (Eds.), *Handbook of health psychology* (pp. 139–174). Mahwah, NJ: Erlbaum.

Terman, L. M., & Oden, M. H. (1947). *The gifted child grows up: Twenty-five years' follow-up of a superior group.* Stanford, CA: Stanford University Press.

Tinsley, B. J. (1992). Multiple influences on the acquisition and socialization of children's health attitudes and behavior: An integrative review. *Child Development, 63,* 1043–1069.

Tucker, J. S., Friedman, H. S., Wingard, D. L., & Schwartz, J. E. (1996). Marital history at mid-life as a predictor of longevity: Alternative explanations to the protective effect of marriage. *Health Psychology, 15,* 94–101.

Twenge, J. M. (2000). The age of anxiety? Birth cohort change in anxiety and neuroticism, 1952–1993. *Journal of Personality and Social Psychology, 79*(6), 1007–1021.

Twenge, J. M. (2001). Birth cohort changes in extraversion: A cross-temporal metaanalysis, 1966–1993. *Personality and Individual Differences, 30,* 735–748.

Twenge, J. M. (2002). Birth cohort, social change, and personality: The interplay of dysphoria and individualism in the 20th century. In D. Cervone & W. Mischel (Eds.), *Advances in personality science* (pp. 196–218). New York: Guilford Press.

Van Heck, G. L. (1997). Personality and physical health: Toward an ecological approach to health-related personality research. *European Journal of Personality, 11,* 415–443.

Wakefield, M., Flay, B., Nichter, M., & Giovino, G. (2003). Effects of anti-smoking advertising on youth smoking: A review. *Journal of Health Communication, 8*(3), 229–247.

Wand, G. S., McCaul, M., Yang, X., Reynolds, J., Gotjen, D., Lee, S., et al. (2002). The mu-opioid receptor gene polymorphism (A188G) alters HPA axis activation induced by opioid receptor blockade. *Neuropsychopharmacology, 26,* 106–114.

Weiss, A., & Costa, P. T. Jr., (2005). Domain and facet personality predictors of all-cause mortality among Medicare patients aged 65 to 100. *Psychosomatic Medicine, 6,* 724–733.

Williams, R. B., Kuhn, C. M., Helms, M. J., Siegler, I. C., Barefoot, J. C., Ashley-Kocy, A., et al. (2004, March). *Central nervous system (CNS) serotonin function and NEO-PI personality profiles.* Presented at the 62nd Annual Meeting of the American Psychosomatic Society, Orlando, FL.

Wills, T. A., Resko, J. A., Ainette, M. G., & Mendoza, D. (2004). Role of parent support and peer support in adolescent substance use: A test of mediated effects. *Psychology of Addictive Behaviors, 18*(2), 122–134.

Wilson, R. S., Mendes de Leon, C. F., Bienias, J. L., Evans, D. A., & Bennett, D. A. (2004). Personality and mortality in old age. *Journal of Gerontology: Psychological Sciences and Social Science, Series B, 59,* 110–116.

Witzig, M. E., Kamarck, T. W., Muldoon, M. F., & Sutton-Tyrrell, K. (2003). *Examining the relationship between conscientiousness and atherosclerosis: The Pittsburgh Healthy Heart Project.* Presented at the 61st Annual Meeting of the American Psychosomatic Society, Phoenix, AZ.

# CHAPTER 10

# Sense of Control and Health

## A Dynamic Duo in the Aging Process

MARILYN McKEAN SKAFF

There is a pervasive assumption that aging has a detrimental effect on an individual's sense of control over her or his life. After all, aging brings irreversible losses and uncontrollable changes that should challenge the belief that one has control. However, this perspective ignores two important factors: that one does not suddenly become old, and that the aging individual is hardly a helpless bystander in the process. As Fred Astaire said, "Old age is like everything else. To make a success of it, you have to start young."

There is no question that aging brings increasing challenges to a person's health, particularly in the prevalence of chronic disease, as well as in the general decline of body systems. In this chapter, I work from the assumption that both health and sense of control change over a lifespan. This perspective suggests that individuals can adapt to the changes that accompany aging in ways that allow them to maintain a sense of control. Furthermore, I take the perspective that sense of control is not only affected by health challenges in later life but it also serves as a resource that affects health; thus, my position is that the relationship between sense of control and health is a reciprocal one and remains dynamic in late life. A lifespan perspective suggests a multidisciplinary, multidimensional, multidirectional, contextual view of control and health (see Baltes, 1987).

A considerable amount of evidence has linked control beliefs to health (e.g., Caplan & Schooler, 2003; Kempen, van Sonderen, & Ormel, 1999; Krause & Shaw, 2000; Marmot, 1999; Mendes de Leon, Seeman, Baker, Richardson, & Tinetti, 1996; Pearlin, Lieberman, Menaghan, & Mullan, 1981; Pill & Stott, 1987). The literature, however, varies in the presumed relationship between control and health. For some (e.g., Pearlin et al., 1981), control has been viewed as a resource that affects the ways individuals react to stressors, including health problems, with control beliefs acting as both mediator and moderator in the relationship between stressors and health outcomes. For others (see DeVellis & DeVellis, 2001), control beliefs are viewed as motivational forces that affect health behaviors and are expected to promote health. Finally, sense of control has been seen as an outcome in its own right (e.g., McAvay, Seeman, & Rodin, 1996; Skaff, Pearlin, & Mullan, 1996). In the context of aging, we might ask how a strong sense of control will interact with health across late life. If control is a resource that people bring with them as they age, we might expect those with a stronger sense of control to enter late life healthier, take better care of themselves, and perhaps face the challenges of aging proactively. However, because health problems and physical decline can occur with aging, we must also ask how health can affect sense of control in late life.

This chapter reviews what we know about control and health in aging in three sections. First, I define control, and discuss models and theories that inform the relationships among control, health, and aging. Next, I discuss some of the influences, including age, on sense of control. Finally, I examine the empirical evidence on the relationship between control and health in late life. In the concluding section, I propose a model for a life-span perspective on control and health.

## DEFINING CONTROL

Definitions of control come from a number of varying disciplinary and conceptual backgrounds, often resulting in very different views of this elephant. Baltes and Baltes (1986) stated that "psychological control refers to a field of study rather than to a singular construct" (p. xviii). Although control is sometimes included under the umbrella of "personality," it is less a trait than a part of the self-concept or a set of beliefs about the self in relation to the environment (Abeles, 1991; Skinner, 1996).

Control beliefs are viewed here as a part of the self-concept, having a basis in childhood experiences, but malleable and responsive to experiences across the lifespan. Influences in early life include socialization, traumatic events, and education (Avison & Cairney, 2003). Throughout life, however, control is susceptible to change due to both positive and negative experiences in major life domains (Pearlin et al., 1981). Social–structural influences operate across the lifespan, both molding the quality of social roles and to some extent influencing the stressors to which individuals are exposed (Avison & Cairney, 2003). In late life, the number of roles one occupies may decrease and, whereas some sources of stress depart, other stressors may arise, challenging one's sense of control.

## DIMENSIONS OF CONTROL

A number of dimensions of control help to characterize the various constructs used in the name of control. These include whether we view control as real or perceived; whether the focus is on a global sense of control or on specific domains of control; whether the beliefs focus on ability to exercise control and/or on environmental contingencies; and whether the emphasis is on the agents, means, or ends of control (Skinner, 1996).

"Control," as used here, refers to perceptions of control, as opposed to "real" control. There is clearly a relationship between the amount of control individuals are able to exercise and their control beliefs. Furthermore, both real and perceived control can affect health. However, the focus in this chapter is on beliefs or "sense" of control. Throughout this chapter, the terms "sense of control," "control," and "control beliefs" are used interchangeably to include the many constructs of control that are used.

Progress has been made in recent years in the study of control, with the recognition that both global and domain-specific control beliefs can be distinguished, and that both can be important in relation to health (Krause & Shaw, 2000; Lachman, 1986a; Skaff, Mullan, Fisher, & Chesla, 2003); that is, individuals may believe they have very different degrees of control over various aspects of their lives. A global sense of control may represent the summing across domains, with some salient domains having more weight in the equation than less important ones. This distinction may become even more important in later life, as individuals exit from social roles and/or lose control in some areas of their lives.

Much of the difference in control constructs across theoretical and disciplinary boundaries arises from different perspectives as to whether the focus should be on individuals' abilities to pursue goals or on their limitations to do so. Skinner (1996) proposed a framework that helps organize and make sense of the myriad constructs that attempt to capture control beliefs. She suggested that concepts of control vary according to how they view the agents, means, and ends of control. The agents involve the individual or group in whose hands the control resides. The agent can be either the individual her- or himself or powerful other(s). The means are the actions or behaviors through which control is exercised, including both cognitive and behavioral actions. The ends include the targets toward which control is exercised, including oneself or the outside world.

## CONTROL CONSTRUCTS

Although there are many control constructs, this chapter focuses on those that have been examined most often in relation to health (see Figure 10.1). In the past, the two most commonly used control constructs, particularly in

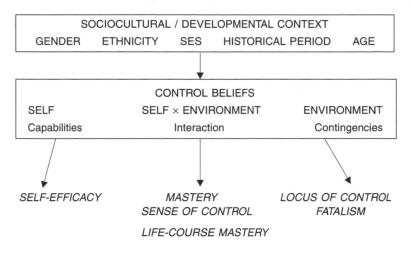

**FIGURE 10.1.** A schematic of control constructs.

relation to health, have been locus of control and self-efficacy. Having its origins in social learning theory, locus of control (LOC) theory focuses on outcome contingencies (Rotter, 1973). LOC reflects beliefs about the way the world works, that is, the degree to which people believe that their outcomes are due to internal or personal influence, or to influences external to the self, such as powerful others, luck, chance, or fate. LOC has been measured both as a general set of beliefs and in relation to specific domains, such as health (Wallston, Wallston, Kaplan, & Maides, 1976). Based on whether individuals believe that control is contingent on their own behavior or on the whim of some outside agent (person, deity, or fate), they are often dichotomized into "internals" and "externals," although the measures used generally reflect a continuum from extreme external to extreme internal. Regarding the relationship of LOC to health, Affleck Tennen, Pfeiffer, and Fifield (1987) offer two perspectives. On the one hand, an external LOC, in the form of surrendering control to a powerful other, might be adaptive where little control is possible, for example, in the case of a terminal illness. On the other hand, believing that control lies in your own hands could result in taking action or at least in looking for aspects of situations that are controllable. Not surprising, the evidence linking health and LOC is mixed, with evidence for both positive and negative effects of internal LOC (Edelstein & Linn, 1987; Peyrot & McMurry, 1985).

Self-efficacy theory also has its roots in social learning theory but focuses more on whether individuals believe they have the capability to produce outcomes (Bandura, 1997; DeVellis & DeVellis, 2001). Bandura (1997) acknowledges the importance of outcome expectancies but believes that the key is whether people believe they are capable of producing the outcomes. He defines *perceived self-efficacy* as "beliefs in one's capabilities to organize and execute the courses of action to produce given attainments" (p. 3). The target may be either internal (self) or external (environment). He also emphasizes that these beliefs are much more potent than objective circumstances, because they provide motivation to act and influence how much effort is put into a behavior.

Self-efficacy is one of the most frequently used measures of control in health-related studies. It is assumed that high self-efficacy should lead individuals to engage in behaviors that positively affect their health. As with LOC, the evidence is mixed, depending upon the measure of self-efficacy used, the target behavior, and the health outcome (e.g., Kempen et al., 1999; Mendes de Leon et al., 1996; Penninx et al., 1998; Schiaffino, Revenson, & Gibofsky, 1991; Schwarzer & Fuchs, 1995; Seeman, Unger, McAvay, & Mendes de Leon, 1999; Skelly, Marshall, Haughey, Davis, & Dunford, 1995), as well as the characteristics of the sample (Skaff et al., 2003).

A group of control constructs that have arisen from both psychology and sociology, including mastery and sense of control, involve both beliefs about the self and about the environment. Sense of control, as Skinner (1996) describes it, "includes a view of the self as competent and efficacious and a view of the world as structured and responsive." (p. 559). Abeles and colleagues (Abeles, 1990; Fung, Abeles, & Carstensen, 1999) describe sense of control as an "umbrella term," involving a schema about the way the world works and the individual's place in it. This model of control incorporates cultural influences on control beliefs, recognizes both global and domain-specific beliefs, and emphasizes the dynamic and dialectical processes at work across contexts and experiences.

Mastery, a global control construct embedded in the stress process model, involves individuals' view of themselves as being able to control the important circumstances of their lives (Pearlin & Schooler, 1978). Mastery is considered an important personal resource related to mental and physical health in many different contexts (Lachman & Prenda-Firth, 2004; Pearlin et al., 1981; Skaff et al., 2003)

Fatalism, another related control construct, has been variously defined as the belief that events in life are beyond one's control (Caplan & Schooler, 2003), as external LOC (Ross, Mirowsky, & Cockerham, 1983), and as a belief in fate governing what happens (Bastida, 1987). In relation to health, it is often assumed that such beliefs lead to lack of action or giving up when faced with health issues. It is frequently measured by the instruments assessing LOC, but scored in the opposite direction.

One new control construct that promises to be useful in a discussion of control and health in late life is life-course mastery, a relatively new construct identified by Pearlin, Nguyen, Schieman, and Milkie (2005). They describe life-course mastery as individuals' views of their control over the exigencies and successes across their lifespan, in essence, the "mediating channel through which the past is connected to the present" (p. 2).

## DEVELOPMENTAL AND SOCIAL INFLUENCES ON CONTROL

To understand how health and sense of control intertwine as people age, we must consider two related questions: First, how is control affected by aging? Second, what other factors influence one's sense of control across the lifespan? Before turning to the empirical literature on changes in control in late life, I examine models and theories of development that might inform expectations.

### Models of Development of Control in Late Life

Although there is currently no lifespan developmental theory of sense of control, several theoretical models might inform us. Much of the literature on control has had a stress and coping focus, so it is not surprising that one of the earliest discussions of changes in control across adulthood and into late life centered around a discussion of the impact of stressors on stability of self-beliefs such as sense of control or mastery. This model suggests that chronic stressors in major life domains have the power, by their very persistence, to wear down people's beliefs about the control they have over their lives. Pearlin and Skaff (1996) described the interactive process linking stress and lifespan development, suggesting that sense of control (mastery) plays a significant role as a personal resource across the lifespan.

Baltes and Baltes (1990) provide a lifespan developmental model for mechanisms that help to explain how people may maintain their sense of control as they age. The three complementary processes of selection, optimization, and compensation (SOC) can be applied to an understanding of means by which people adapt to the challenges to their sense of control. Although this is a lifespan theory, it becomes more relevant as people enter late life. It is based on the concept that, as people age, successful development depends on maximizing gains and minimizing losses. As abilities decline and losses occur, selection involves focusing one's energy on those goals or activities that are most important. This means not only giving up certain goals or valued domains of life but may also involve adding new ones. Optimization involves extra work to perform to potential. Compensation may be necessary to replace old ways of doing things by finding new ways to accomplish a desired goal.

In relation to control beliefs, selection may involve focusing on control in domains that are most important to the individual. Optimization involves the means used to achieve goals, for instance, putting more energy into those domains that are more central. Compensation may involve either cognitive or behavioral adjustments to changes in one's ability to control aspects of life, including shifting focus to domains that are more controllable. The importance of understanding these mechanisms is highlighted in Baltes and Smith's (1999) statement that "work on self and personality in old age has pointed less to age changes and developmental transformations than to understanding the mechanisms that afford the maintenance of personal integrity and well-being in the face of social loss and health constraints" (p. 165). They emphasize that SOC increases in late life, especially compensation.

Building on the Baltes development model, a "lifespan theory of control" has been developed by Schulz and Heckhausen (1999). In this theory, two forms of control are distinguished: Primary control involves the control striving directed toward the environment, with the goal of changing the external environment; secondary control, aimed at internal processes, means changing oneself to adapt to the environment. Primary control, which is seen as having greater adaptive value, increases through young and middle adulthood but declines in late adulthood because of constraints that are encountered. Secondary control, however, increases across the lifespan.

Although this theory takes a lifespan perspective on control, primary and secondary control, as used in this theory, refer not to control beliefs, but rather to control *strategies*, that is, what people *do* to retain or regain control when it is challenged, more closely akin to coping than to control beliefs (Lockenhoff & Carstensen, 2003; Skinner, 1996). For the sake of conceptual clarity, it is crucial to distinguish between people's beliefs about how much they control their world and what they do to exercise control.

In addition, as Baltes and Smith (1999) suggested, internally directed strategies may be more adaptive in late life. A realistic appraisal of one's influence on various domains and an adaptive response to that reality need not be considered an inferior strategy. As Gould (1999) suggests, secondary control may be favored as people age, when they have more time to contemplate their choices. Such a process is consistent with the model of lifespan development of control described by Skinner (1995), in which she suggests that both means and ends of control change across the lifespan; that is, we should expect to see age differences in both the salient domains of control and the strategies that individuals choose to maintain control.

If we view control as a set of malleable beliefs in response to experience rather than as a stable trait, we should expect to see changes in control with aging. Thus, there should be a reciprocal relationship between life experience and control beliefs as people move through the lifespan. In addition, Skinner suggests that, as people age, they may become more philosophical about what they can control. This is a more positive view of the aging process than views that suggest an inevitable decline in control.

# LIFE-STAGE, COHORT, AND SOCIOCULTURAL INFLUENCES ON SENSE OF CONTROL

Taking into account the preceding look at some of the theoretical perspectives that might inform an examination of aging and control, we now consider some empirical evidence on factors that influence variations in sense of control, including age.

## Age, Cohort, and Sense of Control

Does sense of control change with age? There is evidence to suggest that, as people age, their sense of control increases, decreases, and stays the same. There are a number of reasons for this inconsistency, including the confounding of age and cohort, the variety of measures used, the difference between global and domain-specific control, and variability across and within samples studied (Grob, Little, & Wanner, 1999; Lachman & Bertrand, 2001). Much of the evidence comes from cross-sectional studies that compare different age groups, confusing cohort differences with developmental changes. For example, a cross-sequential study by Gatz and Karel (1993) demonstrated that the differences in control observed among three generations of women were more likely due to historical context (the Women's Movement) than to developmental change across the lifespan. Other reasons for equivocal results include the use of different constructs, some of which (e.g., LOC) are not really developmental, whereas others vary in their developmental trajectories (Skinner & Connell, 1986). Indeed, Perlmutter and Eads (1998) and Aldwin (1991) questioned the appropriateness of the measures we use for people in late life. It is also quite likely that global and domain-specific control may vary differently across the lifespan, and that their relationship also varies with age. In addition, the samples used both in cross-sectional and longitudinal research may be nonrepresentative or may ignore sources of variation such as gender, social class, or ethnicity.

Looking at the evidence, both cross-sectional and longitudinal, some of the differences and changes appear as follows: Age is often reported to be negatively related to control, especially when control is measured as a global set of beliefs (Hale & Cochran, 1986; Nurmi, Pullianen, & Salmela-Aro, 1992; Wolinsky, Wyrwich, Babu, Kroenke, & Tierny, 2003; Pearlin et al., 2005). However, a number of studies have shown no age differences in global control (Lachman, 1986a; Lachman & Prenda-Firth, 2004; Reker, Peacock, & Wong, 1987).

Age differences have been found using domain-specific measures. For example, older adults have been found to be lower in intelligence-related control (Lachman, 1986a), as well as control over children and sex lives, but higher in control over work, finances, and marriage (Lachman &

Prenda-Firth, 2004). Lachman and Prenda-Firth also reported an incrcase in constraints on control with age.

Several longitudinal and cross-sequential studies shed some light on the conflicting findings. Lachman (1986b) reported highest efficacy in the oldest (ages 60–67) participants, and stability over 4 years in all age groups. In an 8-year longitudinal study of participants ages 30–59, Brandtstädter and Rothermund (1994) reported that although there were age differences (older adults had a more external LOC), the longitudinal analyses showed no age-related change in externality. They attributed such stability to an accommodative process that involves devaluing specific domains of control.

Gatz and Karel (1993) made a major contribution toward disentangling the effects of aging, cohort, and time of measurement. In a study of three generations, followed over 20 years, they found that the grandparents' control was more external at all times of measurement, but there was also a general increase in internality over time. This latter change they attributed to time of measurement rather than to aging. Specifically, they felt that the self-improvement and autonomy movements of the 1970s and 1980s had an impact on control beliefs in these cohorts. Another important finding of this study was that the cross-sectional difference between middle-aged and older generations was attributable not to aging but due to a cohort effect, especially for female participants. They support this with evidence that the 55- to 70-year-old women in 1971 were more external than both women of the same age in 1991 and men in either time point. They suggested that whereas the Women's Movement gave women more choice, it also made them more aware of disparities in power. Relevant to our focus here, they also found that health is a significant predictor of control beliefs, except in the oldest generation. One of the lessons to be taken from this study involves the importance of attending to factors such as gender, time of measurement, and cohort.

In conclusion, the evidence for developmental changes in sense of control is mixed, depending upon factors such as the measure used, the time frame, and the characteristics of the samples studied. Age differences may be more prevalent than actual age change, although there is little longitudinal evidence to document stability over time. What arises from this evidence is the question of the mechanisms at work, either contributing to stability or explaining change. According to Brandtstädter and Rothermund (1994), as people age, the process of minimizing losses and maximizing gains may be at work in an accommodative process that allows individuals to shift salience from some domains of control that become more challenging to others that are more manageable (consistent with the SOC model). As they put it, "Even when particular goals become unattainable, a sense of control and self-esteem can be maintained by shifting preferences in ways that keep goals commensurate with resources and situational constraints" (p. 271). This might also suggest that individuals who have more domains in which to stake their sense of control might better adapt to threats presented in aging.

Likewise, Fung et al. (1999) suggested that maintaining a strong sense of control means focusing control in a few valued domains. They also stated that "older people may maintain their sense of control by keeping their control beliefs congruent with their environment" (p. 363). They also point out that not only goals and context change with aging, but so may the meaning of control. This would suggest that we need to consider carefully the way we conceptualize and measure control (Perlmutter & Eads, 1998).

## Sociocultural Influences on Sense of Control

As with many of our favorite constructs, much of what we know about control beliefs comes from studies of middle-class European Americans. As our population has become more diverse and cross-cultural studies have become more common, questions have been raised about whether sense of control has the same meaning and manifestations across culturally and economically diverse groups (Azuma, 1984; Bastida, 1987; Kitayama & Markus, 1995; Sastry & Ross, 1998; Schooler, 1990; Skaff & Gardiner, 2002; Varghese & Medinger, 1979). As Kitayama and Markus (1995) pointed out, although the primary model in psychology has been that of the individual self, culture shapes the way individuals view themselves and their world. They used the broadest sense of "culture" to include gender, ethnicity, social class, country of origin, cohort, and historical period. This is made even more relevant for the topic at hand by the fact that health also varies according to many of these aspects of culture, especially socioeconomic status (SES) and ethnicity. Before I address the relationship to health, however, let us consider how cultural frameworks may influence sense of control.

### SES Effects on Sense of Control

Sense of control has repeatedly been shown to vary by social class, including income, education, and work, reflecting the objective conditions in one's life (Kiecolt, 1994; Lachman & Weaver, 1998a; Pearlin et al., 1981, 2005). Ross and Mirowsky (1992) identified the conditions of life that may provide this link, including lack of autonomy on the job, the inability to achieve goals, restricted opportunities, economic dependency, and role overload. Lack of sufficient income can certainly limit the resources needed to exert control over many aspects of life. Education appears to influence sense of control through improved ability to problem-solve (Mirowsky & Ross, 1998; Ross & Mirowsky, 1989). Pearlin et al. (2005) report that autonomy in one's work life during young and middle adulthood is related to life-course mastery, which in turn is related to mastery in late life.

## Gender and Control

Gender is an important social structural variable that definitely has an impact on factors that affect control beliefs, such as economic dependency, restricted opportunities, and the routine nature of jobs and housework (Ross & Sastry, 1999). In general, women have a lower sense of control than do men (Lachman & Prenda-Firth, 2004; Pearlin et al., 2005). However, in this area, we might also expect to find cohort differences as more women reach late life after being employed outside the home and potentially benefiting from the Women's Movement. Future work on variations in domains of control may also contribute to understanding effects of gender on control.

## Ethnic Variations in Meaning and Manifestations of Control

Understanding differences in sense of control across diverse ethnic groups is complicated by the point raised earlier—that both the constructs and their measures have been developed primarily for European Americans, and may not reflect the cultural values and experience of diverse groups. In addition, because of the structure of our society, there is often a socioeconomic confound in studying diverse groups.

One of the ways of conceptualizing control that was mentioned earlier is the primary–secondary control dichotomy. Although Schulz and Heckhausen (1999, p. 139) argued that control striving is "invariant across historical time and diverse cultural settings" Gould (1999) points out that the assumption that primary control is the most adaptive mode of control may not hold in cultures with a more collective view of the self and that emphasize collaborative ways of solving problems. Azuma (1984) described the primary–secondary dichotomy as "quite American." He reported that, in Japan, giving way to the wishes of others is seen as a sign of maturity, and he suggests a much more elaborate view of secondary control. Diaz-Loving and Draguns (1999) described Mexicans as more likely to try to avoid or endure challenges than to confront them directly.

Another control construct that has been used and misused across diverse groups, according to Bastida (1987), is that of fatalism. Differences in fatalism have been reported across both SES levels and racial/ethnic groups, with individuals with lower SES, African Americans, and Latinos usually showing higher levels of fatalism (Ross et al., 1983; Varghese & Medinger, 1979). Latinos, in particular, are often described as holding "fatalistic" views of the world that many assume to be less adaptive—at least from a Northern European American perspective. In discussing fatalism in relation to aging in Latinos, Bastida (1987) prefers to call it "realism." In a study using both qualitative and quantitative methods, she described older Latinos as being able to distinguish between experiences they can and cannot control—an attitude that she sees as adaptive. Varghese and Medinger (1979) described fatalism as an adaptive response to stress in situations of low control, for instance, a lifetime exposure to discrimination and unequal opportunities, allowing individuals to shift the blame for failure from self to outside the self. They do point out that when income is controlled, neither African Americans nor Latinos are more fatalistic than European Americans.

In an attempt to understand differences in the meaning of "sense of control" in older persons across three ethnic groups, I undertook a pilot study using qualitative methods (Skaff, 2004). In both focus groups and individual interviews, I asked Latinos, African Americans, and European Americans, ages 63 to 81, questions about both global control and control across specific domains, including health, across their lifespan, as well as currently. Although there were differences across the groups in some of the barriers to control they described, such as discrimination among African Americans and language difficulties for Latinos, there were far more similarities. In general, all three groups described an increase across their lifespan in sense of control. Some increases in control were attributed to life transitions such as exiting family roles that limited their control over their lives. They also described a growing ability to distinguish between what they could and could not control and a reluctance to waste time and energy on those things they could not control. This does not mean they felt that control was not important or that there were not domains in which they felt they had less control; rather, they were able to maintain a strong sense of control by focusing their energy on those domains in which they did have control (see also Aldwin, 1992).

Understanding variations in control across racial/ethnic groups may help explain disparities in health across diverse groups that have been repeatedly documented (Williams, 1999). Although some of the disparities may be accounted for by differences in SES, others are likely due to persistent experience across the lifespan with racism, discrimination, poor neighborhood environment, poor medical care, and internalization of social stigma (Williams, 1999), which in turn could be expected to have an impact on feelings of control.

## BRINGING TOGETHER CONTROL, HEALTH, AND AGING

This brings us back to our main focus: How are control and health related in aging? The empirical evidence on control and health presented here is limited to studies involving older participants and is organized by the role that sense of control was given in the relationship: (1) control related to health, either directly or as a moderator in the stress process; (2) control related to health through coping or health behaviors; (3) the role of control in adjustment to chronic illness or change in health (as a mediator); and (4) the effects of health on control. The evidence also varies by the operational definition of "health," including general physical and mental health, specific diseases, functional health, and mortality.

## The Effects of Control on Health

Caplan and Schooler (2003) examined two constructs of control in a 20-year longitudinal study. The two measures of control, fatalism (the belief that events in life are beyond one's control) and self-confidence (the belief that one can handle whatever life brings), measured in 1974, were used to predict illness, cognitive difficulty, and functional impairment in 1994. Fatalism and self-confidence predicted cognitive difficulties and disability in ADLs (activities of daily living), and fatalism alone predicted illness. They found that fatalism was positively related to age, and that both fatalism and self-confidence were more predictive of health outcomes for older (65–88 years) than younger (41–64 years) participants. Most striking in this study is that high fatalism and low self-confidence in 1974 predicted functional disability 20 years later.

Additional longitudinal evidence for effects of control beliefs on physical health and functioning comes from a study by Kempen et al. (1999), who examined the effect of four psychological attributes (neuroticism, extraversion, mastery, and general self-efficacy) on functional health 2 years later. Only mastery was predictive of no increase in disability. Mendes de Leon et al. (1996) also reported that low self-efficacy predicts a decline in functioning but, again, the relationship was conditional on whether participants experienced decline in physical performance. In somewhat contradictory findings, Seeman et al. (1999) found that self-efficacy predicted self-reported physical limitations but not physical functioning, 2½ years later.

Menec and Chipperfield (1997) examined perceived control as a moderator of the effects of functional impairment on health and mortality. Their participants were divided into two age groups, young-old (ages 65–79) and old-old (age 80+), and differences were found by age group. Functional impairment appeared to serve as a moderator in the relationship between control and health. In the old-old, control was protective against hospitalization and mortality, but this was true only for those with little functional impairment. For the young-old, there was no interaction between impairment and control. Menec and Chipperfield suggested that for the old-old with less impairment, control beliefs may lead to better health behaviors. They also questioned whether the health-specific measure of control they used was as relevant for the young-old as for the old-old, which might explain why they found no relationship between control and health for the young-old age group.

Although most of the research on control and health in older samples involves global measures of control, Krause and Shaw (2000) used measures of both domain-specific and global control to predict mortality in a sample of participants age 65 and older, followed for 6 years. They further refined domain-specific control by asking participants to indicate their three most important roles. A strong sense of control in the most important domain negatively predicted mortality 6 years later, controlling for smoking, functional disability, and self-related health, but there was no such effect for control in less important domains.

Even in very late life, there is evidence that a strong sense of mastery is related to better physical and mental health. Using longitudinal data from a Swedish sample of oldest-old, Zarit (1996) found that mastery at baseline predicted better functional outcomes 2 years later. He suggests that mastery may reflect an adaptation process that reduces the likelihood of decline in the very old.

## The Effect of Control on Health Behaviors

Much of the health and control literature focuses on a model that suggests sense of control (usually self-efficacy) should activate individuals to engage in health-promoting behaviors (DeVellis & DeVellis, 2001). Schwarzer and Fuchs (1995) found that self-efficacy was related to exercise, but perceived control was not. For older patients with arthritis, Chipperfield and Grenslade (1999) found that low control was related to more physician visits, but only under conditions of higher restrictions due to the disease.

## The Role of Control in Adjustment to Chronic Illness or to Changes in Health

If we view control beliefs as a potential resource with which to face challenges, then sense of control should predict adjustment to both the diagnosis of and living with a chronic illness. Indeed, Felton and Revenson (1984) found that greater health LOC predicted better adjustment to four chronic illnesses: cancer, diabetes, hypertension, and rheumatoid arthritis.

Thompson, Sobolew-Shubin, Galbraith, Schwankovsky, and Cruzen (1993) examined both global and domain-specific control beliefs in relation to recovery from cancer. They found that those with a higher sense of control reported less physical impairment from the disease, more satisfaction with their marriage, and less financial impact from the disease.

## The Effects of Health on Sense of Control

From the evidence presented, it is clear that the relationship between health and control is far from simple, unidirectional, or universal. Penninx et al.

(1996, 1998) found that the relationship between mastery and adjustment to disease varied by chronic disease, and the relationship appeared to be reciprocal in 3,000 individuals ages 55–85. They conclude that more uncontrollable diseases and those resulting in greater functional disability have the greatest impact on both mastery and depression, suggesting that some of the decrease in control and the increase in depression observed in late life may be due to the presence of uncontrollable chronic diseases. In a longitudinal study of changes in domain-specific self-efficacy in a sample age 62 years and older, McAvay, Seeman, and Rodin (1996) reported declines in self-efficacy predicted by baseline health. Also, visits to a physician predicted lower self-efficacy over time. However, the most consistent predictor of decline in self-efficacy across domains was prior depression.

## SUMMARY: WHAT CAN WE SAY ABOUT CONTROL, HEALTH, AND AGING?

Probably the most accurate comment would be "It depends." Cross-sectional studies have been useful in identifying age differences, particularly given the limited longitudinal evidence; however, both are valuable. On the one hand, sense of control is often found to be lower in old age, although cohort differences cannot be overlooked. On the other hand, entering late life with a strong sense of life-course mastery appears to be adaptive (Pearlin et al., 2005).

However, I would like to suggest a pinch of skepticism (or optimism), about decline in control in late life. It is possible, as Perlmutter and Eads (1998) and Aldwin (1991) have suggested, that measures developed generally for younger people are simply not appropriate for those in the later decades of life. We know very little at this point about how domain-specific control beliefs are related to global control, or how their relationship may change with aging. Likewise we have some hypotheses about the process of adaptation in late life, but little empirical evidence of those processes.

One perspective that seems essential to understanding the relationship between control, health, and aging is a lifespan perspective. More knowledge about the trajectory of sense of control across the lifespan, and the factors influencing both lifespan and current control in late life, is essential. Similarly, there is much to be learned about both the antecedents of control and the consequences of control in later life and across diverse groups.

## A MODEL OF A LIFESPAN PERSPECTIVE ON CONTROL AND HEALTH

Figure 10.2 presents a model of the relationship among stress, control beliefs, and health across the lifespan. Modifying and influencing this relationship are the two overriding sets of sociocultural and lifespan influences. Sociocultural influences include income, education, social class, gender, race/ethnicity, and geographical location. These provide the context for the rest of the model and influence the very beliefs that individuals hold regarding the self, the environment, and the relationship between the two. In addition, there is ample evidence that one's location in the social structure has a powerful impact on the stressors to which one is exposed and, in turn, on health status (Adler et al., 1994; Lachman & Weaver, 1998b; Marmot, 1999; Pearlin et al., 2005).

Lifespan influences on the model include both age-related influences, such as normative transitions and changes, and the historical context in which we live our lives. Certainly, the cohort influences on health and control are far from inconsequential (Gatz & Karel, 1993; Skaff, 2006). Evidence for the long-term effects of early childhood experiences suggests that this is an important component of the model (Wheaton, 1983). Furthermore, the trajectories of advantage and/or disadvantage that impact control beliefs and health across the lifespan cannot be overlooked (Pearlin et al., 2005; Ryff, Singer, Love, & Essex, 1998).

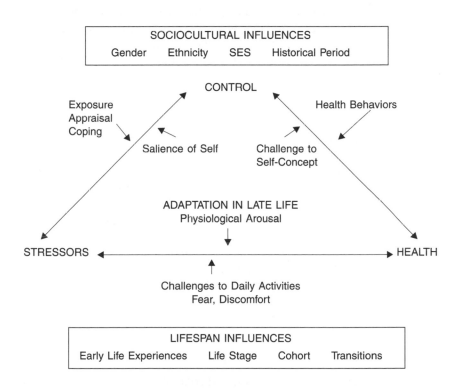

**FIGURE 10.2.** Lifespan model of control and health.

Lying between the sociocultural influences and lifespan factors are the three interactive components of the model: stressors, control, and health. We observe in Figure 10.2 that between each two of these components are double-pointed arrows indicating the reciprocal relationships. Each of the links is labeled with some of the mechanisms that may be at work. In the midst of these relationships is the potential for adaptation.

## Stressors and Control

First, I presented evidence suggesting that control can affect perceived stress, and that stressors can affect sense of control. Among the ways that control affects stress is through its effect on appraisal of stressors and on coping with stressors (Folkman, 1984; Pearlin & Schooler, 1978). Those with greater control are likely to appraise situations as less threatening and their selves as more capable of coping with the stressors. Likewise, greater sense of control has been shown to lead to more effective coping. In addition, it is possible that those higher in control engage in behaviors that allow them to avoid stressful situations or place them in contexts in which stress is less likely.

Stress, in turn, can affect individuals' sense of control. A stressful situation may make the self more salient, raising questions about one's control over important domains in life; that is, conditions of chronic stress, by their very persistence can, over time, wear down individuals' beliefs about control over a specific situation and over their lives in general (Pearlin et al., 1981; Skaff et al., 1996).

## Stressors and Health

The arrow leading from health to stressors in Figure 10.2 represents the impact that health problems can have as a source of stress. By challenging daily activities, increasing discomfort, and raising fear about the future, health problems can become a major stressor in people's lives. Although this is true at any time in the lifespan, it may be particularly poignant in late life, when the problems tend to be more intractable and may be more life threatening.

In the other direction, there is ample evidence that stress does have an impact on health. Although the physiological mechanisms are far from specific, there is an increasing body of knowledge tracking these biological pathways. Evidence on allostatic load has added a lifespan perspective on these links (Ryff et al., 1998).

## Health and Control

The reciprocal effects between health and control operate both directly and indirectly through the stress process. Health problems affect control by challenging self-views. Incorporating chronic illness into the self-concept has been identified as one of the major challenges of coping with the diagnosis of a chronic disease and of late life in general. Especially powerful are those health problems that are not amenable to control and that may also challenge beliefs about the world and its predictability/controllability (Affleck et al., 1987; Caplan & Schooler, 2003; Helgeson, 1992; Penninx et al., 1996; Pitcher & Hong, 1986; Wolinsky & Stump, 1996). Yet even in late life, and in the context of chronic disease, control beliefs can lead to better health behaviors and to more effective coping with illness.

## IMPLICATIONS

Where do we go from here? I would like to suggest four areas where we can focus future investigation, based on the model presented here. First, we need to take a careful look at the constructs and measures of control, matching them to the questions we ask and questioning their appropriateness across diverse groups, including older persons. It seems unwise to ignore the social and cultural context in which people live when we ask them about control over their lives. In response to this gap, Lachman and Prenda-Firth (2004) have added "constraints" to measurement of control.

Second, we know very little about the antecedents of control beliefs. Pearlin's (Pearlin et al., 2005) work on life-course mastery is a step in the right direction in terms of looking at influences across the lifespan. Ideally, both cross-sectional comparisons of influences on sense of control and longitudinal examination of early- and midlife influences on control in late life would help us to understand better people's sense of control as they enter late life.

We know very little about mechanisms of control. By this, I mean both how control affects our well-being, and how people adapt to challenges to their sense of control. How is it that a strong sense of control affects both cognitive and behavioral components of response to stress and avoidance of stressors? Still unexplored are many of the potential social, psychological, and biological pathways through which this component of the self-concept can affect health and well-being. Of particular importance in late life is the question of how individuals go about adapting to the challenges to actual and perceived control that aging brings. I believe SOC theory (Baltes & Baltes, 1990) is promising in this respect. If we can understand how individuals are able to maintain or regain sense of control in situations of low control, then this should also aid us in understanding control in late life.

Finally, only by viewing sense of control from a dynamic, lifespan perspective can we understand current control beliefs and how they operate in individuals' lives. Such a perspective ties together all of the sociocultural influences and individual experiences across the lifespan to explicate the package of beliefs with which individuals traverse late life.

## CONCLUSIONS

Health and sense of control are interactive partners in the aging process. Health problems are a challenge for most aging individuals, but there is evidence that adaptation is quite possible even in very late life (Ryff et al., 1998). Entering later life with a strong sense of control over one's life should prepare the individual to meet the challenges, health and otherwise, that are likely to arise. However, that sense of control has roots in the advantages and disadvantages across an individual's lifespan; thus, we might expect that those who have been more advantaged throughout life would also enter late life at an advantage. This is not to say that individuals cannot and do not adapt to challenges in late life, no matter what earlier life experiences they have faced. In fact, one of the lessons of aging may be what can and cannot be controlled. As one traverses late life, the challenges that arise are increasingly resistant to solution, such as chronic illnesses and, inevitably, death. However, we still know very little about how the process of adapting self-beliefs to current challenges takes place.

Perhaps sense of control does decline in late life. However, before we search for simple interventions, such as increasing scores on a self-efficacy scale, we need to consider whether older persons are simply more realistic about how much they can control. At best, we can help them to gain control over those things that are controllable in their lives. And, we need to take seriously those conditions in our society that contribute to or diminish control across the lifespan. In doing so, we may better understand an important contributor to health and well-being in late life.

## REFERENCES

Abeles, R. P. (1990). Schemas, sense of control, and aging. In J. Rodin, C. Schooler, & K. W. Schaie (Eds.), *Self-directedness: Cause and effects throughout the life course* (pp. 85–94). Hillsdale, NJ: Erlbaum.

Abeles, R. P. (1991). Sense of control, quality of life, and frail older people. In J. E. Birren & J. E. Lubbin (Eds.), *The concept and measurement of quality of life in the frail elderly* (pp. 297–314). San Diego: Academic Press.

Adler, N. E., Boyce, M. A., Cohen, S., Folkman, S., Kahn, R. L., & Syme, S. L. (1994). Socioeconomic status and health: The challenge of the gradient. *American Psychologist, 49*(1), 15–24.

Affleck, G., Tennen, H., Pfeiffer, C., & Fifield, J. (1987). Appraisals of control and predictability in adapting to a chronic disease. *Journal of Personality and Social Psychology, 53*, 273–279.

Aldwin, C. M. (1991). Does age affect the stress and coping process?: The implications of age differences in perceived locus of control. *Journals of Gerontology: Psychological Sciences and Social Sciences, Series B, 46*, P174–P180.

Aldwin, C. M. (1992). Aging, coping, and efficacy: Theoretical framework for examining coping in life-span developmental context. In M. L. Wykle, E. Kahana, & J. Kowal (Eds.), *Stress and health among the elderly* (pp. 96–113). New York: Springer.

Avison, W. R., & Cairney, J. (2003). Social structure, stress, and personal control. In S. H. Zarit, L. I. Pearlin, & K. W. Schaie (Eds.), *Personal control in social and life course contexts* (pp. 127–164). New York: Springer.

Azuma, H. (1984). Secondary control as a heterogeneous category. *American Psychologist, 39*(9), 97–975.

Baltes, M. M., & Baltes, P. B. (Eds.). (1986). *The psychology of control and aging.* Hillsdale, NJ: Erlbaum.

Baltes, P. B. (1987). Theoretical propositions of life-span developmental psychology: On the dynamics between growth and decline. *Developmental Psychology, 23,* 611–626.

Baltes, P. B., & Baltes, M. M. (1990). Psychological perspectives on successful aging: The model of selective optimization with compensation. In *Successful aging: Perspectives from the behavioral sciences* (pp. 1–27). New York: Cambridge University Press.

Baltes, P. B., & Smith, J. (1999). Multilevel and systemic analyses of old age: Theoretical and empirical evidence for a fourth age. In V. L. Bengtson & K. W. Schaie (Eds.), *Handbook of theories of aging* (pp. 153–173). New York: Springer.

Bandura, A. (1997). *Self-efficacy: The exercise of control.* New York: Freeman.

Bastida, E. (1987). Issues of conceptual discourse in ethnic research and practice. In D. E. Gelfand & C. M. Barresi (Eds.), *Ethnic dimensions of aging* (pp. 51–63). New York: Springer.

Brandtstädter, J., & Rothermund, K. (1994). Self-perception of control in middle and later adulthood: Buffering losses by rescaling goals. *Psychology and Aging, 9*(2), 265–273.

Caplan, L. J., & Schooler, C. (2003). The roles of fatalism, self-confidence, and intellectual resources in the disablement process in older adults. *Psychology and Aging, 18*(3), 551–561.

Chipperfield, J. G., & Greenslade, L. (1999). Perceived control as a buffer in the use of health care services. *Journals of Gerontology: Psychological Sciences and Social Sciences, Series B, 54*(3), P146–P154.

DeVellis, B. M., & DeVellis, R. F. (2001). Self-efficacy and health. In A. Baum, T. A. Revenson & J. E. Singer (Eds.), *Handbook of health psychology* (pp. 235–247). Mahwah, NJ: Erlbaum.

Diaz-Loving, R., & Draguns, J. G. (1999). Culture, meaning, and personality in Mexico and in the United States. In Y. T. Lee, C. R. McCauley, & J. G. Draguns (Eds.), *Personality and person perception across cultures* (pp. 103–126). Mahwah, NJ: Erlbaum.

Edelstein, J., & Linn, M. W. (1987). Locus of control and the control of diabetes. *Diabetes Educator, 13,* 51–54.

Felton, B. J., & Revenson, T. A. (1984). Coping with chronic illness: A study of illness controllability and the influence of coping strategies on psychological adjustment. *Journal of Consulting and Clinical Psychology, 52*(3), 343–353.

Folkman, S. (1984). Personal control and stress and coping processes: A theoretical analysis. *Journal of Personality and Social Psychology, 46*(4), 839–852.

Fung, H. H., Abeles, R. P., & Carstensen, L. L. (1999). Psychological control in later life: Implications for life-span development. In J. Brandtstädter & R. M. Lerner (Eds.), *Action and self-development: Theory and research through the life-span* (pp. 345–372). Thousand Oaks, CA: Sage.

Gatz, M., & Karel, M. J. (1993). Individual change in perceived control over 20 years. *International Journal of Behavioral Development, 16*(2), 305–322.

Gould, S. J. (1999). A critique of Heckhausen and Schulz's (1995) life span theory of control from a cross-cultural perspective. *Psychological Review, 106*(3), 597–604.

Grob, A., Little, T. D., & Wanner, B. (1999). Control judgements across the life span. *International Journal of Behavioral Development, 23*(4), 833–854.

Hale, W. D., & Cochran, C. D. (1986). Locus of control across the adult lifespan. *Psychological Reports, 59*, 311–313.

Helgeson, V. S. (1992). Moderators of the relation between perceived control and adjustment to chronic illness. *Journal of Personality and Social Psychology, 63*(4), 656–666.

Kempen, G. I. J. M., van Sonderen, E., & Ormel, J. (1999). The impact of psychological attributes on changes in disability among low-functioning older persons. *Journals of Gerontology: Psychological Sciences and Social Sciences, Series B, 54*(1), P23–P29.

Kiecolt, K. G. (1994). Stress and the decision to change oneself. *Social Psychology Quarterly, 57*(1), 49–63.

Kitayama, S., & Markus, H. R. (1995). Culture and self: Implications for internationalizing psychology. In N. R. Goldberger & J. B. Veroff (Eds.), *The culture and psychology reader* (pp. 366–383). New York: New York University Press.

Krause, N., & Shaw, B. A. (2000). Role-specific feelings of control and mortality. *Psychology and Aging, 15*(4), 617–626.

Lachman, M. E. (1986a). Locus of control in aging research: A case for multidimensional and domain-specific assessment. *Journal of Psychology and Aging, 1*(1), 34–40.

Lachman, M. E. (1986b). Personal control in later life: Stability, change, and cognitive correlates. In M. M. Baltes & P. B. Baltes (Eds.), *The psychology of control and aging* (pp. 207–236). Hillsdale, NJ: Erlbaum.

Lachman, M. E., & Bertrand, R. M. (2001). Personality and the self in midlife. In M. E. Lachman (Ed.), *Handbook of midlife development* (pp. 279–309). New York: Wiley.

Lachman, M. E., & Prenda-Firth, K. M. (2004). The adaptive value of feeling in control during midlife. In O. G. Brim, Jr., C. D. Ryff, & R. C. Kessler (Eds.), *How healthy are we?: A national study of well-being at midlife* (pp. 320–349). Chicago: University of Chicago Press.

Lachman, M. E., & Weaver, S. L. (1998a). The sense of control as a moderator of social class differences in health and well-being. *Journal of Personality and Social Psychology, 74*(3), 763–773.

Lachman, M. E., & Weaver, S. L. (1998b). Sociodemographic variations in the sense of control by domain: Findings from the MacArthur Studies of Midlife. *Psychology and Aging, 13*(4), 553–562.

Lockenhoff, C. E., & Carstensen, L. L. (2003). Is the life span theory of control a theory of development or a theory of coping? In S. H. Zarit, L. I. Pearlin, & K. W.

Schaie (Eds.), *Personal control in social and life course contexts* (pp. 263–280). New York: Springer.

Marmot, M. (1999). Epidemiology of socioeconomic status and health: Are determinants within countries the same as between countries? In N. E. Adler & M. Marmot (Eds.), *Socionomic status and health in industrial nations: Social, psychological and biological pathways* (Vol. 896, pp. 16–29). New York: New York Academy of Sciences.

McAvay, G. J., Seeman, T. E., & Rodin, J. (1996). A longitudinal study of change in domain-specific self-efficacy among older adults. *Journals of Gerontology: Psychological Sciences and Social Sciences, Series B, 51*(5), P243–P253.

Mendes de Leon, C. F., Seeman, T. E., Baker, D. I., Richardson, E. D., & Tinetti, M. E. (1996). Self-efficacy, physical decline, and change in functioning in community-living elders: A prospective study. *Journals of Gerontology: Psychology Sciences and Social Sciences, Series B, 51*(4), S183–S190.

Menec, V. H., & Chipperfield, J. G. (1997). The interactive effect of perceived control and functional status on health and mortality among young-old and old-old. *Journals of Gerontology: Psychological Sciences and Social Sciences, Series B, 52*(3), P118–P126.

Mirowsky, J., & Ross, C. E. (1998). Education, personal control, lifestyle, and health: A human capital hypothesis. *Research on Aging, 20*(4), 415–449.

Nurmi, J., Pulliainen, H., & Salmela-Aro, K. (1992). Age differences in adults' control beliefs related to life goals and concerns. *Psychology and Aging, 7*(2), 194–196.

Pearlin, L. I., Lieberman, M. A., Menaghan, E. G., & Mullan, J. T. (1981). The stress process. *Journal of Health and Social Behavior, 22,* 337–356.

Pearlin, L. I., Nguyen, K. B., Scheiman, S., & Milkie, M. A. (2005). *The life-course origins of mastery.* Unpublished manuscript.

Pearlin, L. I., & Schooler, C. (1978). The structure of coping. *Journal of Health and Social Behavior, 19,* 2–21.

Pearlin, L. I., & Skaff, M. M. (1996). Stress and the life course: A paradigmatic alliance. *Gerontologist, 36*(2), 239–247.

Penninx, B. W., Beekman, J. H., Aartjan, T. F., Ormel, J., Kriegsman, D. M. W., Boeke, A. J. P., et al. (1996). Psychological status among elderly people with chronic diseases: Does type of disease play a part? *Journal of Psychosomatic Research, 40*(5), 521–534.

Penninx, B. W., van Tilbury, T., Boeke, A. J. P., Deeg, D. J. H., Kriegsman, D. M., & van Eijk, J. T. M. (1998). Effects of social support and personal coping resources on depressive symptoms: Different for various chronic diseases? *Health Psychology, 17*(6), 551–558.

Perlmutter, L. C., & Eads, A. S. (1998). Control: Cognitive and motivational implications. In J. Lomeranz (Ed.), *Handbook of aging and mental health: An integrative approach* (pp. 45–67). New York: Plenum.

Peyrot, M., & McMurry, J. F. (1985). Psychosocial factors in diabetes control: Adjustment of insulin-treated adults. *Psychosomatic Medicine, 47,* 542–557.

Pill, R. M., & Stott, N. C. H. (1987). The stereotype of "working-class fatalism" and the challenge for primary care health promotion. *Health Education Research, 2*(2), 105–114.

Pitcher, B. L., & Hong, S. Y. (1986). Older men's perceptions of personal control: The effect of health status. *Sociological Perspectives, 29*(3), 397–419.

Reker, G. T., Peacock, E. J., & Wong, P. T. P. (1987). Meaning and purpose in life and well-being: A life-span perspective. *Journal of Gerontology, 42*(1), 44–49.

Ross, C. E., & Mirowsky, J. (1989). Explaining the social patterns of depression: Control and problem solving—or support and talking? *Journal of Health and Social Behavior, 30*, 206–219.

Ross, C. E., & Mirowsky, J. (1992). Households, employment, and the sense of control. *Social Psychology Quarterly, 55*(3), 217–235.

Ross, C. E., Mirowsky, J., & Cockerham, W. C. (1983). Social class, Mexican culture, and fatalism: Their effects on psychological distress. *American Journal of Community Psychology, 11*(4), 383–399.

Ross, C. E., & Sastry, J. (1999). The sense of personal control: Social–structural causes and emotional consequences. In C. S. Aneshensel & J. C. Phelan (Eds.), *Handbook of the sociology of mental health* (pp. 369–394). New York: Kluwer Academic/Plenum.

Rotter, J. B. (1973). *Social learning and clinical psychology.* New York: Johnson Reprint Corp.

Ryff, C. D., Singer, B., Love, G. D., & Essex, M. J. (1998). Resilience in adulthood and later life: Defining features and dynamic processes. In J. Lomeranz (Ed.), *Handbook of aging and mental health: An integrative approach* (pp. 69–96). New York: Plenum.

Sastry, J., & Ross, C. E. (1998). Asian ethnicity and the sense of personal control. *Social Psychology Quarterly, 61*(2), 101–120.

Schiaffino, K. M., Revenson, T. A., & Gibofsky, A. (1991). Assessing the impact of self-efficacy beliefs on adaptation to rheumatoid arthritis. *Arthritis Care and Research, 4*(4), 150–157.

Schooler, C. (1990). Individualism and the historical and social–structural determinants of people's concerns over self-directedness and efficacy. In J. Rodin, C. Schooler, & K. W. Schaie (Eds.), *Self-directedness: Causes and effects throughout the life course* (pp. 19–49). Hillsdale, NJ: Erlbaum.

Schulz, R., & Heckhausen, J. (1999). Aging, culture, and control: Setting a new research agenda. *Journals of Gerontology: Psychological Sciences and Social Sciences, Series B, 54*(3), P139–P145.

Schwarzer, R., & Fuchs, R. (1995). Changing risk behaviors and adopting health behaviors: The role of self-efficacy beliefs. In A. Bandura (Ed.), *Self-efficacy in changing societies* (pp. 259–288). Cambridge, UK: Cambridge University Press.

Seeman, T. E., Unger, J. B., McAvay, G., & Mendes de Leon, C. F. (1999). Self-efficacy beliefs and perceived declines in functional ability: Macarthur Studies of Successful Aging. *Journals of Gerontology: Psychological Sciences and Social Sciences, Series B, 54*(4), P214–P222.

Skaff, M. M. (2004, November). *A life span view of control: Individuals' reflections on agents, means, and targets.* Presented at the annual meeting of the Gerontological Society of America. Washington, DC.

Skaff, M. M. (2006). The view from the driver's seat: Sense of control in the baby boomers at midlife. In S. K. Whitbourne & S. L. Willis (Eds.), *The baby boomers grow up: Contemporary perspectives on middle age.* Mahwah, NJ: Erlbaum.

Skaff, M. M., & Gardiner, P. (2002). Cultural variations in meaning of control. In S. H. Zarit, L. I. Pearlin, & K. W. Schaie (Eds.), *Personal control in social and life course contexts* (pp. 83–103). New York: Springer.

Skaff, M. M., Mullan, J. T., Fisher, L., & Chesla, C. A. (2003). A contextual model of control beliefs, behavior, and health: Latino and European Americans with Type 2 diabetes. *Psychology and Health, 18*(3), 295–312.

Skaff, M. M., Pearlin, L. I., & Mullan, J. T. (1996). Transitions in the caregiving career: Effects on sense of mastery. *Psychology and Aging, 11*(2), 247–257.

Skelly, A. H., Marshall, J. R., Haughey, B. P., Davis, P. J., & Dunford, R. G. (1995). Self-efficacy and confidence in outcomes as determinants of self-care practices in inner city women with non-insulin-dependent diabetes. *Diabetes Educator, 21*(1), 38–46.

Skinner, E. A. (1995). *Perceived control, motivation, and coping.* Thousand Oaks, CA: Sage.

Skinner, E. A. (1996). A guide to constructs of control. *Journal of Personality and Social Psychology, 71*(3), 549–570.

Skinner, E. A., & Connell, J. P. (1986). Control understanding: Suggestions for a developmental framework. In M. M. Baltes & P. B. Baltes (Eds.), *The psychology of control and aging* (pp. 35–69). Hillsdale, NJ: Erlbaum.

Thompson, S. C., Sobolew-Shubin, A., Galbraith, M. E., Schwankovsky, L., & Cruzen, D. (1993). Maintaining perceptions of control: Finding perceived control in low control circumstances. *Journal of Personality and Social Psychology, 64*(2), 293–304.

Varghese, R., & Medinger, F. (1979). Fatalism in response to stress among the minority aged. In D. E. Gelfand & A. J. Kutzik (Eds.), *Ethnicity and aging: Theory, research, and policy* (pp. 96–116). New York: Springer.

Wallston, B. S., Wallston, K. A., Kaplan, G. D., & Maides, S. A. (1976). Development and validation of the health locus of control (HLC) scale. *Journal of Consulting and Clinical Psychology, 44*(4), 580–585.

Wheaton, B. (1983). Stress, personal coping resources, and psychiatric symptoms. *Journal of Health and Social Behavior, 24*, 208–229.

Williams, D. R. (1999). Race, socioeconomic status, and health: The added effects of racism and discrimination. In N. E. Adler & M. Marmot (Eds.), *Socioeconomic status and health in industrial nations: Social, psychological, and biological pathways* (Vol. 896, pp. 173–188). New York: New York Academy of Sciences.

Wolinsky, F. D., & Stump, T. E. (1996). Age and the sense of control among older adults. *Journals of Gerontology: Psychological Sciences and Social Sciences, Series B, 51*(4), S217–S220.

Wolinsky, F. D., Wyrwich, K. W., Babu, A. N., Kroenke, K., & Tierny, W. M. (2003). Age, aging, and the sense of control among older adults: A longitudinal reconsideration. *Journals of Gerontology: Psychological Sciences and Social Sciences, Series B, 58*(4), S212–S220.

Zarit, S. H. (1996). Continuities and discontinuities in very late life. In V. L. Bengtson (Ed.), *Adulthood and aging: Research on continuities and discontinuities* (pp. 46–65). New York: Springer.

# CHAPTER 11

# Coping, Health, and Aging

CAROLYN M. ALDWIN, LORIENA A. YANCURA,
and DARIA K. BOENINGER

As detailed in Chapter 1, this volume, not only the nation but the world in general is facing a demographic transition in which the numbers of older adults will rise dramatically in the next couple of decades. With this transition will come an increase in health problems and many other types of stressors related to aging, such as losses—of friends, loved ones, health, and mobility. Because coping is thought to mitigate the adverse health effects of stress, coping capacity and resources are an important component of optimal aging (Aldwin & Gilmer, 2004). Thus, the focus of this chapter is on whether coping, defined as behavioral and cognitive efforts to regulate both environmental stressors and negative emotional reactions, is more or less efficacious at mitigating the effects of stress in late life.

The question of whether the effects of coping strategies change with age is complex, and breaks down into a number of subquestions that first need to be addressed. The most basic of these appears to be whether coping changes with age. However, closer inspection reveals that the answer to this question depends on a number of things, including what types of coping are assessed—or rather, the underlying assumption system about the nature of coping. Even if coping strategies do change with age, it is possible that this is only because the types of stressors faced by older adults change. Alternatively, changes in coping strategies could reflect changes in the way stress is appraised. All of this is further complicated by the fact that very few purely developmental studies of coping exist: most studies occur within the context of individuals coping with chronic health problems, and developmental issues are not directly addressed but must be teased out, where possible. Thus, this chapter addresses general age-related changes in the stress process, as well as age-related changes in coping and adaptation, before seeking to address the main question: whether the effect of coping changes with age, drawing in part upon the health psychological literature on coping with chronic illness, as well as the caregiving literature.

## CHANGES IN STRESS AND STRESS VULNERABILITY WITH AGE

### Aging and Vulnerability to Stress

Both normal, age-related changes in specific physiological systems and disease-related changes increase older adults' vulnerability to physiological stressors. Although nearly all physiological systems show these changes, our discussion involves only those most directly implicated in the stress response: the nervous system, the endocrine system, and the immune system. Age-related changes in the hypothalamus influence the hypothalamic–pituitary–adrenal (HPA) axis, which is involved in regulation of the stress response. Decreases in the sensitivity of the hypothalamus to glucocorticoids, or stress hormones, may be due to the pathogenic effects of prolonged glucocorticoid exposure (see Epel, Burke, & Wolkowitz, Chapter 7, this volume; Gruenewald & Kemeny, Chapter 6, this volume; Sapolsky, 1992, 1998). These changes in the brain influence many other systems in the body, notably the endocrine system.

Age-related changes in the endocrine system involve changes in levels of circulating glucocorticoids and sex hormones. As mentioned earlier, changes in the hypothalamus may result in increased levels of cortisol in the blood, which may result in the impaired clearance of cortisol, thus prolonging the physiological stress response. Changes in blood levels of sex hormones are related to female menopause and male andropause. Both of these physiological events involve a crossover of hormone concentration curves in which levels of sex hormones (estrogen in females and testosterone in males) decline with age, and follicle-stimulating hormone (FSH) and luteinizing hormone (LH) increase with age. This crossover in the endocrine system in turn influences immune function because sex hormones contribute toward thymic involution (Fabris, Mocchegiani, & Provinciali, 1997), contributing to poorer immune responses.

Aging in the cells of the immune system may be related to an increased rigidity of lymphocyte cell membranes that results in the inability of specific receptors to bind to antigens or hormones (Guidi et al., 1998). There may also be irregularities in the transduction of signals between the nucleus and the cell membrane, which might also interfere with antigen and hormone binding. There are also changes in specific types of immune cells, primarily in T-cells, to a lesser extent in β-cells, and to a minor extent in macrophages and dendritic cells (Alder & Nagel, 1994; Wick, Jansen-Durr, Berger, Blasko, & Grubeck-Loebstein, 2000).

Many of the changes in T-cell function with age are related to involution of the thymus. By the fifth decade of life, most of human thymic tissue is replaced by fat cells (Wick et al., 2000). The thymus serves an extremely important function, because it converts lymphocytes into T-cells, which supply specific responses to antigen invasion (cellular immunity). Thymic involution results in decreased overall numbers of mature T-cells (DiGiovanna, 2000). Changes in the numbers of specific types of T-cells with age are difficult to detect, because the T-cell cascade is a temporally complex process (Antel & Minuck, 1994). However, the asymmetrical nature of thymic involution (Chakravarti & Abraham, 1999) suggests that age-related changes may involve decreased numbers of helper T-cells (CD4+) relative to suppressor T-cells (CD8+). The ratio of CD4+ to CD8+ is a marker of the immune system's ability to maintain homeostasis. A high CD4+:CD8+ ratio indicates an overzealous immune response, which can lead to autoimmune problems.

These changes promote the heightened susceptibility of older adults to physical stressors. They are less able to regulate their body temperature than are younger adults, and are thus more vulnerable to heat waves, as several tragic events in Chicago, Europe, and New Orleans have illustrated so vividly. Age-related changes in responses to epinephrine and norepinephrine may make it more difficult to regulate blood pressure (see Epel et al., Chapter 7, and Cooper, Katzel, & Waldstein, Chapter 8, this volume). Older immune systems are also less able to mount effective challenges to pathogens (see Gruenewald & Kemeny, Chapter 6, this volume), although with age, there is an increase in memory T-cells. In effect, older immune systems have more experience and are thus able to respond more quickly to known pathogens (Miller, 1996). Indeed, biological gerontologists have argued that the decreased ability of cells to regulate their responses to stress is a hallmark of the aging process (for a review, see Aldwin & Gilmer, 2004).

However, it is still an open question whether older adults are more vulnerable to psychosocial stress. Mroczek and Almeida (2004) found that older adults are more vulnerable to psychosocial stress, although Aldwin, Sutton, Chiara, and Spiro (1996) found no differences in psychological symptom responses to psychosocial stressors. Johnson, Backlund, Sorlie, and Loveless (2000) found that the effects of bereavement on mortality were stronger in middle age than in late life, even controlling for concordance in health behavior habits. Several studies have found that stress interferes with cognitive functioning (Neupert, 2003); however, others have found no interactions between stress and age on cognition (Elias, Elias, D'Agostino, & Wolf, 2000; VonDras, Powless, Olson, Wheeler, & Snudden, 2005).

There are some emerging findings with regard to aging and cardiovascular reactivity (CVR; see Cooper et al., Chapter 8, this volume). For example, Uchino, Holt-Lunstad, Bloor, and Campo (2005) reported age differences in CVR to stress, some of which may be due to disease status. Older adults with hypertension have greater CVR in response to stress; however, age still has independent effects on CVR (Jennings et al., 1997). Thus, differential vulnerability to stress may very well depend on both disease status and the particular type of outcome under study. More research is needed to clarify whether there is increased vulnerability to psychosocial stress with age.

## Does Type of Stress Change with Age?

Whether stress changes with age depends, in part, upon how it is conceptualized and measured. There are a number of different ways of assessing stress in every day life, including trauma (extremely serious events involving death or threats to life), life events (e.g., marriage, divorce, widowhood), chronic role strain (e.g., poverty, poor marriages, stressful work conditions), and microstressors (events that are assessed on a daily or even hourly basis).

Age-related patterns of change in stressors depend upon whether one examines lifetime prevalence or what has happened in the recent past. For example, we know that lifetime prevalence of trauma increases with age. Not surprisingly, the longer one lives, the more likely it is that one will be exposed to trauma (Norris, 1992). The assessment of life events in the past year, however, is a different matter. On most inventories, older adults report fewer stressful life events, primarily because most life event inventories consist of items that young adults are more likely to experience, such as births, marriages, graduations, job change, arrests, and so on. However, various instruments have been developed to assess events that are more likely to be experienced by older adults, such as deaths of friends, retirement, widowhood and illness of self or family. On these types of instruments, there is relatively little age-related change (Aldwin, 1990). Thus, many life events tend to be age-graded. Furthermore, it is generally accepted in lifespan developmental psychology that experiencing age-graded events off-time tend to be far more stressful than doing so on-time. Thus, having a child may be much more difficult at 13 or 50 than at 25; retiring at age 30 due to poor health or at the end of an athletic career may be more stressful than retiring at 65, after careful preparation and planning.

As far as we are able to determine, no studies have examined whether there are age-related differences in chronic role strain. Again, we hypothesize that the type of chronic role strain varies by age. Younger adults are more likely than older adults to experience role strain due to poverty, parenting, and poor working conditions, whereas the latter are more likely to be taking care of chronically ill relatives or experiencing chronic illness themselves. However, these types of chronic role strain may be self-limiting in young adulthood. Most (but not all) poor younger people grow out of poverty; troubled marriages end in divorce; and most people who are unhappy with their jobs find alternative employment. However, older adults may experience long-term chronic role strain, such as taking care of a spouse with Alzheimer's disease, which may last for years, if not decades (see Fortinsky, Tennen, Frank, & Affleck, Chapter 12, this volume). Furthermore, poverty-stricken older adults are not likely to get out of poverty (Crown, 2001). Thus, Aldwin et al. (1996) hypothesized that the nature of stressors shifts in later life, from episodic to chronic stressors.

How microstressors change with age is quite surprising. Most studies show that, in general, the number of minor problems or hassles that are reported on a daily or weekly basis decrease with age, with some notable exceptions, such as those due to health (Aldwin et al., 1996; Aldwin & Levenson, 2001; Almeida & Horn, 2004; Chiriboga, 1997). The reason for this is unclear. The most logical answer is that as the number of social roles decrease with age, so do hassles. Thus, by exiting work and parenting roles, one avoids the types of hassles associated with those roles. However, this does not explain why hassles linearly decrease from young adulthood to midlife—a time of greatly increased responsibility. Some of this may be due to cohort effects; more recent cohorts in general report more stressors (Chiriboga, 1997). With notable exceptions, there are very few longitudinal studies of stress with age, and even fewer that try to disentangle the effect of age versus cohort effects.

The problem with retrospective stress measures is that they tend to reflect personal biases. For example, a variety of studies have revealed gender differences in the reporting of stress and coping processes. However, studies that used ecological momentary assessments (EMAs), in which individuals are paged throughout the day and asked to record immediate experiences, often show no differences between the genders in stress reporting or coping (for a review, see Aldwin, in press). It would be extremely interesting to use this methodology to determine whether there are age differences in hassles using EMA procedures, but, to our knowledge, no published studies exist which have done this.

There may be systematic, age-related changes in the manner in which older individuals appraise stress, however. Stress appraisals can take many forms, including assessments of the type of stressor (e.g., harm/loss, threat, or challenge), the degree of controllability or responsibility for the stressor, and its stressfulness. Aldwin et al. (1996) examined age differences in the first type of appraisal, and found that older adults were no more likely than middle-age ones to use harm/loss or threat appraisals, contrary to the view of aging that focuses on the amount of loss older adults face. However, they were also less likely to report challenges, although nearly half of even the oldest group (age 80+) did so. Boeninger, Shiraishi, Aldwin, and Spiro (2003) also found fewer appraisals with age, even controlling for personality, and this appraisal pattern contributed to the lower perceived stress levels.

Controllability of stressors, a more complex issue, was reviewed by Skaff (Chapter 10, this volume) and is not addressed here. However, Aldwin (1991) did find that older adults were less likely to say they were responsible for either the occurrence or the management of their problems, although there were no age differences in the amount of problem-focused coping, suggesting that this denial of responsibility was a way of managing emotional distress and did not constitute frank denial.

There do appear to be age differences in perceived stress, with older adults reporting fewer stressors overall and less subjective stress in response to their everyday problems than younger adults (e.g., Aldwin, 1991; Aldwin et al., 1996; Chang, 2002). As we shall see, this is in line with a conservation model of both aging (Baltes, Staudinger, & Lindenberger, 1999) and coping (Hobfoll, 2002) If older people are more vulnerable to stress, then minimizing the existence of problems could well be adaptive.

## Do Coping Strategies Change with Age?

Not surprisingly, the answer to whether coping strategies change with age also depends upon the conceptualization and measurement of coping strategies. Briefly, the myriad approaches to coping can be condensed into two types: styles versus processes. Coping styles may include defense mechanisms, such as denial or projection, or they may be based on information processing (approach–avoidance) or personality processes, and are assumed to be relatively stable across time and situations. In contrast, process measures focus on strategies that are used in particular situations, and are viewed as responsive to situational demands. Process measures may focus on a recent problem, a problem that occurred during the past day (daily diary studies), or may be assessed using "real time" measures (ecological momentary assessments). Many have argued that there is little empirical evidence for coping styles; studies that have looked for changes in coping across situations have generally found them, although there is a little evidence of consistency in emotion-focused coping across situations (Aldwin, in press; Folkman & Moskowitz, 2004). The lifespan developmental theorists who have started to examine age-related changes in coping and other adaptive processes typically work within a coping styles framework, whereas the health psychologists have typically examined coping processes. Thus, this brief review is divided into these two approaches.

### Changes in Coping Styles

Early studies focused on whether coping ability decreases with age, with some arguing that older copers are more passive (Gutmann, 1974), whereas others argued that older adults become more adept, using fewer "immature" or "neurotic" defense mechanisms (Vaillant, 1977, 2000). In a cross-sectional study, Whitty (2003) confirmed that middle-aged and older adults are more likely to use mature defenses such as suppression and sublimation. There is some longitudinal support for decreases in less-adaptive strategies such as projection with age, coupled with increases in repression/denial (Costa, Zonderman, & McCrae, 1991).

Recent theories in lifespan development have focused on changes in goal structures with age, with attendant changes in coping strategies, most of which are predicated on declines in resources and the need to conserve them. For example, the Freund and Baltes (1998) selection, optimization, and compensation theory is based on the premise that, with age, individuals become increasingly selective in focusing their efforts. Some activities or goals lose salience, either due to their unattainability or lack of sufficient resources to maximize all goals, with individuals refocusing their efforts on fewer goals. For the latter, individuals compensate for any deficits they may have and optimize their remaining capacities. This is similar to Brandtstädter's (1999) hypothesized shift in goal structure with age, which argues that younger individuals engage in more tenacious goal pursuit, whereas older individuals need to be more flexible in their goals. There is a similar shift in coping with age, from assimilative (problem-focused coping) to accommodative (emotion-focused coping). For example, Rothermund and Brandtstädter (2003) found that compensatory actions to cope with physical deficits were common until the age of 70 or so, at which time older individuals switched to a more accommodative mode. Indeed, they argued that failure to shift in terms of goal structure and coping to age-appropriate modes results in poorer well-being in late life.

Carstensen, Mikels, and Mather (2006) also focus on changes in motivation, but in a way that is more similar to Golub and Langer's (Chapter 2, this volume) call for a more positive perspective on goal setting in later life. Carstensen et al. propose that meaning becomes more central with age. Older adults are more selective in their activities with age, but not necessarily due to any sense of deficit; rather, they wish to spend their time in meaningful occupations and with loved ones. They may be also more interested in selecting environments that promote emotion regulation; Carstensen et al. therefore hypothesized that older adults' coping is more focused on the regulation of both emotional and behavioral responses. This suggests that meaning making (see Park & Blumberg, 2002) may become more salient in later life (see Gatz, Harris, & Turk-Charles, 1995).

## Changes in Coping Processes

Some early studies found decreases in problem-focused coping with age (Folkman, Lazarus, Pimley, & Novacek, 1987), whereas others showed that older adults use similar levels of problem-focused coping (Aldwin, 1991; Felton & Revenson, 1984). In part, whether older adults use less problem-focused coping depends on the type of situation with which they are coping. Given that older adults are more likely to be coping with bereavement, the type of situation they face may confound attempts at identifying age-related changes (Aldwin, in press; Folkman & Moskowitz, 2004).

More recent studies have shown that older adults perceive themselves as being effective copers in later life (Aldwin et al., 1996; Whitty, 2003), even when coping with chronic health problems and loss (Zautra & Wrabetz, 1991). Surprisingly, even impaired older adults have been shown to generate novel strategies when coping with new problems, and their ability to do so may be predictive of successful aging (Brennan & Cardinali, 2000).

From the perspective of adult development and aging research, it would be fair to say that older adults may be more judicious in their use of coping strategies, often in the service of conserving energy (Baltes et al., 1999; Hobfoll, 2002). However, meaning may become more central, as might maintenance of close ties to loved ones (Carstensen et al., 2006). Although older people often perceived themselves to be just as effective copers as younger individuals, to our knowledge, there are no studies that directly examine the interaction between age and coping strategies on either health or well-being outcomes. However, many of the studies on older people have actually been in the health psychology literature, either in the context of caregiving or of coping with chronic illness. Thus, we provide a brief review of that literature for hints on age-related changes in coping efficacy.

## AGING AND COPING STUDIES
## IN HEALTH PSYCHOLOGY

### Coping and Caregiving

Much of the literature on coping and health outcomes in older adult populations has been in the context of the caregiving relationship. Overall, caregiving is believed to place a significant burden on the psychological and physical health of caregivers. Physical health symptoms reported by caregivers have been demonstrated to increase by one-third over the course of the first year of caregiving (Shank-McElroy & Strobino, 2001). A recent review of the literature on the influence of coping on the chronic stress of caregiving concluded that caregivers were somewhat more likely to develop health problems than noncaregivers, but that this effect was stronger for self-reported global health, stress hormones and antibodies than for specific disease outcomes (Vitaliano, Zhang, & Scanlan, 2003). Specifically, in samples of older adults, perceived caregiving stress has been positively associated with levels of interleukin-6 (Kiecolt-Glaser, McGuire, Robles, & Glaser, 2002) and nerve growth factor (NGF) (Hadjiconstantinou et al., 2001), and negatively associated with proliferative responses to concanavalin A (ConA) and phytohemagglutinin (PHA) (Cacioppo et al., 1998), suggesting greater general inflammatory responses but poorer specific immune responses.

Some evidence also suggests that coping may buffer between the stress and health relationship in caregivers, but this appears to differ among the methods and measurements used in the studies, and the preexisting health and personality characteristics of the caregivers (Hooker, Monahan, Shifren, & Hutchinson, 1992). One prospective study of middle-aged and elderly caregivers for heart transplant recipients over 1 year postsurgery classified caregivers into five temporal clusters, depending upon the nature and direction of the caregivers' health. Cluster membership was predicted by both coping styles and preexisting health status (Dew et al., 1998). These results not only indicate that coping has an effect on the physical health outcomes of caregivers, but also demonstrate the importance of other influences. Vitaliano et al. (2003) noted that the relationship between caregiving and health is moderated by the resources and vulnerabilities of the caregiver, which include coping and other health factors that are certainly an important to consider for older caregivers.

Studies assessing the influence of coping on self-reported health in field settings have demonstrated beneficial effects of coping on both mortality and global health outcomes in samples of older caregivers. Wives who used hospice care to help them cope with caregiving for their critically ill spouses were significantly less likely to die themselves within 18 months of the deaths of their spouses than were those who did not use hospice care (Christakis & Iwashyna, 2003). Subjective support, avoidant coping, active coping, and appraisal have all been shown to influence self-report physical health outcomes in samples of elderly caregivers (Bakas & Burgener, 2002; Musil & Ahmad, 2002).

The influence of coping on the physical health of elderly caregivers has also been assessed using proximal health indicators, such as lipids and proliferative measures of immune function. In a sample of older male caregivers, triglycerides were negatively predicted by anger-in (anger suppression) and positively predicted by avoidance coping, whereas high-density lipoprotein cholesterol (HDL-c) was negatively predicted by anger-control and positively predicted by anger-in (Vitaliano, Russo, & Niaura, 1995). One very interesting study found an interaction between perceived stress and coping on both ConA and PHA in elderly caregivers. Active coping was positively related to these proximal measures of immune function in conditions of high, but not low, perceived stress (Stowell, Kiecolt-Glaser, & Glaser, 2001). However, another study in a similar sample found that anger expression was negatively related to mitogen responses in caregivers but not controls. This second study also reported a significant relationship between depressed mood and change in PHA over 15–18 months (Scanlan, Vitaliano, Zhang, Savage, & Ochs, 2001). Thus, whereas coping has been shown to have an effect on proximal health outcomes in caregivers, this effect is not always evident and may be influenced by affective variables. Note also that none of these studies compared the efficacy of coping across age groups, so no conclusions can be drawn as to age-related changes in coping efficacy. However, the finding that the effects of coping on health have been shown in older caregiving samples suggests that at least some of the protective influences of coping in later life are preserved.

## Coping with Illness

The other major source of studies on coping in late life can be found in the health psychology literature on coping with the types of chronic illnesses typically seen in later life, namely, arthritis, heart disease, and multiple chronic illnesses.

### Arthritis

Of the over 400 articles on coping and arthritis reviewed for this chapter, fewer than 50 reported age differences on any measure. Most of those studies examined age differences in outcomes or adjustment to illness, from which coping can only be inferred. Only a handful reported the associations between age and coping. An interesting pattern of associations between age and health outcomes emerges from these studies that highlight differences between osteoarthritis (OA) and rheumatoid arthritis (RA). For physical functioning, two studies reported decreased functioning with age for OA (Brenes, Rapp, Rejeski, & Miller, 2002; Rapp, Rejeski, & Miller, 2000). For RA, however, four studies revealed no age differences (Bartlett, Piedmont, Bilderback, Matsumoto, & Bathon, 2003; Evers, Kraaimaat, Geenen, & Bijlsma, 1997, 2003a, 2003b; Keefe et al., 1991), and one that did find correlations with age and disability demonstrated that these associations with age disappeared once illness duration and activity were controlled (Chorus, Miedema, Boonen, & Van Der Linden, 2003).

In one of the rare studies explicitly investigating age differences in coping and outcomes for RA, Chorus et al. (2003) discovered that age positively predicted greater quality of life, until coping variables were entered into their model. This suggests that the older adults' better adaptation resulted from better coping but does not address whether coping efficacy changes with age. Among a large sample of OA patients over age 65, no correlations between age and coping surfaced (Rapp et al., 2000), nor did Keefe et al. (1991) find significant correlations between age and coping in a smaller sample of 55 RA patients. In another study of OA patients (mostly women), older patients used less selection, optimization, and compensation than did younger adults (Gignac, Cott, & Badley, 2002), contrary to that predicted by the Freund and Baltes's (1998) model reviewed earlier. The authors posit that older adults may not have as many options for paring activities as do younger adults, and that they conserve energy by not engaging in as much optimization.

Watkins, Shifren, Park, and Morrell (1999) explicitly investigated direct and moderating effects of age on coping strategies. They found that middle-aged and older adults used more catastrophizing and praying/hoping when they had mild pain; for severe pain, age did not predict coping strategy, because these approaches were more likely used by all age groups. Young adults also used more self-statements during mild pain than did older adults. In contrast to some research finding that passive/negative emotion-focused coping strategies relate to greater pain (e.g., Keefe et al., 1997), the older adults in this study rated their condition as less severe than did the middle-aged adults, and did not report greater pain, although they reported greater fatigue. Evers et al. (2003a, 2003b) found that passive pain coping strategies predicted RA pain only in the early phases (first 3 years) of the disease, which may help explain the Watkins et al. (1999) findings. Thus, severity of illness may overwhelm any age effects in choice of coping, but, as in the caregiving literature, no studies examined differential efficacy of coping in earlier and later life.

## Heart Disease

As with research on patients with arthritis, only a handful of studies report associations between coping and age among cardiac patients. Whereas the bulk of studies on arthritis—especially RA—include mostly female participants, the bulk of studies on coping in cardiac patients include mostly male patients. Differences between men and women in adjustment and coping surface consistently in the literature (see Tamres, Janicki, & Helgeson, 2002), and these differences should be kept in mind as this review proceeds.

In a qualitative study of 62 patients, older participants were more likely to discuss avoidance and acceptance regarding their disease than those who were younger than 65. Positive reframing appeared about equally between the age groups (Buetow, Goodyear-Smith, & Coster, 2001). The only other studies to report coping and age associations specifically among cardiac patients found no age differences in coping (Murberg, Furze, & Bru, 2004; Shen, McCreary, & Myers, 2004), although they only looked at overall associations with positive and negative coping (instead of subscales). These findings are particularly striking in the Murberg et al. (2004) study, which found that disengagement coping predicted mortality across 6 years.

As with research on arthritis, the literature lacks much information on how age relates to coping among cardiac patients. Given that cardiac patients appear to experience better adjustment and more coping resources with age (Barefoot et al., 2000; Plach, Napholz, & Kelber, 2001, Rankin, 2002; Shen et al., 2004), future research should explore whether coping mediates between the stress of cardiac illness and long-term outcome.

### Chronic Illness—Multiple

In a sample of adults with chronic illness, Zautra and Wrabetz (1991), after controlling for multiple confounds, found age unrelated to coping efficacy or negative changes as a result of health stressors. Age was inversely related to negative changes around loss events. Felton and Revenson (1987) undertook an ambitious investigation of age differences in coping across multiple chronic illnesses. After controlling for illness type and other confounds, they found that use of emotional expression as a coping strategy linearly decreased with age. They also discovered that older adults were least likely to seek information as the seriousness of their disease increased. Thus, age demonstrated both direct and moderating effects on coping with chronic illness. These authors concluded that the differences most likely stemmed from cohort effects. Certainly, future research should try to delineate this further and control for cohort effects to assess whether the observed differences are truly developmental in nature rather than sociohistorical.

## SUMMARY

In conclusion, there is little evidence to suggest that older adults are poorer copers than younger adults; indeed, some evidence suggests that older adults, in some arenas at least, do better than younger adults. There is some evidence to suggest that they may be more likely to conserve energy when they cope, and some intriguing suggestions that they may be more interested in meaning making, although, clearly, empirical studies are needed in this area. The few studies that do examine coping and health outcomes in older adults find effects of coping on physiogical processes, as well as adaptation to illness. However, few studies in health psychology directly examine the question of whether the impact of coping changes with age, although Rothermund and Brandtstädter (2003) suggest that the use of age-appropriate coping strategies is associated with better psychological outcomes. It may be that in late life, chronic illness overwhelms the impact of psychosocial factors on health outcomes. For example, one study that did examine coping and the metabolic syndrome in later life found that positive coping predicted better outcomes only in those individuals who did not have cardiovascular disease (Yancura, Aldwin, & Spiro, 2005). Given the importance of psychosocial factors in the development of optimal aging, future studies that examine how coping changes with age and whether different strategies are more or less efficacious in later life are imperative.

## REFERENCES

Adler, W. H., & Nagel, J. E. (1994). Acquired immunodeficiency syndrome in the elderly. *Drugs and Aging, 4*, 410–416.

Aldwin, C. M. (1990). The Elders Life Stress Inventory: Egocentric and nonegocentric stress. In M. A. P. Stephens, J. H. Crowther, S. E. Hobfoll, & D. T. Tennenbaum (Eds), *Stress and coping in later-life families* (Series in applied psychology; pp. 49–69). Washington, DC: Hemisphere.

Aldwin, C. M. (1991). Does age affect the stress and coping process?: Implications of age differences in perceived control. *Journal of Gerontology, 46*, 174–180.

Aldwin, C. M. (in press). *Stress, coping, and human development: An integrative perspective*. New York: Guilford Press.

Aldwin, C. M., & Gilmer, D. F. (2004). *Health, illness, and optimal aging: Biological and psychosocial perspectives*. Thousand Oaks, CA: Sage.

Aldwin, C. M., & Levenson, M. R. (2001). Stress, coping, and health at mid-life: A developmental perspective. In M. E. Lachman (Ed.), *The handbook of midlife development* (pp. 188–214). New York: Wiley.

Aldwin, C. M., Spiro, A., III, & Park, C. L. (2006). Health, behavior, and optimal aging: A lifespan developmental perspective. In J. Birren & K. W. Schaie (Eds.), *Handbook of the Psychology of Aging* (6th ed., pp. 85–104). San Diego: Academic Press.

Aldwin, C. M., Sutton, K. J., Chiara, G., & Spiro, A., III. (1996). Age differences in stress, coping, and appraisal: Findings from the Normative Aging Study. *Journals of Gerontology: Psychological Sciences and Social Sciences, Series B, 51*, 179–188.

Almeida, D. M., & Horn, M. C. (2004). Is daily life more stressful in middle adulthood? In O. G. Brim, C. D. Ryff, & R. C. Kessler (Eds.), *How healthy are we?: A national study of well-being at mid-life* (pp. 425–451). Chicago: University of Chicago Press.

Antel, J. P., & Minuck, J. (1994). Neuroimmunology of aging. In M. L. Albert & J. E. Knoefel (Eds.), *Clinical neurology of aging* (2nd ed., pp. 121–135). London: Oxford University Press.

Bakas, T., & Burgener, S. C. (2002). Predictors of emotional distress, general health, and caregiving outcomes in family caregivers of stroke survivors. *Topics in Stroke Rehabilitation, 9*(1), 34–45.

Baltes, P. B., Staudinger, U. M., & Lindenberger, U. (1999). Lifespan psychology: Theory and application to intellectual functioning. *Annual Review of Psychology, 50*, 471–507.

Barefoot, J. C., Brummett, B. H., Clapp-Channing, N. E., Siegler, I. C., Vitaliano, P. P., Williams, R. B., et al. (2000). Moderators of the effect of social support on depressive symptoms in cardiac patients. *American Journal of Cardiology, 86*, 438–442.

Bartlett, S. J., Piedmont, R., Bilderback, A., Matsumoto, A. K., & Bathon, J. M.

(2003). Spirituality, well-being, and quality of life in people with rheumatoid arthritis. *Arthritis and Rheumatology, 49,* 778–783.

Boeninger, D. K., Shiraishi, R. W., & Aldwin, C. M. (May, 2003). *Associations of age, personality, and stressor type with primary stress appraisal.* Poster presented at the APA/UC Health Psychology Conference, San Bernadino, CA.

Brandtstädter, J. (1999). The self in action and development: Cultural, biosocial and ontogenetic bases of intentional self-development. In J. Brandtstädter & R. M. Lerner (Eds.), *Action and self-development: Theory and research through the life span* (pp. 37–66). Thousands Oaks, CA: Sage.

Brenes, G. A., Rapp, S. R., Rejeski, W. J., & Miller, M. E. (2002). Do optimism and pessimism predict physical functioning? *Journal of Behavioral Medicine, 25,* 219–231.

Brennan, M., & Cardinali, G. (2000). The use of preexisting and novel coping strategies in adapting to age-related vision loss. *Gerontologist, 40,* 327–334.

Buetow, S., Goodyear-Smith, F., & Coster, G. (2001). Coping strategies in the self-management of chronic heart failure. *Family Practice, 18,* 117–122.

Cacioppo, J. T., Poehlmann, K. M., Kiecolt-Glaser, J. K., Malarkey, W. B., Burleson, M. H., Berntson, G. G., et al. (1998). Cellular immune responses to acute stress in female caregivers of dementia patients and matched controls. *Health Psychology, 17*(2), 182–189.

Carstensen, L. L., Mikels, J. A., & Mather, M. (2006). Aging and the intersection of cognition, motivation and emotion. In J. Birren & K. W. Schaie (Eds.), *Handbook of the psychology of aging* (6th ed., pp. 343–362). San Diego: Academic Press.

Chakravarti, B., & Abraham, G. N. (1999). Aging and T-cell-mediated immunity. *Mechanisms of Ageing and Development, 108,* 183–206.

Chiriboga, D. A. (1997). Crisis, challenge, and stability in the middle years. In M. E. Lachman & J. B. James (Eds.), *Multiple paths of midlife development* (pp. 293–343). Chicago: University of Chicago Press.

Chorus, A. M., Miedema, H. S., Boonen, A., & Van Der Linden, S. (2003). Quality of life and work in patients with rheumatoid arthritis and ankylosing spondylitis of working age. *Annals of Rheumatic Disease, 62,* 1178–1184.

Christakis, N. A., & Iwashyna, T. J. (2003). The health impact of health care on families: A matched cohort study of hospice use by decedents and mortality outcomes in surviving, widowed spouses. *Social Science and Medicine, 57*(3), 465–475.

Costa, P. T., Zonderman, A. B., & McCrae, R. R. (1991). Personality, defense, coping, and adaptation in older adulthood. In E. M. Cummings, A. L. Greene, & K. H. Karraker (Eds.), *Life-span developmental psychology: Perspectives of stress and coping* (pp. 277–293). Hillsdale, NJ: Erlbaum.

Crown, W. (2001). Economic status of the elderly. In R. H. Binstock & L. K. Goerge (Eds.), *Handbook of aging and the social sciences* (5th ed., pp. 352–368). San Diego: Academic Press.

Dew, M. A., Goycoolea, J. M., Stukas, A. A., Switzer, G. E., Simmons, R. G., Roth, L. H., et al. (1998). Temporal profiles of physical health in family members of heart transplant recipients: Predictors of health change during caregiving. *Health Psychology, 17*(2), 138–151.

DiGiovanna, A. G. (2000). *Human aging: Biological perspectives.* New York: McGraw-Hill.

Elias, M., Elias, P., D'Agostino, R., & Wolf, P. (2000). Comparative effects of age and blood pressure on neuropsychological performance. In S. Manuck, R. Jennings, B. Rabin, & A. Baum (Eds.), *Health, behavior, and aging* (pp. 199–224). Mahwah, NJ: Erlbaum.

Evers, A. W., Kraaimaat, F. W., Geenen, R., & Bijlsma, J. W. (1997). Determinants of psychological distress and its course in the first year after diagnosis in rheumatoid arthritis patients. *Journal of Behavioral Medicine, 20,* 489–504.

Evers, A. W., Kraaimaat, F. W., Geenen, R., Jacobs, J. W., & Bijlsma, J. W. (2003a). Stress–vulnerability factors as long-term predictors of disease activity in early rheumatoid arthritis. *Journal of Psychosomatic Research, 55*(4), 293–302.

Evers, A. W., Kraaimaat, F. W., Geenen, R., Jacobs, J. W., & Bijlsma, J. W. (2003). Pain coping and social support as predictors of long-term functional disability and pain in early rheumatoid arthritis. *Behavioral Research Therapy, 41,* 1295–1310.

Fabris, N., Mocchegiani, E., & Provinciali, M. (1997). Plasticity of neuroendocrine–thymus interactions during aging. *Experimental Gerontology, 32,* 415–419.

Felton, B. J., & Revenson, T. A. (1984). Coping with chronic illness: A study of illness controllability and the influence of coping strategies on psychological adjustment. *Journal of Consulting and Clinical Psychology, 52,* 343–353.

Felton, B. J., & Revenson, T. A. (1987). Age differences in coping with chronic illness. *Psychology and Aging, 2,* 164–170.

Folkman, S., Lazarus, R. S., Pimley, S., Novacek, J. (1987). Age differences in stress and coping processes. *Psychology and Aging, 2,* 171–184.

Folkman, S., & Moskowitz, J. T. (2004). Coping: Pitfalls and promise. *Annual Review of Psychology, 55,* 745–774.

Freund, A. M., & Baltes, P. B. (1998). Selection, optimization, and compensation as strategies of life management: Correlations with subjective indicators of successful aging. *Psychology and Aging, 13*(4), 531–543.

Gignac, M. A., Cott, C., & Badley, E. M. (2002). Adaptation to disability: Applying selective optimization with compensation to the behaviors of older adults with osteoarthritis. *Psychology and Aging, 17,* 520–524.

Guidi, L., Tricerri, A., Frasca, D., Vangeli, M., Errani, A. R., & Bartoloni, C. (1998). Psychoneuroimmunology and aging. *Gerontology, 44*(5), 247–261.

Gutman, D. L. (1974). Alternatives to disengagement: The old men of the Highland Druze. In R. A. LeVine (Ed.), *Culture and personality: Contemporary readings* (pp. 232–245). Chicago: Aldine.

Hadjiconstantinou, M., McGuire, L., Duchemin, A. M., Laskowski, B., Kiecolt-Glaser, J., & Glaser, R. (2001). Changes in plasma nerve growth factor levels in older adults associated with chronic stress. *Journal of Neuroimmunology, 116*(1), 102–106.

Hobfoll, S. E. (2002). Social and psychological resources and adaptation. *Review of General Psychology, 6,* 307–324.

Hooker, K., Monahan, D., Shifren, K., & Hutchinson, C. (1992). Mental and physical health of spouse caregivers: The role of personality. *Psychology and Aging, 7*(3), 367–375.

Jennings, J. R., Kamarck, T., Manuck, S., Everson, S.A., Kaplan, G., & Salonen, J. T. (1997). Aging or disease?: Cardiovascular reactivity in Finnish men over the middle years. *Psychology and Aging, 12,* 225–238.

Johnson, J. V., Backlund, E., Sorlie, P. D., & Loveless, C. A. (2000). Marital status and mortality: The National Longitudinal Mortality Study. *Annals of Epidemiology, 10*, 224–238.

Keefe, F. J., Affleck, G., Lefebvre, J. C., Starr, K., Caldwell, D. S., & Tennen, H. (1997). Pain coping strategies and coping efficacy in rheumatoid arthritis: A daily process analysis. *Pain, 69*(1–2), 35–42.

Keefe, F. J., Caldwell, D. S., Martinez, S., Nunley, J., Beckham, J., & Williams, D. A. (1991). Analyzing pain in rheumatoid arthritis patients: Pain coping strategies in patients who have had knee replacement surgery. *Pain, 46*, 153–160.

Kiecolt-Glaser, J. K., McGuire, L., Robles, T. F., & Glaser, R. (2002). Psychoneuro-immunology: Psychological influences on immune function and health. *Journal of Consulting and Clinical Psychology, 70*, 537–547.

Miller, R. A. (1996). The aging immune system: Primer and prospectus. *Science, 273*, 70–74.

Mroczek, D. K., & Almeida, D. M. (2004). The effect of daily stress, personality, and age on daily negative affect. *Journal of Personality, 72*, 355–378.

Murberg, T. A., Furze, G., & Bru, E. (2004). Avoidance coping styles predict mortality among patients with congestive heart failure: A 6-year follow-up study. *Personality and Individual Differences, 36*, 757–766.

Musil, C. M., & Ahmad, M. (2002). Health of grandmothers: A comparison by caregiver status. *Journal of Aging and Health, 14*(1), 96–121.

Neupert, S. D. (2003). Daily stressors and memory failures in a naturalistic setting: Findings from the Normative Aging Study. *Dissertation Abstracts International: Section B, Sciences and Engineering, 64*(5–B), 2419.

Norris, F. H. (1992). Epidemiology of trauma: Frequency and impact of different potentially traumatic events on different demographic groups. *Journal of Consulting and Clinical Psychology, 60*, 409–418.

Park, C. L., & Blumberg, C. J. (2002). Disclosing trauma through writing: Testing the meaning-making hypothesis. *Cognitive Therapy and Research, 26*(5), 597–616.

Plach, S. K., Napholz, L., & Kelber, S. T. (2001). Differences in anxiety and role experiences between three age groups of women with heart disease. *Archives of Psychiatric Nursing, 15*, 195–199.

Rankin, S. H. (2002). Women recovering from acute myocardial infarction: Psychosocial and physical functioning outcomes for 12 months after acute myocardial infarction. *Heart and Lung, 31*, 399–410.

Rapp, S. R., Rejeski, W. J., & Miller, M. E. (2000). Physical function among older adults with knee pain: The role of pain coping skills. *Arthritis Care Research, 13*, 270–279.

Rothermund, K., & Brandtstädter, J. (2003). Coping with deficits and losses in later life: From compensatory action to accommodation. *Psychology and Aging, 18*, 896–905.

Sapolsky, R. (1992). *Stress, the aging brain, and the mechanisms of neuron death*. Cambridge, MA: MIT Press.

Sapolsky, R. (1998). *Why zebras don't get ulcers: An updated guide to stress, stress-related diseases, and coping*. New York: Freeman.

Scanlan, J. M., Vitaliano, P. P., Zhang, J., Savage, M., & Ochs, H. D. (2001). Lymphocyte proliferation is associated with gender, caregiving, and psychosocial variables in older adults. *Journal of Behavioral Medicine, 24*, 537–559.

Shanks-McElroy, H. A., & Strobino, J. (2001). Male caregivers of spouses with Alz-
    heimer's disease: Risk factors and health status. *American Journal of Alzheimer's
    Diseases and Other Dementias, 16*(3), 167–175.
Shen, B. J., McCreary, C. P., & Myers, H. F. (2004). Independent and mediated contri-
    butions of personality, coping, social support, and depressive symptoms to phys-
    ical functioning outcome among patients in cardiac rehabilitation. *Journal of
    Behavioral Medicine, 27,* 39–62.
Stowell, J. R., Kiecolt-Glaser, J. K., & Glaser, R. (2001). Perceived stress and cellular
    immunity: When coping counts. *Journal of Behavioral Medicine, 24,* 323–339.
Tamres, L. K., Janicki, D., & Helgeson, V. E. (2002). Sex differences in coping behav-
    ior: A meta-analytic review and an examination of relative coping. *Personality
    and Social Psychology Review, 6,* 2–30.
Uchino, B. N., Holt-Lunstad, J., Bloor, L. E., & Campo, R. A. (2005). Aging and car-
    diovascular reactivity to stress: Longitudinal evidence for changes in stress reac-
    tivity. *Psychology and Aging, 20*(1), 134–143.
Vaillant, G. (1977). *Adaptation to life: How the best and the brightest came of age.*
    Boston: Little, Brown.
Vaillant, G. (2002). *Aging well: Surprising guideposts to a happier life.* Boston: Little,
    Brown.
Vitaliano, P. P., Russo, J., & Niaura, R. (1995). Plasma lipids and their relationships
    with psychosocial factors in older adults. *Journals of Gerontology: Psychologi-
    cal Sciences and Social Sciences, Series B, 50,* P18–P24.
Vitaliano, P. P., Zhang, J., & Scanlan, J. M. (2003). Is caregiving hazardous to one's
    physical health?: A meta-analysis. *Psychological Bulletin, 129*(6), 946–972.
VonDras, D. D., Powless, M. R., Olson, A. K., Wheeler, D., & Snudden, A. L. (2005).
    Differential effects of everyday stress on the episodic memory test performances
    of young, mid-life, and older adults. *Aging and Mental Health, 9*(1), 60–70.
Watkins, K. W., Shifren, K., Park, D. C., & Morrell, R. W. (1999). Age, pain, and cop-
    ing with rheumatoid arthritis. *Pain, 82,* 217–228.
Whitty, M. T. (2003). Coping and defending: Age differences in maturity of defense
    mechanisms and coping strategies. *Aging and Mental Health, 7,* 123–132.
Wick, G., Jansen-Durr, P., Berger, P., Blasko, I., & Grubeck-Loebstein, B. (2000). Dis-
    eases of aging. *Vaccine, 18,* 1567–1583.
Williams, R. B. (2000). Psychological factors, health, and disease: The impact of aging
    and the life cycle. In S. B. Manuck, R. Jennings, B. S. Rabin, & A. Baum (2000).
    *Behavior, health, and aging* (pp. 135–151). Mahwah, NJ: Lawrence Erlbaum.
Yancura, L., Aldwin, C.M., & Spiro, A. III. (2005, December). *The pathways among
    stress, coping, affect, and the metabolic syndrome differ between men with and
    without a history of cardiovascular disease.* Poster presented at the annual con-
    vention of the Gerontological Society of America, Orlando, FL.
Zautra, A. J., & Wrabetz, A. B. (1991). Coping success and its relationship to psycho-
    logical distress for older adults. *Journal of Personality and Social Psychology,
    61,* 801–810.

# CHAPTER 12

# Health and Psychological Consequences of Caregiving

RICHARD H. FORTINSKY, HOWARD TENNEN,
NATALIE FRANK, and GLENN AFFLECK

Families and friends are the foundation of long-term care for community-dwelling older persons with chronic illnesses and disabilities in the United States. National survey data reveal that nearly 75% of all such older adults rely solely on family members and other informal sources for support, whereas fewer than 10% receive help exclusively from formal or paid service providers (Noelker & Whitlatch, 2005). This chapter focuses on family caregivers, because they comprise the vast majority of informal caregivers; only about 10% of frail older adults rely exclusively on friends, neighbors, and other unpaid nonkin for help to remain in their homes (Barker, 2002). Within the family, individuals primarily responsible for ongoing care are most likely to be spouses or, if older adults are widowed, adult children. Adult daughters tend to provide personal care and emotional support, whereas adult sons tend to provide financial and legal advice. When these family members are not available, siblings, nieces and nephews, and grandchildren often step in to provide primary assistance (Noelker & Whitlatch, 2005).

With the growth of human service options for disabled older persons over the past few decades, many policymakers have been concerned that families would abdicate their responsibilities to their relatives in favor of publicly funded health and social services. However, numerous investigations of this so-called "substitution effect" have consistently shown that families do not reduce their involvement when formal services are introduced (Penning, 2002). This chapter examines the extensive health and psychological consequences of family caregiving to older adults, psychological theories commonly used to explain caregiving strategies and consequences, and interventions designed to alleviate these consequences.

## NATIONAL FAMILY CAREGIVER PROFILE:
## SOCIODEMOGRAPHICS AND MAGNITUDE OF CARE

Findings from a recently completed national study shed light on the current sociodemographic composition of family caregivers in the United States (National Alliance for Caregiving and American Association of Retired Persons [AARP], 2004). Caregivers were operationally defined as respondents who reported assisting another person age 18 years or older with at least one personal care activity of daily living (ADL; e.g., bathing, dressing) or instrumental activity of daily living (e.g., preparing meals, shopping) "to help them take care of themselves." This study found that 79% of self-defined caregivers helped adults age 50 or older (i.e., older adults), and that 83% helped family members. Sociodemographic characteristics of these family caregivers to older adults yielded the following profile: mean age = 47 years; 63% female; 74% European American, 11% black or African American, 10% Hispanic or Latino, 4% Asian American; 63% married; 57% employed full-time or part-time. One in four caregivers reported that the older adult they cared for (mean age = 75 years) had Alzheimer's disease or other type of dementia, whereas equal proportions reported that the older adult had the main problem of cancer, diabetes, or heart disease (9% each).

The magnitude of caregiving was reported in an article comparing caregivers to older adults with or without Alzheimer's disease or another type of dementia (Ory, Hoffman, Yee, Tennstedt, & Schulz, 1999). Both caregiver groups had been providing care for a mean of 5 years, but caregivers to older adults with dementia were more likely to be spouses and provided more hours of care per week (17 hours vs. 12.5 hours), compared to caregivers to older adults without dementia. More than half of all caregivers reported helping older adults with all instrumental activities of daily living (IADLs), and at least one-third helped with all personal care ADLs. Caregivers to older adults with dementia were more likely than their counterparts to provide help with every personal care ADL and nearly every IADL. These results indicate that all caregivers to older adults provide extensive care, week in and week out, and that having an older adult with dementia is often associated with a greater magnitude of care responsibilities.

## PSYCHOLOGICAL, SOCIAL, AND HEALTH
## CONSEQUENCES OF CAREGIVING

Caregiver health has attracted considerable attention in recent years, as it has become apparent that caregivers are at increased risk for psychological and physical morbidity, and impaired social functioning, and that their health affects their ability to care for an elderly family member. Research in this area has focused on documenting caregivers' risks for emotional and health impairments, and determining the factors associated with health and well-being among individuals who care for an older family member.

## Psychological Adjustment

It is now well established that compared to their noncaregiving peers, caregivers suffer from poorer emotional health. Caregivers complain of overall distress, report lower psychological well-being, and experience a stronger sense of being weighed down by life's burdens (Canadian Study of Health and Aging Working Group, 2002). Several reviews have documented high levels of depressive and anxious symptoms among caregivers, and higher rates of clinical depression and anxiety disorders (Bookwala, Yee, & Schulz, 2000). Many caregivers experience a loss of personal control over their lives, combined with a sense that everyday demands are overwhelming. Tied to their perceived loss of control, caregivers describe feeling trapped by their caregiving role, a general sense of helplessness, and at times feeling paralyzed by even the most mundane daily tasks (Schulz & Williamson, 1991).

## Social Adjustment

In addition to psychological distress, caregivers display relatively poor social adjustment, an important indicator of overall adjustment among individuals confronted with stressful life circumstances. Caring for an older adult is associated with perceived loss of social support, a constricted social life, social isolation, and compromised relationships with other family members, whom caregivers often believe are failing to put forth sufficient effort to relieve their burden (Ory et al., 1999; National Alliance for Caregiving and AARP, 2004).

Family caregivers frequently turn to their elderly relative's physician for support both during and between office visits. Yet they do not feel that their support needs are being met (Beisecker, Chrisman, & Wright, 1997). Physicians may not fully appreciate the importance of supplying this type of support, or they may view themselves as adequately and effectively performing this role. Studies have demonstrated that caregivers rate physicians fairly low on providing advice about dementia symptom management and community resources; physicians also often fail to connect caregivers with available support services in the community (Fortinsky, 1998, 2001). Future work in this area would provide valuable insights by clarifying the comparative roles of social support provided by health professionals and other types of support in facilitating caregivers' efforts to adapt to caregiving demands.

## Physical Health

Although the empirical connection between exposure to chronic stress and illness risk has been established (see Cohen, Kessler, & Underwood-

Gordon, 1997), only recently have investigators begun to document the mechanisms through which chronic stress creates the conditions for physical illness. Vitaliano, Zhang, and Scanlan (2003) offer a dual-pathway model to explain the stress–illness relationship. Through one path, chronic stressors produce psychosocial distress (described earlier), which in turn affects stress hormones by way of the hypothalamic–pituitary–adrenal axis. Repeated arousal and dysregulation set the stage for pathophysiological reactions (see McEwen, 2000). The second path depicts chronic caregiver stress initiating and maintaining health-threatening behaviors such as poor diet, sleep disturbance, and substance use, which in turn influence health outcomes. Vitaliano and colleagues (2003) speculated that these two pathways increase cardiovascular, metabolic, and immunological risk.

A growing body of empirical findings now documents the health consequences of family caregiving for an older adult relative (Vitaliano, 1997). Compared to their noncaregiving peers, caregivers experience poorer self-reported health, more physical symptoms, and more illnesses and disabilities identified through objective assessments (Schulz et al., 1995; Beach, Schulz, Yee, & Jackson, 2000), and long-term caregivers' self-rated health appears to deteriorate over time (Skaff, Pearlin, & Mullan, 1996).

Individuals who care for the elderly suffer a higher prevalence of diagnosable physical disabilities than do noncaregivers (Schulz et al., 1995); have numerous somatic complaints (Moritz, Kasl, & Berkman, 1989); demonstrate a high prevalence of respiratory problems (Fuller-Jonap & Haley, 1995), relatively high rates of angina pectoris (Schulz & Beach, 1999), and higher rates of diabetes, hay fever, back problems, and chronic physical aches and pains than noncaregivers (Jutras & Lavoie, 1995); higher levels of chronic illnesses; and greater use of medications to treat physical complaints (e.g., Pruchno & Potashnik, 1989; Kiecolt-Glaser, Dura, Speicher, Trask, & Glaser, 1991). Even after controlling for age, gender, and race, caregivers report higher rates of backaches, insomnia, arthritis, rectal problems, and hearing problems, and they are more likely to report at least two or more health problems compared to noncaregivers. Substantial memory problems have also been found among caregivers (Lichtenberg, Manning, & Turkheimer, 1992). These memory deficits might further compromise caregivers' ability to fulfill the demands of their role and their capacity to care for themselves.

Vitaliano et al. (2003) reviewed 23 well-designed studies that evaluated various indicators of health outcomes among individuals caring for elderly adults with dementia or related cognitive impairments. They found that, compared to noncaregivers, caregivers reported poorer global health; a greater number of somatic complaints; higher rates of chronic illness; more use of medications for health-related distress; higher rates of health care utilization, including clinic and physician visits, and hospital stays; and poorer perceived global health.

Vitaliano et al.'s (2003) meta-analysis included only well-designed cross-sectional studies; therefore, causal inference regarding the temporal sequence between psychological and physical health effects of caregiving remains compromised. As we demonstrate in our discussion of caregiver coping, reliance on cross-sectional designs was commonplace in the caregiving literature until recently. A smaller number of investigations have begun to focus on improving understanding of the relationship between psychosocial and physical health, as well as on moderators of the association between caregiving and these health domains.

## RELATIONSHIPS BETWEEN AND CORRELATES OF PSYCHOSOCIAL AND PHYSICAL HEALTH

A well-replicated relationship has been observed between psychosocial and physical health among caregivers. Poorer self-rated health is associated with elevated depressive and anxious symptoms during the entire course of the caregiving experience (Beach et al., 2000; Schulz et al., 1995). Relatively little is known, however, about the conditions, personal characteristics, or mediators of this relationship. We now describe some of the psychological, contextual, cultural, and physiological factors that may be involved in the relationships among caregiving, well-being, and health outcomes.

In their study of caregivers of patients with dementia, Fortinsky, Kercher, and Burant (2002) evaluated whether perceived self-efficacy, the belief that one can perform a specific behavior or task (Bandura, 1990), was related to depressive symptoms and health problems. They found that higher levels of perceived self-efficacy for helping a loved one with symptom management was associated with fewer depressive symptoms, whereas higher levels of perceived self-efficacy for locating and utilizing community support services predicted fewer physical health problems.

Numerous studies have demonstrated the positive association between psychosocial and physical health among caregivers and have reliably documented person factors related to both. Indicators of poor mental health are associated with corresponding impairments in self-rated physical health (Hooker, Monahan, Bowman, Frazier, & Shifren, 1998). Specific psychosocial difficulties, including greater prevalence of psychiatric symptoms; higher level of neuroticism; perceived lack of control over life; more depressive symptoms; low levels of perceived self-efficacy; less satisfaction in role-related decision making; poorer social functioning; and dissatisfaction with emotional support, perceived stress, and low levels of optimism have all been related to poor self-rated general physical health (Li, Seltzer, & Greenberg, 1997; Miller, Campbell, Farran, Kaufman, & Davis, 1995; Smerglia & Deimling, 1997; Bookwala & Schulz, 1998). These associations, however, are not unique to the lives of caregivers. Moreover, shared method variance haunts studies that rely on self-reported distress and self-reported physical health. Relatively few studies have examined the relationship between psychological and health outcomes among caregivers over time, and few have attempted to differentiate the correlates, mediators, and moderators of these associations.

## CONTEXTUAL FACTORS INFLUENCING ADAPTATION TO CAREGIVING

In view of the array of populations being cared for, differences in the caregiving environment and caregivers themselves, and the inconsistent findings regarding relationships between caregiving and health outcomes, investigators have examined a number of contextual factors to determine how they might influence caregiver well-being or modify (moderate) the association between caregiver stress and adaptational outcomes. These studies have evaluated caregiver gender, ethnic identity, relationship to care recipient, living arrangements, time demands, outside employment, perception as the primary caregiver, income, and type of disability and behavior problems of care recipients (Vitaliano et al., 2003; Schulz et al., 1995; Bookwala et al., 2000).

### Sociodemographic Characteristics

Caregiver gender is perhaps the most widely studied caregiver factor in relation to well-being. Wife caregivers appear to experience more subjective burden and depression than do husband caregivers (Bookwala & Schulz, 2000). The increased burden experienced by women caregivers appears to be due to women's more direct personal care provision, their greater employment strain when trying to negotiate family caregiving and work demands, and the relatively fewer resources available to help them in their caregiving role compared to the resources of men caregivers (Kramer & Kipnis, 1995). In a review of 30 empirical studies, Yee and Schulz (2000) found that women caregivers were more likely than men caregivers to report psychiatric symptoms including depression and anxiety, and lower life satisfaction. These investigators suggested that the observed gender differences might be related to women spending more time in caregiving overall, and in direct caregiving tasks. Women, they speculated, view themselves as less able to obtain informal assistance and are less willing than men to relinquish the caregiver role.

Gender differences have also been found in caregivers' physical well-being. Women caregivers report more somatic complaints than do men caregivers (Schulz et al., 1995), and in a study of spousal caregivers, wives experienced more physical health strains than husbands (Miller, 1990). These differences were related to women spending more time caregiving. The meta-analysis by Vitaliano and colleagues (2003) revealed that women caregivers of elders with dementia reported poorer global health than did men caregivers or noncaregivers of either gender; however, they cautioned that women are more likely to recognize and report health problems in many stressful situations. Thus, these gender differences in self-reported health are not unique to the caregiving context (Barsky, Peekna, & Borus, 2001).

Ethnic group differences in response to caregiving have been reported in numerous studies (see Dilworth-Anderson, Williams, & Gibson, 2002; and Pinquart & Sorensen, 2005, for comprehensive reviews). Dilworth-Anderson and Anderson (1994) concluded that although African American caregivers may have fewer economic resources than European American caregivers, they may have greater spiritual resources, which facilitate better adjustment to the stress associated with caregiving for the elderly members of their community. In a more detailed examination involving a comparison of African American, European American, and Puerto Rican caregivers, Calderon and Tennstedt (1998) found that European American women, and African American and Puerto Rican men, reported more frustration and anger regarding their caregiving situation, whereas African American and Puerto Rican women were more likely to manifest somatic complaints.

The relationship of the caregiver to the care recipient and the family member's place of residence are also associated with caregiver physical and psychological health. For example, family caregivers report fewer depressive symptoms when their relative is living in an institution, even when that relative exhibits significant disability and dysfunction, compared with caregivers of less severely disabled family members who live at home (Grunfeld, Glossop, McDowell, & Danbrook, 1997). Spouse caregivers, and caregivers residing with the family member being cared for, reported higher levels of distress than did adult child caregivers and those residing away from the family member receiving care (Berg-Weger, Rubio, & Tebb, 2000).

Finally, it is unclear how and why caregiving differentially impacts older caregivers compared to younger caregivers. Caregivers of persons with dementia are older than caregivers of older adults without dementia, and they provide more hours of care per week (Ory et al., 1999). They are also more likely to be spouses. Older caregivers report greater psychological morbidity (Cullen, Grayson, & Jorm, 1997) and poorer self-reported physical health than younger caregivers (Vitaliano et al., 2003; Vitaliano, Young, & Zhang, 2004). Vitaliano et al. (2003) speculated that the physical illnesses and disabilities associated with aging may be exacerbated by psychosocial stress, leading older caregivers to report more health-related caregiving consequences than do younger caregivers. Alternatively, older caregivers may suffer greater consequences, because they are more likely to be spouses and to provide greater amounts of care than do younger caregivers. Future studies should more carefully isolate independent age effects on caregivers by controlling for relationship to care recipient and amount of care provided.

## Caregivers' Own Health Conditions

Finally, Vitaliano et al. (2003, 2004) offer evidence that coexisting health conditions may modify caregiving effects on health. For example, they note that although natural killer cell activity is comparable for caregivers and noncaregivers who have not had cancer, caregivers who have had cancer have lower natural killer activity than do noncaregivers who have had cancer. Thus, caregivers with a cancer history are at particular risk for tumor growth. Similarly, whereas caregiver status is not related to blood pressure reactivity among individuals with normal blood pressure, hypertensive caregivers demonstrate greater reactivity than noncaregiving hypertensive individuals. This places hypertensive caregivers at unique risk for coronary events. These and other moderated effects begin to capture the complex relationship between caregiving and health.

Studies based on longitudinal designs have begun to emerge in the literature. Vitaliano et al. (2004) highlighted several prospective studies that followed caregivers and noncaregivers who did not have major health problems at the start of the study. Shaw et al. (1997) found that caregivers with the greatest caregiving load were more likely to develop a health problem over the following 1–6 years than were noncaregivers or caregivers who provided less assistance to a family member. Schulz and Beach (1999) reported that strained caregivers had a higher death rate than noncaregivers over an average of 4 years. Vitaliano et al. (2002) found that over 30 months, men who were caregivers were more likely to develop heart disease than men who were not caregivers. Although their sample was relatively small, these and other longitudinal findings strengthen our causal inferences in linking caregiving with health risks.

One study has begun to elaborate a biochemical mechanism that places caregivers at greater risk for compromised immune functioning in response to their experience of chronic stress. Kiecolt-Glaser et al. (2003) followed spousal caregivers of patients with dementia and noncaregivers for 6 years, and found that caregivers showed a considerably higher rate of increase in interleukin 6 (IL-6)—an increase that was comparable for former caregivers (whose spouse had died) and continuing caregivers. Overproduction of IL-6, a proinflammatory cytokine, is associated with a wide range of illnesses associated with aging, including arthritis, cardiovascular disease, and Type II diabetes. Caregiving studies that use longitudinal designs, that consider effect modifiers, and that attempt to measure biochemical and behavioral mechanisms hold the greatest promise of uncovering the conditions and processes through which caregiving affects health.

## Dementia as a Contextual Factor in Caregiving

Cognitive, behavioral, and affective deterioration associated with the progression of dementia is especially challenging for family caregivers (Ory et al., 1999), who are faced with managing their family member's wandering, agitation, hallucinations, memory loss, confusion, disorientation, emotional distress, and dangerous and embarrassing behavior (Bourgeois,

Schulz, & Burgio, 1996). Caregivers of persons with dementia display relatively high rates of psychiatric illness, particularly elevated levels of depressive symptoms and emotional strain (Schulz et al., 1995; Ory et al., 1999). The problem behaviors these patients display are closely linked to distress and depression in their caregivers. This relationship between patient problem behavior and caregiver distress appears to be stronger for women (Schulz & Williamson, 1991). It is easy to imagine a mutually escalating cycle in which patients with Alzheimer's disease who live with highly distressed caregivers are more likely to have intensified behavior problems, agitation, and aggression (Dunkin & Anderson-Hanley, 1998) because the patient and the caregiver exacerbate each other's symptoms.

Ory et al. (1999) identified two differences between caregivers of patients with and without dementia. Caregivers of patients with dementia experienced higher degrees of perceived emotional and physical strain, as well as more severe physical problems that caused considerable distress, compared with caregivers of patients without dementia. These differences were retained after controlling for gender, race, education, and income. Caregivers of patients with dementia also displayed more compromised social adjustment than caregivers of patients without dementia, abandoning social activities and spending less time with friends and family. These reactions in turn create the conditions for estrangement and further social isolation.

The severity of the family member's disability and accompanying behavior problems are reliable predictors of caregiver health. Cullen et al. (1997) demonstrated that older adults' levels of dementia-related disability and disturbed behavior accounted for most of the variation in their caregivers' reports of physical and emotional well-being. Caregivers with more demands on their time, those who identified themselves as the primary caregiver, and older caregivers were most adversely affected. Nagaratnam, Lewis-Jones, Scott, and Palazzi (1998) found that older family members' behavior problems predicted the greatest amount of psychological burden for caregivers, whereas the older family members' aggression was most closely linked to their caregivers' distress. As the patients' dysfunction and problem behaviors increased during the progressive course of their illness, their caregivers experienced more depressive symptoms and a greater sense of being burdened (Schulz & Williamson, 1991).

## COPING WITH THE DEMANDS OF PROVIDING CARE FOR AN OLDER FAMILY MEMBER

The empirical literature on caregiver coping echoes the broader coping literature in its limited study designs, compromised measurement strategies, and imprecise conceptualizations. Therefore, rather than review the conflicting and inconclusive pattern of findings from this substantial and complex literature, we highlight the major problems found in studies of coping with the demands of caring for an elderly relative, with a focus on dementia caregiving. We then examine one particular coping effort, *finding benefits*, to underscore several potential directions for studying coping as it unfolds over extended periods of time in the daily lives of caregivers of older adults.

Gottlieb and Wolfe's (2002) critical review of the literature on coping with family caregiving to individuals with dementia identified a number of widespread methodological and conceptual problems. Mirroring the broader coping literature, all of the studies in Gottlieb and Wolfe's review measured coping via a coping checklist (see Coyne & Gottlieb, 1996, for a trenchant critique). These coping checklists not only varied in the specific aspects of coping assessed, but all also required recollection of coping efforts. As Gottlieb and Wolfe (2002) noted, retrospection of coping strategies is particularly problematic in the context of caregiving, because caregivers face many stressors and are thus likely to conflate how they coped with any particular stressor. The caregiver's emotional state at the time may also influence recall of coping efforts (Salovey & Birnbaum, 1989).

Gottlieb and Wolfe (2002) conjectured that the most consistent finding in the studies they reviewed, the positive relationship between coping through *wishful thinking* and psychological distress, may actually reflect an effort on the part of caregivers to explain their distress. Indeed, Ross's (1989) concept of implicit theories of stability and change suggests that when a coping researcher asks caregivers to report strategies used to cope with a particular aspect of caregiving, caregivers recreate their response to the encounter by reflecting on their current status, their theory of change, and a model of how they respond to caregiving demands. If they are currently distressed or feeling ineffective, according to Ross's theory, they are likely to infer that they used ineffective coping strategies. This reconstructive process may well have led to the replicable "discovery" that coping through wishful thinking "predicts" lower levels of caregiver distress. The broader literature on autobiographical memory (Singer & Salovey, 1993) posits myriad processes that may conspire to distort the recollection of personally relevant experiences and behavior, including how accurately one remembers his or her efforts to cope with the demands of caring for an older family member.

Gottlieb and Wolfe (2002) also documented an extensive reliance on cross-sectional study designs in family caregiving studies. Remarkably, *all* of the studies they reviewed used cross-sectional designs (see Powers, Gallagher-Thompson, & Kraemer, 2002, for a more recent exception). Although the language of regression analysis offers the appearance that coping predicts psychological and health outcomes, it is easy to imagine multiple scenarios in which health and emotional well-being affect the ways in which caregivers cope with the demands of their caregiver role. Gottlieb and Wolfe (2002) identified several other major problems in the literature on coping with family caregiving. Few studies specified the stressor that the caregivers were to focus on in reporting their coping efforts, and none of the studies reminded participants to focus on a particular period of time, despite compelling evidence that people describe their coping strategies based in large part on the time frame they have in mind (Stone, Greenberg, Kennedy-Moore, & Newman, 1991). Despite considerable evidence that personality influences coping choices (Suls, David, & Harvey, 1996), none of the studies reviewed related individual factors such as perceptual styles or personality characteristics to caregivers' coping responses.

## COPING AS A DAILY PROCESS

Gottlieb and Wolfe (2002) also encouraged investigators to adopt study designs that would capture coping close to its real-time occurrence and enable observation of coping as it unfolds over time. Daily process designs (Tennen & Affleck, 1996; Tennen, Affleck, Armeli, & Carney, 2000) might overcome numerous methodological limitations that emerged from their review: (1) Daily process studies are microlongitudinal and focus on the temporal unfolding of coping and adaptational outcomes; (2) their close to real-time orientation limits the recall error and bias that have plagued the caregiver coping literature; (3) these designs also track coping processes that might unfold rapidly in daily life; (4) daily process designs, by their very nature, require participants to focus on a particular time frame and a particular stressor; (5) the structure of daily process designs is idiographic–nomothetic (Tennen & Affleck, 1996); and (6) the logic of the data-analytic strategies used in these studies embeds daily processes within the person and contextual factors related to coping that thus far have been excluded from the family caregiver literature (see Affleck, Zautra, Tennen, & Armeli, 1999).

Although we are unaware of any study that has examined the daily coping efforts of family caregivers, we offer as an example of the promise of daily coping studies an investigation of how perceived benefits in the experience of chronic pain affected day-to-day psychological well-being. In a study of women with fibromyalgia, a chronic pain syndrome with unknown etiology, Affleck and Tennen (1996; Tennen & Affleck, 1999) examined the deliberate daily use of benefit cognitions, which they called *benefit-reminding*, and used a self-monitoring methodology to determine how benefit-reminding unfolds day to day.

The time-intensive self-monitoring methodology used in this study involved a combination of a nightly structured diary, with a computer-assisted, "real-time" assessment of pain intensity and mood several times each day. One item on the nightly questionnaire asked participants to describe how much that day they had reminded themselves of some of the benefits that have come from living with their chronic pain. Whereas 33 of 89 participants never reminded themselves of benefits, the remainder reported benefit-reminding on average 24 of the 30 study days. Some who had cited many benefits on an initial questionnaire never reminded themselves of these benefits during the subsequent month of daily recording. On the other hand, some who had cited only one benefit on the questionnaire also reported benefit-reminding on many days.

The design of this study enabled a within-person analysis of day-to-day differences in benefit-reminding, with day-to-day variation in pain and mood. Tennen and Affleck (1996) discovered that days characterized by more benefit-reminding did not differ in pain intensity, but they were accompanied by improved mood—specifically, increased levels of pleasant, aroused, and aroused–pleasant mood. All three mood dimension scores combined were found to be correlated with benefit-reminding frequency. Thus, on days when these chronic pain sufferers made greater efforts to remind themselves of the benefits that have come from their illness, they were especially more likely to experience pleasurable mood, regardless of their pain intensity on these days. It is easy to imagine how benefit-reminding among family caregivers might ease that day's emotional toll and actually engender positive mood.

The findings we have described fully support Gottlieb and Wolfe's (2002) call for family caregiving studies that examine particular ways of coping, such as finding benefits, and studies that turn to methods that track coping as it unfolds day to day, and those that employ longitudinal designs. Such study designs and methods promise to uncover the mechanisms through which caregiving demands lead to psychological and physical health outcomes, how coping efforts moderate the association between demands and health, and how coping unfolds in family caregivers' daily lives.

## FINDING BENEFITS IN THE BURDEN OF FAMILY CAREGIVING

Gottlieb and Wolfe (2002) concluded their review of the coping with family caregiving literature with a call for studies that examine particular ways of coping, such as finding benefits, rather than measuring many varied strategies simultaneously. We now describe the promise of examining the psychological and health consequences of benefit-finding as a coping strategy among family caregivers. We also demonstrate the virtues of daily process designs for studies of family caregiving that focus on benefit-finding or any other way of coping.

One way that individuals bring meaning to adversity is by finding some benefit or gain that would not have accrued otherwise. Individuals facing adversity frequently report benefits in their negative experiences (Affleck &

Tennen, 1996). Benefit-finding has been linked to psychological and physical health, and it plays a prominent role in theories of cognitive adaptation to threatening circumstances (Janoff-Bulman, 1992; Taylor, 1983).

Most of the studies reviewed by Gottlieb and Wolfe (2002) indirectly assessed benefit-finding nested within the Ways of Coping Checklist (WOCC; Folkman & Lazarus, 1988) and other coping measures. For example, the "Positive Reappraisal" subscale of the WOCC includes the items "Changed or grew as a person in a good way", "Rediscovered what is important in life," and "I was inspired to do something creative." More recently, studies of family caregiving have begun to follow Gottlieb and Wolfe's (2002) advice by focusing specifically on benefit-finding as a coping strategy (e.g., Rapp & Chao, 2000).

The majority of individuals who face threatening circumstances, including invasive medical treatment, life-threatening illness, chronic disability, HIV infection, rape, sexual abuse, accident, and natural disaster, appear to endorse at least some benefit (Tennen & Affleck, 2002). Longitudinal studies, although quite rare, seem to suggest that benefit-finding predicts subsequent psychological and health outcomes, a finding that is consistent with the literature on the health benefits of finding positive meaning (Folkman, Chesney, Collette, Boccellari, & Cooke, 1996).

Davis, Nolen-Hoeksema, and Larson (1998) conducted a prospective study of individuals whose parent, spouse, partner, child, or sibling was in hospice care. Seventy-three percent reported that they had found something positive in the experience, and their specific responses were consistent with those reported in cross-sectional studies of benefit-finding, including personal growth, new life perspective, strengthening family bonds, and support from others. Davis et al. examined whether finding a benefit 6 months following the loss predicted distress 7 months later. They found that benefit-finding predicted less distress at 13 months, even after controlling for the extent to which the loss "made sense." These investigators also found that it was not the number of benefits that held predictive value, but rather whether *any* benefit was endorsed.

In their study of mothers whose infants were in a newborn intensive care unit, Affleck, Tennen, and Rowe (1991) asked their participants whether they had found any benefits from their child's hazardous delivery and hospitalization. Seventy-five percent of these mothers cited at least one benefit, including improved relationships with family and friends, the importance of keeping life's problems in perspective, increased empathy, positive changes in their personality, and the certainty that their child was now even more precious to them. Benefit-finding not only predicted mothers' own well-being but also their child's developmental test scores 18 months later. This finding has particular relevance for caregivers of older family members, because it suggests that by extracting some benefit or gain from the caregiving experience, caregivers may be contributing to the health of the family member in their care.

Another demonstration that objective health outcomes can be predicted from earlier benefit-finding comes from a long-term study of men who survived a first heart attack (Affleck, Tennen, Croog, & Levine, 1987). Seven weeks after their initial heart attack, 58% of these men cited benefits, including anticipated changes in lifestyle, increased enjoyment, valued lessons about the importance of health behavior, and positive changes in their values and life philosophies. Eight years later (and controlling for age, socioeconomic status, and the severity of the initial attack), those men who had reported benefits were in better cardiac health and were less likely to have suffered another attack. That benefit-finding anticipated long-term health outcomes is especially noteworthy for the study of family caregivers, in view of the significant health consequences associated with caring for an older family member.

In a study of AIDS-related mortality among bereaved HIV-seropositive men who had been caregivers, Bower, Kemeny, Taylor, and Fahey (1998) found that benefit-finding anticipated CD4 T lymphocyte (helper T-cell) decline. Benefit-finding was also associated with a lower rate of AIDS-related mortality over the next 4–9 years. And the prospective relationship between benefit-finding and mortality was fully mediated by CD4 slope (i.e., the lower rate of AIDS-related mortality among those who had reported benefits was due to their less rapid decline in CD4 lymphocytes). This pattern of findings, in which benefit-finding appears to affect immunological functioning, which in turn affects mortality, seems particularly relevant to Kiecolt-Glaser et al.'s (2003) description of immune dysregulation among family caregivers that can linger for years after they end their caregiver role. It seems reasonable to speculate that benefit-finding moderates the prospective association between caregiver stress and compromised immune functioning.

## PSYCHOLOGICAL THEORIES COMMONLY USED TO EXPLAIN CAREGIVING STRATEGIES AND CONSEQUENCES

### Stress and Coping Theory

Despite the methodological limitations of coping research outlined earlier, the dominant paradigm used by social and behavioral scientists in family caregiver research is based on the stress and coping model (Lazarus, 1966), developed most creatively in the work of Pearlin and colleagues (e.g., Pearlin & Schooler, 1978; Pearlin, Mullan, Semple, & Skaff, 1990). In elaborating on the stress process underlying family care for relatives with dementia, Pearlin and colleagues presented a conceptual model linking the background and context of stress, the immediate sources of stress, mediators of stress (coping and social support), and the outcomes or manifestations of stress. Proponents of the stress and coping model have examined relationships between personality characteristics of caregivers and their coping styles (Hooker, Frazier, & Monahan, 1994). They also have articulated the impact of caregiver burden and coping styles on physical and mental health and well-being measures (Pruchno & Resch, 1989). Another valuable contribution of this paradigm has been the development a wide array of family caregiver outcomes based on self-reported symptoms, as well as physiological measures of health and well-being (Kiecolt-Glaser et al., 1991; Ory et al., 1999; Schulz et al., 1995).

This line of research has helped to underscore the practical value to family caregivers of developing coping skills to address the stresses associated with having cognitively and behaviorally impaired older relatives. The importance of social support as a stress buffer also helps explain why family caregivers turn to physicians for support (Silliman, 1989). Unfortunately, research thus far has shown that physicians provide only modest levels of emotional and informational support to family caregivers (Fortinsky, 2001). Little is known about the extent to which other health professionals provide support to caregivers.

## Self-Efficacy Theory

The distinguishing feature of self-efficacy is its reliance on behavior-specific domains to describe how certain or confident individuals believe they are in taking specific actions. In the context of chronic illness, perceived self-efficacy presumes that individuals have the capacity to assume control over their situations by learning about key aspects of care (Bandura, 1990; Lorig, Mazonson, & Holman, 1993). For example, measures of self-efficacy for pain management, exercise, and medication management have been devised for persons with arthritis (Lorig et al., 1993) or osteoporosis (Horan, Kim, Gendler, Froman, & Patel, 1998).

Much less work has adapted the concept and measurement of self-efficacy to family caregivers of persons with chronic illness. Equipped with adequate knowledge about chronic disease and disability management, caregivers could become "psychological activists" (Thoits, 1994), proactively shaping their lives as caregivers. The paradigm of social learning and self-efficacy, therefore, could fruitfully complement the stress and coping theoretical approach to understanding caregiving and its consequences. Family caregiver self-efficacy is especially important to consider when older relatives have Alzheimer's disease or another dementia, because as this disease process progresses, the caregiving career increasingly includes responsibility for carrying out specific care and care management behaviors (Aneshensel, Pearlin, Mullan, Zarit, & Whitlatch, 1995). Measures of family caregiver mastery and competence have been developed (Lawton, Kleban, Moss, Rovine, & Glicksman, 1989; Pearlin et al., 1990), but these represent global constructs, without reference to specific behaviors.

Several investigators have begun developing more domain-specific measures of family caregiver self-efficacy. For example, a measurement approach for "coping efficacy" among caregivers of persons with dementia focused on how often caregivers reported ways of dealing with stressors (Gignac & Gottlieb, 1996). Haley and colleagues (1996) briefly described a measure of family caregiver self-efficacy (i.e., confidence) in managing dementia-related problems. Zeiss and colleagues (1999) reported on the development and testing of caregiver self-efficacy scales covering two domains: caregiver self-care and problem solving to cope with the daily challenges of caregiving. A revised version of these scales was also tested for reliability and validity, covering three domains: obtaining respite, responding to disruptive patient behaviors, and controlling upsetting thoughts (Steffen, McKibbin, Zeiss, Gallagher-Thompson, & Bandura, 2001). Finally, caregiver self-efficacy measures incorporating the domains of dementia symptom management and community support service use have also been developed and tested (Fortinsky et al., 2002). Future research should employ such measures of caregiver self-efficacy as outcomes to help judge the effectiveness of caregivers' encounters with primary care physicians and other health care professionals.

## Cognitive-Behavioral Problem-Solving Theory

Cognitive-behavioral problem-solving theory is based on the premise that problems must be defined in the individual's own terms, that the individual's thinking and feeling about the problem must be clarified, and that problems must be reframed in more positive ways, paving the way to consider productive problem-solving strategies (Burgio, Solano, Fisher, Stevens, & Gallagher-Thompson, 2003; Goldstein & Noonan, 1999). Cognitive-behavioral problem-solving treatment strategies assume a relationship among beliefs, emotions, and behavior; therefore, beliefs about an experience impact how an individual will behave in that situation (Burgio et al., 2003). For example, many ethnic/minority individuals have negative beliefs about the use of community-based health and social services originating from past experiences and a desire to keep problems private, within the family system. Beliefs associated with this learned mistrust of formal services must be identified and acknowledged before problem solving can begin.

## EMPIRICALLY TESTED INTERVENTIONS TO HELP REDUCE HEALTH AND PSYCHOLOGICAL CONSEQUENCES

Numerous models of group-based and individual–family caregiver interventions have been developed and tested to relieve the burdens of caregiving and to educate families about dementia and other chronic illnesses. A recent review of these interventions found that family caregivers showed the best health outcomes when education and counseling support were offered together (Sorensen, Pinquart, & Duberstein, 2002). This review noted the lack of inclusion of ethnic and racial/minority groups in caregiver intervention studies, even though dementia strikes members of ethnic and racial/minority groups at least as commonly as Whites in the general population (Sorensen et al., 2002), and despite findings that family caregivers from ethnic and racial/minority groups have been found to be less likely than whites to use community-based services to support their own care (Dillworth-Anderson, Williams, & Gibson, 2002; Williams & Dillworth-Anderson, 2002). Several caregiver intervention studies published following this review did include members of ethnic and racial/minority groups in randomized trials, and all found that psychological outcomes such as depression and coping skills could be positively affected in ethnic and racial/minority groups as well as in whites, using carefully implemented intervention protocols (Burgio, Stevens, Guy, Roth, & Hayley, 2003; Eisdorfer, Czaja, Loewenstein, Rubert, Arguelles, Mitrani, et al., 2003; Gallagher-Thompson, Coon, Solano, Ambler, Rabinowitz, & Thompson, 2003; Gitlin, Winter, Corcoran, Dennis, Schinfeld, & Hauck, 2003). Whether or not these controlled research results can be replicated in practice with diverse ethnic and racial/minority groups awaits further study.

Another meta-analysis of interventions designed specifically for family caregivers of older adults with dementia found that the most beneficial outcomes were a reduction in psychological morbidity in caregivers and increased likelihood that nursing home admission could be delayed (Brodaty, Green, & Koschera, 2003). Interventions that provided individualized flexibility depending on caregivers' needs, and those that attempted to involve both the person with dementia and the caregiver, were more likely to achieve beneficial outcomes (Brodaty et al., 2003).

## CONCLUSIONS

Several conclusions may be drawn based on this review of literature on health and psychological consequences of caring for older family members with chronic illnesses and disabilities. First, more prospective, longitudinal study designs utilizing methodologies, such as daily process approaches, are sorely needed in caregiving research to illuminate coping patterns and potentially positive aspects of caregiving, such as benefit-finding. Second, translational studies exploring links among immunological markers of stress, self-reported caregiver stress, and specific health outcomes among caregivers would build upon the work pioneered by Kiecolt-Glaser and Vitaliano (Kiecolt-Glaser et al., 1991, 1996, 2003; Vitaliano, 1997; Vitaliano et al., 2002, 2003, 2004). Third, interventions that integrate components from the major psychological theoretical schools of thought might be especially effective in relieving negative consequences of caregiving, particularly interventions that combine self-efficacy with cognitive-behavioral problem-solving components. Finally, all of these types of studies should maximize caregiver diversity to enhance external validity, particularly in terms of racial and ethnic background of caregivers and their older relatives, and in terms of the type of chronic disease and level of disability of older adults cared for by family members.

## REFERENCES

Affleck, G., & Tennen, H. (1996). Construing benefits from adversity: Adaptational significance and dispositional underpinnings. *Journal of Personality, 64,* 899–922.

Affleck, G., Tennen, H., Croog, S., & Levine, S. (1987). Causal attribution, perceived benefits, and morbidity following a heart attack: An eight-year study. *Journal of Consulting and Clinical Psychology, 55,* 29–35.

Affleck, G., Tennen, H., & Rowe, J. (1991). *Infants in crises: How parents cope with newborn intensive care and its aftermath.* New York: Springer-Verlag.

Affleck, G., Zautra, A., Tennen, H., & Armeli, S. (1999). Multilevel daily process designs for consulting and clinical psychology: A preface for the perplexed. *Journal of Consulting and Clinical Psychology, 67,* 746–754.

Aneshensel, C. S., Pearlin, L. I., Mullan, J. T., Zarit, S. H., & Whitlatch, C. J. (1995). *Profiles in caregiving: The unexpected career.* San Diego: Academic Press.

Bandura, A. (1990). Self-efficacy mechanism in physiological activation and health-promoting behavior. In J. Madden (Ed.), *Neurobiology of learning, emotion, and affect* (pp. 229–269). New York: Raven Press.

Barker, J. C. (2002). Neighbors, friends, and other nonkin caregivers of community-living dependent elders. *Journals of Gerontology: Psychological Sciences and Social Sciences, Series B, 57,* S158–S167.

Barsky, A. J., Peekna, H. M., & Borus, J. F. (2001). Somatic symptom reports in women and men. *Journal of General Internal Medicine, 16,* 266–275.

Beach, S. R., Schulz, R., Yee, J. L., & Jackson, S. (2000). Negative and positive health effects of caring for a disabled spouse: Longitudinal findings from the caregiver health effects study. *Psychology and Aging, 15,* 259–271.

Beisecker, A. E., Chrisman, S. K., & Wright, L. J. (1997). Perceptions of family caregivers of persons with Alzheimer's disease: Communication with physicians. *American Journal of Alzheimer's Disease, 12,* 73–83.

Berg-Weger, M., Rubio, D. M., & Tebb, S. S. (2000). Living with and caring for older family members: Issues related to caregiver well-being. *Journal of Gerontological Social Work, 33,* 47–62.

Bookwala, J., & Schultz, R. (1998). The role of neuroticism and mastery in spouse caregivers' assessment of and response to a contextual stressor. *Journals of Gerontology: Psychological Sciences and Social Sciences, Series B, 53,* 155–164.

Bookwala, J., & Schultz, R. (2000). A comparison of primary stressors, secondary stressors, and depressive symptoms between elderly caregiving husbands and wives: The Caregiver Health Effects study. *Psychology and Aging, 15,* 607–616.

Bookwala, J., Yee, J. L., & Schulz, R. (2000). Caregiving and detrimental mental and physical health outcomes. In G. M. Williamson, D. R. Shaffer, & P. A. Parmelee (Eds.), *Physical illness and depression in older adults: A handbook of theory, re-*

search, and practice. (pp. 93–131). Dordrecht, the Netherlands: Kluwer Academic.

Bourgeois, M. S., Schulz, R., & Burgio, L. (1996). Interventions for caregivers of patients with Alzheimer's disease: A review and analysis of content, process, and outcomes. *International Journal of Aging and Human Development, 43*(1), 35–92.

Bower, J. E., Kemeny, M. E., Taylor, S. E., & Fahey, J. L. (1998). Cognitive processing, discovery of meaning, CD4 decline, and AIDS-related mortality among bereaved HIV-seropositive men. *Journal of Consulting and Clinical Psychology, 66*, 979–986.

Brodaty, H., Green, A., & Koschera, A. (2003). Meta-analysis of psychosocial interventions for caregivers of people with dementia. *Journal of the American Geriatrics Society, 51,* 657–664.

Burgio, L. D., Solano, N., Fisher, S. E., Stevens, A., & Gallagher-Thompson, D. (2003). Skill building: Psychoeducational strategies. In D. W. Coon, D. Gallagher-Thompson, & L. W. Thompson (Eds.), *Innovative interventions to reduce dementia caregiver distress* (pp. 119–138). New York: Springer.

Burgio, L., Stevens, A., Guy, D., Roth, D. L., & Hayley, W. E. (2003). Impact of two psychosocial interventions on white and African-American family caregivers of individuals with dementia. *Gerontologist, 43*, 568–579.

Calderon, V., & Tennstedt, S. L. (1998). Ethnic differences in the expression of caregiver burden: Results of a qualitative study. *Journal of Gerontological Social Work, 30*, 159–178.

Canadian Study of Health and Aging Working Group. (2002). Patterns of health effects of caring for people with dementia: The impact of changing cognitive and residential status. *Gerontologist, 42*, 643–652.

Cohen, S., Kessler, R. C., & Underwood-Gordon, L. (Eds.). (1997). *Measuring stress: A guide for health and social scientists.* New York: Oxford University Press.

Coyne, J. C., & Gottlieb, B. H. (1996). The mismeasure of coping by checklist. *Journal of Personality, 64*, 959–991.

Cullen, J. S., Grayson, D. A., & Jorm, A. F. (1997). Clinical diagnoses and disability of cognitively impaired older persons as predictors of stress in their carers. *International Journal of Geriatric Psychiatry, 12*(10), 1019–1028.

Davis, C. G., Nolen-Hoeksema, S., & Larson, J. (1998). Making sense of loss and benefiting from the experience: Two construals of meaning. *Journal of Personality and Social Psychology, 75*, 561–574.

Dilworth-Anderson, P., & Anderson, N. B. (1994). Dementia caregiving in Blacks: A contextual approach to research. In B. Lebowitz, E. Light, & G. Neiderehe (Eds.), *Mental and physical health of Alzheimer's caregivers* (pp. 385–409). New York: Springer.

Dilworth-Anderson, P., Williams, I. C., & Gibson, B. E. (2002). Issues of race, ethnicity, and culture in caregiving research: A 20-year review. *Gerontologist, 42,* 237–272.

Dunkin, J. J., & Anderson-Hanley, C. (1998). Dementia caregiver burden: A review of the literature and guidelines for assessment and intervention. *Neurology, 5*, S53–S60.

Eisdorfer, C., Czaja, S. J., Loewenstein, D. A., Rubert, M. P., Arguelles, S., Mitrani, V. B., et al. (2003). The effect of a family therapy and technology based intervention on caregiver depression. *Gerontologist, 43*, 514–531.

Folkman, S., Chesney, M., Collette, L., Boccellari, A., & Cooke, M. (1996). Postberevement depressive mood and its preberevement predictors in HIV+ and HIV-gay men. *Journal of Personality and Social Psychology, 70,* 336–348.

Folkman, S., & Lazarus, R. S. (1988). *The Ways of Coping Questionnaire.* Palo Alto, CA: Consulting Psychologists Press.

Fortinsky, R. H. (1998). How linked are physicians to community support services for their patients with dementia? *Journal of Applied Gerontology, 17,* 482–500.

Fortinsky, R. H. (2001). Health care triads and dementia care: Integrative framework and future directions. *Aging and Mental Health, 5,* S35–S48.

Fortinsky, R. H., Kercher, K., & Burant, C. J. (2002). Measurement and correlates of family caregiver self efficacy for managing dementia. *Aging and Mental Health, 6,* 153–160.

Fuller-Jonap, F., & Haley, W. E. (1995). Mental and physical health of male caregivers of a spouse with Alzheimer's disease. *Journal of Aging and Health, 7*(1), 99–118.

Gallagher-Thompson, D., Coon, D. W., Solano, N., Ambler, C., Rabinowitz, Y., & Thompson, L. W. (2003). Change in indices of distress among Latino and Anglo female caregivers of elderly relatives with dementia: Site-specific results from the REACH national collaborative study. *Gerontologist, 43,* 580–591.

Gignac, M. A., & Gottlieb, B. H. (1996). Caregivers' appraisals of efficacy in coping with dementia. *Psychology and Aging, 11,* 214–225.

Gitlin, L. N., Winter, L., Corcoran, M., Dennis, M., Schinfeld, S., & Hauck, W. (2003). Effects of the home environment skill-building program on the caregiver–care recipient dyad: Six-month outcomes from the Philadelphia REACH initiative. *Gerontologist, 43,* 532–546.

Goldstein, E., & Noonan, M. (1999). *Short-term treatment and social work practice: An integrative perspective.* New York: Free Press.

Gottlieb, B. H., & Wolfe, J. (2002). Coping with family caregiving to persons with dementia: A critical review. *Aging and Mental Health, 6,* 325–342.

Grunfeld, E., Glossop, R., McDowell, I., & Danbrook, C. (1997). Caring for elderly people at home: The consequences to caregivers. *Canadian Medical Association Journal, 157*(8), 1101–1105.

Haley W. E., Roth, D. L., Coleton, M. I., Ford, G. R., West, C. A. C., Collins, R. P. et al. (1996). Appraisal, coping, and social support as mediators of well-being in black and white family caregivers of patients with Alzheimer's disease. *Journal of Consulting and Clinical Psychology, 64,* 121–129.

Hooker, K., Frazier, L. D., & Monahan, D. J. (1994). Personality and coping among caregivers of spouses with dementia. *Gerontologist, 34,* 386–392.

Hooker, K., Monahan, D. J., Bowman, S. R., Frazier, L. D., & Shifren, K. (1998). Personality counts for a lot: Predictors of mental and physical health of spouse caregivers in two disease groups. *Journals of Gerontology: Psychological Sciences and Social Sciences, Series B, 53,* 73–85.

Horan, M. L., Kim, K. K., Gendler, P., Froman, R. D., & Patel, M. D. (1998). Development and evaluation of the Osteoporosis Self-Efficacy Scale. *Research in Nursing and Health, 21,* 395–403.

Janoff-Bulman, R. (1992). *Shattered assumptions: Towards a new psychology of trauma.* New York: Free Press.

Jutras, S., & Lavoie, J. P. (1995). Living with an impaired elderly person: The informal caregivers' physical and mental health. *Journal of Aging and Health, 7*(1), 46–73.

Kiecolt-Glaser, J. K., Dura, J. R., Speicher, C. E., Trask, O. J., & Glaser, R. (1991). Spousal caregivers of dementia victims: Longitudinal changes in immunity and health. *Psychosomatic Medicine, 53,* 345–362.

Kiecolt-Glaser, J. K., Glaser, R., Gravenstein, S., Malarkey, W. B., & Sheridan, J. (1996). Chronic stress alters the immune response to influenza virus vaccine in older adults. *Proceedings of the National Academy of Sciences, USA, 93*(7), 30–43.

Kiecolt-Glaser, J. K., Preacher, K. J., MacCallum, R. C., Atkinson, C., Malarkey, W. B., & Glaser, R. (2003). Chronic stress and age-related increases in the prominflammatory cytokine IL-6. *Proceedings of the National Academy of Sciences of the United States of America, 100*, 9090–9095.

Kramer, B. J., & Kipnis, S. (1995). Eldercare and work role conflict: Toward an understanding of gender differences in caregiver burden. *Gerontologist, 35*, 340–348.

Lawton, M. P., Kleban, M. H., Moss, M., Rovine, M., & Glicksman, A. (1989). Measuring caregiving appraisal. *Journals of Gerontology: Psychological Sciences and Social Sciences, Series B, 44*, P61–P71.

Lazarus, R. S. (1966). *Psychological stress and coping process.* New York: McGraw-Hill.

Lichtenberg, P. A., Manning, C. A., & Turkheimer, E. (1992). Memory dysfunction in depressed spousal caregivers. *Clinical Gerontologist, 12*(1), 77–80.

Li., L. W., Seltzer, M. M., & Greenberg, J. S. (1997). Social support and depressive symptoms: Differential patterns in wife and daughter caregivers. *Journals of Gerontology: Psychological Sciences and Social Sciences, Series B, 52*, S200–S211.

Lorig, K. R., Mazonson, P. D., & Holman, H. R. (1993). Evidence suggesting that health education for self management in patients with chronic arthritis has sustained health benefits while reducing health care costs. *Arthritis and Rheumatism, 36*, 439–446.

McEwen, B. S. (2000). The neurobiology of stress: From serendipity to clinical relevance. *Brain Research, 886*, 172–189.

Miller, B. (1990). Gender differences in spouse caregiver strain: Socialization and role expectations. *Journal of Marriage and the Family, 52*, 311–321.

Miller, B., Campbell, R. T., Farran, C. J., Kaufman, J. R., & Davis, L. (1995). Race, control, mastery, and caregiver distress. *Journals of Gerontology: Psychological Sciences and Social Sciences, Series B, 50*, S374–S382.

Moritz, D. J., Kasl, S. V., & Berkman, L. F. (1989). The health impact of living with a cognitively impaired elderly spouse: Depressive symptoms and social functioning. *Journals of Gerontology: Psychological Sciences and Social Sciences, Series B, 44*(1), S17–S27.

Nagaratnam, N., Lewis-Jones, M., Scott, D., & Palazzi, L. (1998). Behavioral and psychiatric manifestations in dementia patients in a community: Caregiver burden and outcome. *Alzheimer's Disease and Associated Disorders, 12*(4), 330–334.

National Alliance for Caregiving & AARP. (2004). *Caregiving in the U.S.* Retrieved from www.caregiving.org on May 10, 2004.

Noelker, L. S., & Whitlatch, C. J. (2005). Informal caregiving. In C. J. Evashwick (Ed.), *The continuum of long-term care* (3rd ed., pp. 29–47). Clifton Park, NY: Thomson Delmar Learning.

Ory, M. G., Hoffman, R. R., Yee, J. L., Tennstedt, S., & Schulz, R. (1999). Prevalence and impact of caregiving: A detailed comparison between dementia and non-dementia caregivers. *Gerontologist, 39*, 177–185.

Pearlin, L. I., Mullan, J. T., Semple, S. J., & Skaff, M. M. (1990). Caregiving and the stress process: An overview of concepts and their measures. *The Gerontologist, 30*, 583–584.

Pearlin, L. I., & Schooler, C. (1978). The structure of coping. *Journal of Health and Social Behavior, 19*, 2–21.

Penning, M. J. (2002). Hydra revisited: Substituting formal for self- and informal in-home care among older adults with disabilities. *Gerontologist, 42*, 4–16.

Pinquart, M., & Sorensen, S., (2005). Ethnic differences in stressors, resources, and psychological outcomes of family caregiving: A meta-analysis. *Gerontologist, 45*, 90–106.

Powers, D. V., Gallagher-Thompson, D., & Kraemer, H. C. (2002). Coping and depression in Alzheimer's caregivers: Longitudinal evidence of stability. *Journals of Gerontology: Psychological Sciences and Social Sciences, Series B, 57*, P205–P211.

Pruchno, R. A., & Potashnik, S. L. (1989). Caregiving spouses: Physical and mental health in perspective. *Journal of the American Geriatrics Society, 37*, 697–705.

Pruchno, R. A., & Resch, N. L. (1989). Mental health of caregiving spouses: Coping as mediator, moderator, or main effect? *Psychology and Aging, 4*, 454–463.

Rapp, S. R., & Chao, D. (2000). Appraisals of strain and gain: Effects on psychological well-being of caregivers of dementia patients. *Aging and Mental Health, 4*, 142–147.

Ross, M. (1989). Relation of implicit theories to the construction of personal histories. *Psychological Review, 96*, 341–357.

Salovey, P., & Birnbaum, D. (1989). Influence of mood on health-relevant cognitions. *Journal of Personality and Social Psychology, 57*, 539–551.

Schulz, R., & Beach, S. R. (1999). Caregiving as a risk factor for mortality: The caregiver health effects study. *Journal of the American Medical Association, 282*, 2215–2219.

Schulz, R., O'Brien, A. T., Bookwala, J., & Fleissner, K. (1995). Psychiatric and physical morbidity effects of dementia caregiving: Prevalence, correlates, and causes. *The Gerontologist, 35*, 771–791.

Schulz, R., & Williamson, G. M. (1991). A 2-year longitudinal study of depression among Alzheimer's caregivers. *Psychology and Aging, 6*, 569–578.

Shaw, W. S., Patterson, T. L., Semple, S. J., Ho, S., Irwin, M. R., Hauger, R. L., et al. (1997). Longitudinal analysis of multiple indicators of health decline among spousal caregivers. *Annals of Behavioral Medicine, 19*, 101–109.

Silliman, R. A. (1989). Caring for the frail older patients: The doctor–patient–family caregiver relationship. *Journal of Genereal Internal Medicine, 4*, 237–241.

Singer, J. A., & Salovey, P. (1993). *The remembered self: Emotion and memory in personality.* New York: Free Press.

Skaff, M. M., Pearlin, L. I., & Mullan, J. T. (1996). Transitions in the caregiving career: Effects on sense of mastery. *Psychology and Aging, 11*, 247–257.

Smerglia, V. L., & Deimling, G. T. (1997). Care-related decision-making satisfaction and caregiver well-being in families caring for older members. *Gerontologist, 37*, 658–665.

Sorensen, S., Pinquart, M., & Duberstein, P. (2002). How effective are interventions with caregivers?: An updated meta-analysis. *Gerontologist, 42*, 356–372.

Steffen, A. M., McKibbin, C., Zeiss, A. M., Gallagher-Thompson, D., & Bandura, A. (2001). The revised scale for caregiving self-efficacy: Reliability and validity studies. *Journals of Gerontology: Psychological Sciences and Social Sciences, Series B, 57*, P74–P86.

Stone, A. A., Greenberg, M. A., Kennedy-Moore, E., & Newman, M. G. (1991). Self-report, situation-specific coping questionnaires: What are they measuring? *Journal of Personality and Social Psychology, 61*, 648–658.

Suls, J., David, J. P., & Harvey, J. H. (1996). Personality and coping. *Journal of Personality, 64,* 711–735.

Taylor, S. E. (1983). Adjustment to threatening events: A theory of cognitive adaptation. *American Psychologist, 38,* 1161–1173.

Tennen, H., & Affleck, G. (1996). Daily processes in coping with chronic pain: Methods and analytic strategies. In M. Zeidner & N. S. Endler (Eds.), *Handbook of coping* (pp. 151–177). New York: Wiley.

Tennen, H., & Affleck, G. (1999). Finding benefits in adversity. In C. R. Snyder (Ed.), *Coping: The psychology of what works* (pp. 279–304). New York: Oxford University Press.

Tennen, H., & Affleck, G. (2002) Benefit-finding and benefit-reminding. In C. R. Synder & S. Lopez (Eds.), *The handbook of positive psychology* (pp. 584–597). New York: Oxford University Press.

Tennen, H., Affleck, G., Armeli, S., & Carney, M. A. (2000). A daily process approach to coping: Linking theory, research, and practice. *American Psychologist, 55,* 626–636.

Thoits, P. A. (1994). Stressors and problem solving: The individual as psychological activist. *Journal of Health and Social Behavior, 35,* 143–159.

Vitaliano, P. P. (1997). Physiological and physical concomitants to caregiving: Introduction to special issue. *Annals of Behavioral Medicine, 19,* 75–77.

Vitaliano, P. P., Scanlan, J. M., Zhang, J., Savage, M. V., Hirsch, I., & Siegler, I. C. (2002). A path model of chronic stress, the metabolic syndrome, and coronary heart disease. *Psychosomatic Medicine, 64,* 418–435.

Vitaliano, P. P., Young, H. M., & Zhang, J. (2004). Is caregiving a risk factor for illness? *Current Directions in Psychological Science, 13,* 13–16.

Vitaliano, P. P., Zhang, J., & Scanlan, J. M. (2003). Is caregiving hazardous to one's physical health?: A meta-analysis. *Psychological Bulletin, 129,* 946–972.

Williams, S. W., & Dilworth-Anderson, P. (2002). Systems of social support in families who care for dependent African-American elders. *Gerontologist, 42,* 224–236.

Yee, J. L., & Schulz, R. (2000). Gender differences in psychiatric morbidity among family caregivers: A review and analysis. *Gerontologist, 40,* 147–164.

Zeiss, A. M., Gallagher-Thompson, D., Lovett, S., Rose, J., & McKibbin, C. (1999). Self-efficacy as a mediator of caregiver coping: Development and testing of an assessment model. *Journal of Clinical Geropsychology, 5,* 221–230.

# CHAPTER 13

# Psychosocial Stress, Emotion Regulation, and Resilience among Older Adults

MARY C. DAVIS, ALEX J. ZAUTRA,
LISA M. JOHNSON, KATE E. MURRAY,
*and* HEATHER A. OKVAT

A common view of the changes wrought by aging is reflected in Bette Davis's famous statement that "old age is no place for sissies." This view focuses on the negative repercussions of dealing with age-related physical and psychological changes that require some level of adaptation, often quite substantial. Physical capacity declines and risk for the development of chronic and disabling diseases, such as arthritis, increases. Moreover, the experience of psychosocial stressors including the loss of loved ones and peers also occurs at greater levels as individuals get older. This focus on age-related losses suggests that growing older is best characterized as an inexorable descent into a life of ever-increasing limitation.

Another, more optimistic view draws on the observation that many older individuals maintain full and active lives up until the very end of life. Perhaps most important given the high prevalence of age-related illnesses, even those with significant health concerns can continue to be engaged in life despite their physical limitations. What characteristics determine an individual's resilience in the face of challenges associated with aging and permit recovery from difficulty and preservation of capacity over the long term? A hint is offered in the words of 19th-century author Thomas Aldrich: "To keep the heart unwrinkled, to be hopeful, kindly, cheerful, reverent, that is to triumph over old age."

## POSITIVE EMOTIONS AND AGING

Aldrich's observation is aligned with accruing research evidence that points to a capacity to sustain positive emotions as an important factor in promoting optimal functioning and high quality of life among older adults. Perhaps not surprisingly, a steady diet of positive emotion is related to increased psychological health and well-being (e.g., Affleck & Tennen, 1996). Recent data point to the impact of positive affect on physical health outcomes as well (e.g., Moskowitz, 2003; Ostir, Ottenbacher, & Markides, 2004). In one example, the Nun Study (Danner, Snowdon, & Friesen, 2001), researchers examined the relation between the emotional content in handwritten autobiographies recorded in early young adulthood and mortality some six decades later in a sample of 180 Catholic nuns. These autobiographies were coded for the expression of positive, negative, or neutral emotional experiences. Sixty years later, mortality among nuns in the lowest quartile of positive emotional expression was 2.5 times higher than the mortality of those in the highest quartile, a difference that translated into approximately an additional 7 years of life in the group of nuns with the greatest positive emotional expression.

How might positive emotions impact on health? In their review of the literature, Salovey, Rothman, Detweiler, and Steward (2000) described the physiological, cognitive, social, and behavioral pathways linking emotional states to physical health outcomes. At the physiological level, positive emotions are related to more adaptive cardiovascular and immune system responses (e.g., Cohen, Doyle, Turner, Alper, & Skoner, 2003). Positive emotions are also related to more abundant cognitive resources, including greater feelings of self-efficacy and increased willingness to process threatening information thoroughly, at least in some circumstances. With regard to social and behavioral pathways, a more positive emotional style relates to an increased ability to elicit social support from the environment and to higher levels of health-promoting behavior.

A key area of interest in research on resilient emotions has been on uncovering changes in the experience of emotions across the lifespan. The bulk of available data suggest that there is a small but reliable increase in positive emotions as individuals get older (Mroczek & Kolarz, 1998; Carstensen, Pasupathi, Mayr, & Nesselroade, 2000). In addition, there appears to be a significant decrease in the experience of negative emotions, such that the highest levels of negative emotions occur in the early adult years and gradually decline until about age 60, when they level off (Carstensen et al., 2000). Corresponding findings are evident in research on emotional expression. In data gleaned from over 3,000 individuals who participated in studies regarding disclosure of emotional events in their lives, age was related to use of more positive affect and fewer negative affect words (Pennebaker & Stone, 2004). The changes in emotional experiences associated with aging appear to be reflected in changes in the functioning of brain regions associated with emotion processing. For example, Mather and colleagues (2004) used functional magnetic resonance imaging (fMRI) to examine the brain activation patterns in younger and older adults while they viewed positive, negative, and neutral emotional pictures. Among older adults, activation of the amygdala, a brain structure that plays a central role in integrating emotional experiences, was more pronounced in viewing positive versus negative pictures, whereas among younger adults, degree of activation was similar across the positive and negative pictures.

Given the shift toward the experience of more positive and less negative emotion that occurs with age, we might expect that personality attributes associated with emotional experiencing also change. Although early theories suggested that personality characteristics are highly heritable and essentially "fixed" by age 30 (McCrae & Costa, 1999), there is increasing evidence that not only does personality change over the course of a lifetime, but the changes may be also most pronounced in adulthood (Srivastava, John, Gosling, & Potter, 2003). Reliable changes across the lifespan have been observed in some of the traits described by the five-factor model of personality, including decreases in neuroticism and increases in conscientiousness (Srivastava et al., 2003). Of the Big Five personality attributes, neuroticism arguably has the clearest associations with elevated negative affects (and low positive affect; e.g., Mroczek & Kolarz, 1998), including depressive and anxiety symptoms, and unhappiness (e.g., Hayes & Joseph, 2003). Moreover, exposure to negative emotional stimuli yields increased brain activation in the left temporal cortex, the extent of which is associated with neuroticism (Canli et al., 2001). In contrast, exposure to positive emotional stimuli is associated with increased activity of the right temporal cortex, activation that correlates with extraversion rather than neuroticism (Canli et al., 2001; Canli, 2004). Fewer data are available regarding the emotional concomitants of conscientiousness, but there is evidence that conscientiousness is related to higher ratings of life satisfaction and of subjective well-being (Hayes & Joseph, 2003). Thus, the decrease in neuroticism and increase in conscientiousness that occur over the lifespan correspond to the increased positive affect and decreased negative affect observed among older relative to younger adults.

Accruing evidence, then, suggests that the balance of emotional experiencing shifts with age. These findings coincide with Carstensen's socioemotional selectivity theory of functioning in adulthood, which posits that affect becomes much more salient to individuals as they get older and become more adept at regulating their emotions (Carstensen, Isaacowitz, & Charles, 1999). With aging comes a recognition of a foreshortened future, and under these perceived time constraints, individuals shift their goals to find emotional satisfaction and meaning in their existing relationships.

Therefore, despite other setbacks in life, such as psychological and physical hardships, older adults seek positive emotional experiences (and avoid negative experiences) to a greater extent than do younger adults. Their social networks become smaller, but their experience of social integration within these relationships becomes greater (Carstensen et al., 1999).

Older adults become adroit at not only attending to positive emotions but also appreciating the fleeting nature of their emotions. They are able to focus on interpreting the larger meaning of the situations they encounter, and to value both the positive and negative aspects of their experiences. Positive and negative emotions become less tightly bound together, reflecting greater complexity of emotional experiencing (Carstensen et al., 2000). As development proceeds, individuals are able to achieve greater emotional differentiation and regulation over time, despite declines in cognitive and physical functioning associated with aging. This prepares older adults to manage additional challenges and to maintain their physical and psychological functioning even when they encounter setbacks. Our own work, described below, builds on the theory that sustaining affective differentiation may be an important key to resilience over the lifespan, particularly in the face of challenges such as pain and stress.

## EMOTIONAL COMPLEXITY AND RESILIENCE DURING STRESS IN CHRONIC PAIN

Although emotional complexity differs between people (e.g., Carstensen et al., 2000), we have argued that it also varies within people over time, a perspective reflected in the dynamic model of affect (DMA; e.g., Reich, Zautra, & Davis, 2003; Zautra, Smith, Affleck, & Tennen, 2001). The processing of emotion always occurs in an environmental context. In a safe and predictable environment, individuals process information from multiple sources, including emotional inputs, to develop an adaptive response. This complex processing demands substantial resources but provides a complex and nuanced assessment of the current demands imposed by the environment. Thus, in calm and predictable times, individuals acquire information arising from both negative and positive features of a situation. In these circumstances, positive and negative affective registers provide the broadest range of information, allowing maximal flexibility in developing the most favorable response on a moment-to-moment basis. In times of low stress, then, positive and negative affects should be relatively uncorrelated.

During times of stress and uncertainty, resources to engage in complex, time-consuming processing are no longer available. The press is toward more simplified and rapid judgments that allow for quick responses designed to alleviate the discomfort of the situation. Negative information takes precedence at the expense of positive, and attention narrows to focus on the immediate demands and potential threats to well-being. As a consequence, during times of stress, positive and negative affects fuse to become a simple bipolar dimension, reflected in a high inverse relationship between the two.

The DMA posits that stressful contexts influence affective information processing to some extent for all individuals, and indeed, in work examining affective dynamics among healthy individuals, we have found evidence consistent with the prediction (e.g., Zautra, Reich, Davis, Potter, & Nicolson, 2000), as have other investigators (Pruchno & Meeks, 2004). Yet the model may be especially relevant for individuals managing chronic pain. Chronic pain, a common medical condition found in aging adults (Wijeratne, Shome, Hickie, & Koschera, 2001), has an affective component (Fernandez & Turk, 1992; Melzak & Wall, 1965). Typically, patients with chronic pain experience greater elevations in negative affective states, such as depression and anxiety. The link between pain and negative affect is well established across a range of medical conditions, including osteoarthritis and fibromyalgia (Affleck, Tennen, Urrows, & Higgins, 1992; Zautra et al., 2001). Cognitive resources may already be stretched to the limit for patients with pain, particularly when they are distressed (Hart, Wade, & Martelli, 2003). Not surprisingly, patients with chronic pain are more likely than healthy individual to report a tendency to process information in a simple fashion (Reich, Zautra, & Potter, 2001). Many of the difficulties with emotions that accompany stress, in fact, are also apparent among those in chronic pain (Fernandez & Turk, 1992; Melzak & Wall, 1965). These findings are consistent with the notion that the chronic pain condition itself may serve as a stressor, reducing the individual's capacity for information processing and shrinking affective experiences.

One approach to test the DMA in patients with pain is to examine whether the relation between positive affect (PA) and negative affect (NA) shifts during episodes of pain. If pain functions as a stressor, PA and NA should become more highly related when pain levels are high. We explored this possibility in a study of women with rheumatoid arthritis or osteoarthritis who were interviewed weekly for 12 weeks regarding their experience of pain, PA, and NA (Zautra et al., 2001, Study 1), using multilevel modeling to examine within-person changes in PA–NA relations. Consistent with past research, weekly increases in pain and decreases in PA each predicted weekly increases in NA (both $p$'s < .001). Of particular relevance for the current question, changes in PA and pain interacted to predict changes in NA ($p$ < .01). Just as the DMA would predict, increases in weekly pain were related to a stronger inverse relationship between weekly PA and NA.

A similar pattern emerged in a sample of female pain patients diagnosed with fibromyalgia, a widespread pain syndrome of unknown etiology that affects approximately 4% of adult women (Lawrence et al., 1998). Patients with fibromyalgia reported on their pain and affect three times per day for 30 consecutive days (Zautra et al., 2001, Study 2). Multilevel modeling again yielded an interaction between changes in daily PA and pain in the prediction of NA ($p < .01$), indicating that PA had a stronger inverse relationship with NA when pain was high, a pattern that is in line with the findings for patients with rheumatoid arthritis. Thus, in two samples of patients assessed across differing time frames, we demonstrated that affective states appear to become less differentiated with the stress of increased pain. We have since replicated these findings in a second study of patients with fibromyalgia and osteoarthritis (Zautra, Fasman, et al., 2005).

## INDIVIDUAL DIFFERENCES
## IN EMOTIONAL COMPLEXITY

Are there differences between individuals in the ability to sustain affective differentiation during difficult times, such that some people are more able to sustain affective differentiation? In our work, we probed for individual differences in the within-subject correlations between affects, and found evidence that all participants do not show the same pattern of relationships between PA and NA. We concluded that dispositional factors may account for individual differences in the slopes linking PA and NA (Zautra, Berkhof, & Nicolson, 2002). Of particular relevance to the ability to sustain affective differentiation are skills related to emotion regulation. A number of aspects of emotion regulation are likely to play a role, including the ability to identify, understand, process, and express one's emotions. Because it represents an early link in the chain of emotional regulation processes, we have also tested whether the ability to be clear about emotional experiences moderates the constriction of affective experiences that occurs during stressful experiences. Based on the DMA, we reasoned that increased skills in understanding one's emotions should relate to greater differentiation during stress between NA and PA among individuals in chronic pain.

We examined whether patients in pain had the ability to label their own emotions, termed mood clarity (Salovey & Mayer, 1990), related to affect differentiation over time (Zautra et al., 2001). After providing ratings of their mood clarity, participants completed 12 weekly assessments of affect and pain. Multilevel modeling permitted us to examine whether between-person differences in mood clarity affected within-person slopes between NA and PA. As would be predicted by the DMA, higher levels of mood clarity were related to weaker associations between PA and NA in this sample experiencing the chronic stress of pain. The role of trait-level understanding of one's emotions in promoting affective differentiation may not be straightforward, however, because we did not replicate our findings in a second sample of patients with pain (Zautra et al., 2001, Study 2). Nevertheless, mood clarity may prove to be an important moderator of stress-related responses. For example, Salovey, Stroud, Woolery, and Epel

(2002) reported that greater mood clarity is associated with lower levels of depression and social anxiety, and lower cortisol secretion during stressful days among healthy young adults. These results suggest that those who have more clarity of mood seem to manage stress more adaptively and recover from stress more easily, both physiologically and psychologically, than individuals with less mood clarity.

Among other stable dimensions of emotional experiencing that may contribute to the ability to sustain affective complexity is the person's capacity to experience positive emotions. As noted earlier, positive affectivity may promote resilience by facilitating expansive and complex information processing that presumably includes processing of emotions (Fredrickson & Joiner, 2002; Hobfoll, 1989). Thus, individuals who are high in PA may be able to draw on these psychological resources to promote adaptive coping during times of pain and stress. Recently, we tested this possibility in a sample of women with osteoarthritis and/or fibromyalgia who completed 10 to 12 weekly interviews regarding pain, interpersonal stress, NA, and PA (Zautra, Johnson, & Davis, 2005). In multilevel models, we examined the relation between stable, between-person differences in average level of PA, and the experience of NA during weeks of pain and stress. Individuals who experienced greater average PA over the weeks of assessment were less likely to show elevated NA both during high pain weeks and weeks in which they encountered high levels of interpersonal conflict. Thus, those individuals whose dispositions were characterized by high PA were more emotionally resilient in the face of both increased bodily pain and mounting interpersonal conflict.

The evidence to this point suggests that not only does affective differentiation vary within individuals over time, but also the degree of differentiation of affective states varies between people. As we have noted, advantages are significant for individuals who are able to maintain clarity about their emotions, and who evince positive emotions despite the natural tendency to experience negative emotions during times of difficulty. Emotionally complex individuals do not restrict their focus; rather, they broaden their mind-sets and counter negative stimuli with positive emotions. These skills may make them better able, relative to those with poorer emotion regulation skills, to adapt to the negative emotions that they experience during difficulty, potentially circumventing future painful episodes.

## DOES POSITIVE AFFECT
## PROMOTE EMOTIONAL REGULATION?

If well-developed emotion regulation skills are a key to resilience in the face of pain and other stressors, then efforts to enhance emotion regulation should promote adaptation among vulnerable populations. The accessibility of positive emotions during stress is an especially promising target for change, particularly among individuals who are vulnerable because they have few positive affective resources. Chronic pain patients with fibromyalgia may represent just such a vulnerable group: Patients with fibromyalgia report lower levels of PA compared to others in chronic pain (e.g., Davis, Zautra, & Reich, 2001). What is more, they appear to respond to stressful interpersonal events with a greater loss of positive emotions than their counterparts—patients with osteoarthritis. We examined weekly levels of PA and NA in conjunction with reports of pain, positive events, and everyday stressors in patients with osteoarthritis or fibromyalgia (Zautra, Fasman, et al., 2005). We found deficits in PA levels among patients with fibromyalgia compared to those with osteoarthritis. Upon closer examination, we were able to identify the source of that deficit: a relatively greater decline in PA in the fibromyalgia compared with the osteoarthritis sample during weeks of high pain and stress. The fibromyalgia sample was not anhedonic, however. In response to positive events, patients with fibromyalgia showed elevations in PA of the same magnitude as that of the comparison group. These data suggest that emotion regulation strategies that accentuate the positive may indeed be effective in patients with chronic pain in general and are particularly well-suited for patients with fibromyalgia.

Positive affective experiences may benefit emotion complexity as well. In an ongoing study of patients with rheumatoid arthritis we examined the role of positive interpersonal events in the day-to-day management of PA and NA (Zautra, Affleck, Tennen, Reich, & Davis, 2005). Men and women with rheumatoid arthritis kept daily diaries of their pain, stress, and affective health for 30 days. We computed composite indices of day-to-day changes in PA and changes in NA, daily stress, and pain exacerbations across the 30 days, and looked at the relationships among these variables. In support of the DMA model, stressful events had the expected effect of constricting affective experiencing. We also found that positive events had the opposite influence. On days when the patient reported a higher frequency of positive interpersonal experiences, not only was PA higher but the relationship between PA and NA was also less constricted. Complexity favors those with a steady diet of positive experiences.

Positive emotions influence physiological responses to stress as well (Fredrickson, 2001). The negative emotions that are commonly experienced during times of stress are typically associated with increased physiological arousal, including elevations in heart rate and blood pressure levels. The presence of positive emotions during stressful times may decrease the experience of negative emotions and downregulate the automatic physiological reactions associated with NA. Consequently, positive emotions can aid in dampening physiological stress responses and speeding recovery from a stressful event, allowing one to return more quickly to baseline physiological levels. In fact, Fredrickson and Levenson (1998) reported that cardiovascular recovery following stress is more rapid when individuals are exposed to positive compared to neutral or negative emotional stimuli.

## BEYOND CHRONIC PAIN: POSITIVE EMOTION, EMOTIONAL COMPLEXITY, AND STRESSORS OF AGING

Our understanding of the benefits of emotional complexity for health and well-being has implications for those confronting age-related challenges other than chronic pain. Several aging populations may be especially vulnerable to chronic stressors and, hence, be at risk of emotional simplification, as well as physical and psychological complications, that may accompany these conditions. A common experience for older adults is caregiving for loved ones who may be ill or dying, a situation that is especially poignant among those providing care for patient with Alzheimer's disease (AD). These caregivers often take responsibility for tending to most basic needs of a patient with dementia, whose prognosis is one of continued decline, possibly over a period spanning many years (see Fortinsky, Tennen, Frank, & Affleck, Chapter 12, this volume). In such circumstances, the DMA would predict that the chronic strain of caregivers limits their cognitive and affective resources, fueling less complex emotional processing.

In fact, available data bear this prediction out. In an investigation of older adults, Robinson-Whelen, Cheongtag, MacCallum, and Kiecolt-Glaser (1997) compared caregivers of patients with AD to those who were not caregivers on ratings of optimism, pessimism, and affective symptoms. Consistent with the DMA, optimism and pessimism were largely independent among noncaregivers but were strongly inversely related among caregivers. Moreover, optimism was negatively related to NA and symptoms of depression and anxiety only among caregivers of patients with AD. Thus, the chronic stress of caregiving appears to degrade the boundaries between PA and NA experiences, resulting in less complex emotion processing. In a recent study, Pruchno and Meeks (2004) looked directly at the relationship between PA and NA states for older women who were still caring for their adult children with developmental disabilities. Those women with high levels of caregiving stress showed a more tightly interwoven affective system, with PA and NA more inversely correlated in comparison to a control sample without the chronic stress of caregiving. The authors of these studies have noted, and we agree, that their results indicate that people living with chronic stress, like these caregivers, are less able to sustain the complex but ultimately hopeful view that both good and bad experiences can be expected to occur in the future.

Cognitive simplification and narrowing of thought also occurs among individuals dealing with anxiety, potentially restricting their ability to consider a variety of options for coping (Derryberry & Tucker, 1994). With limited cognitive resources to cope, people may resort to less effective strategies, such as rumination or catastrophizing rather than problem solving and cognitive reframing, fueling continued psychological disturbance over time. This narrowed perception of possibilities likely limits the consideration of the full range of options to manage such difficulty, and may prove a useful target for intervention.

Ong and his colleagues (in press) have examined the flip side of this question: the extent to which older adults with a profile of resilience show a broader range of affective choices during stress. After first administering a battery of personality measures that included a measure of resilience, they assessed daily fluctuations in stress, and PA and NA among older adult widows. For older adults who scored high on resilience, elevations in PA tended to persist from one day to the next, and to reduce the level of stress reported on subsequent days. The authors also explicitly examined the relationship between PA and NA during days of elevated stress. Older adults with high resilience showed the least affective constriction during stress, a finding that was replicated in two additional samples of older adults.

The experience of positive emotional states may also expand cognitive processing of an ambiguous or threatening situation, such as the possibility that one may have a serious health condition, allowing one to confront rather than retreat from the stressor. This kind of active coping would engage more personal and psychological resources, allowing one to be more resilient in the face of such a stressor and to recover more quickly (Fredrickson, 1998; Salovey et al., 2000). In some instance, such a response may be life saving, for example, seeking help for a critical health condition. The experience of positive emotions, then, appears to have not only beneficial effects directly on our health but also indirect effects through the mechanisms of coping and recovery when we are confronted with a stressor or a potential health problem.

Although being able to engage positive emotions during stressful times, when our resources are taxed, may alleviate acute responses to stress, the long-term benefits of the cultivation of these positive emotions may not be so obvious. Fredrickson (2001) posits that positive emotions are worth cultivating as a means to achieve psychological growth and improved well-being over the long term. Positive emotions may propel an "upward spiraling" toward emotional well-being, where the more positive emotions one has, the more likely one is able to cope more effectively and create more positive emotions in the future (Fredrickson & Joiner, 2002). This kind of capacity building may be responsible for the kinds of effects recently observed in a longitudinal study of the onset of frailty with 1,558 Hispanic older adults (Ostir et al., 2004). Healthy older adults who reported greater happiness, enjoyment of life, and hopefulness at the initial interviews were significantly less likely to be classified as frail during the 7-year follow-up assessment.

## ENHANCING EMOTIONAL RESILIENCE

Most of us react to the events in our lives out of habit, guided by our mental heuristics rather than thoughtful reflection that leads to a conscious choice between a range of options. That a choice exists is, much of the time, completely out of our awareness, and never more so than when we are stressed. If simplified processing of affectively laden information contributes to poor adaptation in the face of pain and other stressors that often accompany aging, then intervention efforts directed at enhancing individuals' ability to process affect with greater complexity may prove useful, especially during times of pain and stress, when NA tends to dominate.

Many methods are available to self-regulate behavior and emotions, but the most widely used is arguably cognitive-behavioral therapy (CBT). Traditional CBT applied in the treatment of one of the most common health problems of aging, chronic pain, attempts to enhance patients' sense of mastery over pain by focusing on the development of pain coping skills. It incorporates a range of specific techniques, including biofeedback, relaxation training, cognitive restructuring and distraction, and activity pacing. CBT is regarded as the most effective behavioral intervention available for the treatment of chronic pain conditions, but empirical support for these claims is uneven. In fact, a recent review found that despite some improvements in pain management, CBT does not reduce mood symptoms in patients with pain (Nicassio & Greenberg, 2001). Some evidence suggests that CBT may sometimes be worse than control conditions in alleviating depressive symptoms, and even exacerbate depressive symptoms despite improvements in pain (e.g., Bradley et al., 1987). These findings are perhaps not surprising given that CBT interventions have not typically included a focus on both PA and NA, or on the development of affective complexity.

An emerging treatment approach, mindfulness meditation, has been garnering empirical support over the past decade for the treatment of health problems, including pain, depression, and anxiety (Baer, 2003; Kabat-Zinn, Lipworth, & Burney, 1985; Segal, Williams, & Teasdale, 2002; Teasdale, Segal, & Williams, 1995; Teasdale et al., 2002), and offers a unique contrast to the use of traditional CBT (see Golub & Langer, Chapter 2, this volume). Mindfulness promotes greater emotional regulation by increasing nonjudgmental awareness and acceptance of current experiences, including emotions, sensations, and cognitions (e.g. Kabat-Zinn, 1994; Segal et al., 2002). This approach encourages effortful processing of mental events, in contrast to the automatic processing that occurs during pain and other stressors. Habitual responses that may act to intensify negative arousal, such as avoidance, catastrophizing, and helplessness, are limited, and tolerance of negative emotional arousal is increased. When a difficult or painful experience emerges, individuals are encouraged to attend to this experience with deliberateness, and to hold it in awareness with an accepting, nonjudgmental frame of mind. Similar to traditional CBT, dysfunctional thought patterns are identified, but rather than promoting attempts to neutralize such thoughts through the processes of reframing and reappraisal, a mindful approach promotes detached observation. Mindfulness may help to increase tolerance of difficult emotions and, through exposure, to transform such emotions into innocuousness. Anxiety symptoms and panic sensations, for example, typically amplify emotional reactivity, a cycle that may be interrupted by halting the automatic tendency to avoid the sensations, and instead intentionally observing the sensations without judgment (Kabat-Zinn et al., 1992). By fostering objective awareness of feelings, thoughts, behaviors, and choices, mindfulness attempts to help individuals be more cognizant of the whole range of choices available to them at any given moment.

An optimal outgrowth of a mindful treatment approach for those in chronic pain or stress would be an increase in their emotional complexity, such that patients would be able to sustain access to positive affective resources despite the experience of pain and other stressors. Thus, greater attention to a variety of experiences in the moment facilitates awareness that PA may be present, even during arousal of NA states. Patients learn that the experience of pain and other stressors does not preclude the experience of PA engagement. Consistent with the DMA, greater access to PA may facilitate more adaptive, flexible responses to current circumstances, with the potential to enhance well-being and functional health.

During trying times, when PA and NA are strongly related, the ability to continue to laugh and experience pleasure may make the powerful negative emotions less overwhelming. During times of low pain and stress, when PA and NA represent separate dimensions, the ability to enhance positive emotions could serve to "broaden and build" the resources for coping with flare-ups of pain and increase overall life satisfaction (Fredrickson, 1998). Developing a variety of supportive relationship and sources of pleasure could prove invaluable in sustaining an individual through a major health crisis.

In fact, more mindful individuals are more aware of and better able to describe their emotions than their less mindful counterparts, and report higher levels of positive affect (Brown & Ryan, 2003). Moreover, recent evidence gleaned from healthy individuals points to significant neurophysiological changes with mindfulness training that are consistent with a "broadening" of PA resources. Davidson and colleagues (2003) assessed patterns of brain electrical activity in response to positive and negative emotion induction in a group of 41 healthy adults, randomly assigned either to participation in an 8-week mindfulness meditation training program or a wait-list control group, with assessments occurring at both pre- and postintervention. The authors posited that those assigned to mindfulness meditation would show increased left-sided activation, a pattern associated with increased positive affectivity. The findings were consistent with this prediction. The mindfulness group had greater relative left-sided brain activation posttreatment in general, and in response to both the positive and negative mood inductions compared to the wait-list control group. Of particular relevance for our discussion of affective dynamics in chronic pain and stress are the increases in left-sided activation that occurred in response to the experience of negative emotion among those trained to increase awareness and acceptance of internal experiences, including their emotions.

The findings suggest that an intervention that enhances emotional skills may increase the ability of individuals to preserve positive engagement during their experience of pain and stress, and to respond to these negative events more adaptively by finding positive emotional features embedded within the negative (Zautra, 2003).

Although a mindfulness meditation intervention has been applied to the treatment of chronic pain and other medical conditions (e.g., Kabat-Zinn et al., 1985), its effect on affective dynamics in these populations has yet to be explored. In our view, successful aging hinges on the ability to sustain positive emotion during difficult life circumstances, including declines in health. The growing research evidence for the relation between mindfulness and well-being suggests that the cultivation of mindfulness may represent one avenue to promote affective differentiation. As findings accumulate from controlled studies that include appropriate control groups, any distinct benefits of mindfulness interventions should be brought into sharper focus. Our research team is in the midst of a clinical trial of patients with rheumatoid arthritis to examine the impact of a mindfulness-based intervention on aspects of resilience, including affective complexity.

## CONCLUDING COMMENTS

The ability to maintain an awareness of our positive emotions in the face of life's inevitable difficulties, including challenges to health, may be a hidden key to resilience as we age. Stressful situations appear to magnify the influence of positive emotions not only on healthy behaviors but also on neuroimmune processes that restore physiological balance following disturbing events. Dynamic models of affect regulation, such as those we have discussed here, offer new ways to examine health-related effects of emotion by proposing an integration of stress and emotion in daily life. This approach lays out a set of testable hypotheses governing how emotions set the stage for good and also poor health across the lifespan. We hope that our work encourages future research using cutting edge approaches to increase our understanding of this exceedingly complex domain of human functioning.

# REFERENCES

Affleck, G., & Tennen, H. (1996). Daily processes in coping with chronic pain: Methods and analytic strategies. In M. Zeidner & N. Endler (Eds.), *Handbook of coping* (pp. 151–180). New York: Wiley.

Affleck, G., Tennen, H., Urrows, S., & Higgins, P. (1992). Neuroticism and the pain–mood relation in rheumatoid arthritis: Insights from a prospective daily study. *Journal of Consulting and Clinical Psychology, 60,* 119–126.

Baer, R. A. (2003). Mindfulness training as a clinical intervention: A conceptual and empirical review. *Clinical Psychology: Science and Practice, 10,* 125–143.

Bradley, L. A., Young, L. D., Anderson, K. O., Turner, R. A., Agudelo, C. A., McDaniel, L. K., et al. (1987). Effects of psychological therapy on pain behavior or rheumatoid arthritis patients. *Arthritis and Rheumatism, 30,* 1105–1114.

Brown, K. W., & Ryan, R. M. (2003). The benefits of being present: Mindfulness and its role in psychological well-being. *Journal of Personality and Social Psychology, 84,* 822–848.

Canli, T. (2004). Functional brain mapping of extraversion and neuroticism: Learning from individual differences in emotion processing. *Journal of Personality, 72,* 1105–1132.

Canli, T., Zhao, Z., Desmond, J. E., Kang, E., Gross, J., & Gabrieli, J. D. E. (2001). An fMRI study of personality influences on brain reactivity to emotional stimuli. *Behavioral Neuroscience, 115,* 33–42.

Carstensen, L. L., Isaacowitz, D. M., & Charles, S. T. (1999). Taking time seriously: A theory of socioemotional selectivity. *American Psychologist, 54,* 165–181.

Carstensen, L. L., Pasupathi, M., Mayr, U., & Nesselroade, J. R. (2000). Emotional experience in everyday life across the adult life span. *Journal of Personality and Social Psychology, 79,* 644–655.

Cohen, S., Doyle, W. J., Turner, R. B., Alper, C. M., & Skoner, D. P. (2003). Emotional style and susceptibility to the common cold. *Psychosomatic Medicine, 65,* 652–657.

Danner, D. D., Snowdon, D. A., & Friesen, W. V. (2001). Positive emotions in early life and longevity: Findings from the Nun Study. *Journal of Personality and Social Psychology, 80,* 804–813.

Davidson, R. J., Kabat-Zinn, J., Schumacher, J., Rosenkranz, M., Muller, D., Santorelli, S. F., et al. (2003). Alterations in brain and immune function produced by mindfulness meditation. *Psychosomatic Medicine, 65,* 564–570.

Davis, M. C., Zautra, A. J., & Reich, J. W. (2001). Vulnerability to stress among women in chronic pain from fibromyalgia and osteoarthritis. *Annals of Behavioral Medicine, 23,* 215–226.

Derryberry, D., & Tucker, D. M. (1994). Motivating the focus of attention. In P. M. Neidenthal & S. Kitayama (Eds.), *The heart's eye: Emotional influences in perception and attention* (pp. 167–196). San Diego: Academic Press.

Fernandez, E., & Turk, D. C. (1992). Sensory and affective components of pain: Separation and synthesis. *Psychological Bulletin, 112,* 205–212.

Fredrickson, B. L. (1998). What good are positive emotions? *Review of General Psychology, 2,* 300–319.

Fredrickson, B. L. (2001). The role of positive emotions in positive psychology. *American Psychologist, 56,* 218–226.

Fredrickson, B. L., & Joiner, T. (2002). Positive emotions trigger upward spirals toward emotional well-being. *Psychological Science, 13*, 172–175.

Fredrickson, B. L., & Levenson, R. W. (1998). Positive emotions speed recovery from the cardiovascular sequelae of negative emotions. *Cognition and Emotion, 12*, 191–220.

Hart, R. P., Wade, J. B., & Martelli, M. F. (2003). Cognitive impairment in patients with chronic pain: The significance of stress. *Current Pain and Headache Reports, 7*, 116–226.

Hayes, N., & Joseph, S. (2003). Big Five correlates of three measures of subjective well-being. *Personality and Individual Differences, 34*, 723–727.

Hobfoll, S. E. (1989). Conservation of resources: A new attempt at conceptualizing stress. *American Psychologist, 44*, 513–524.

Kabat-Zinn, J. (1994). *Wherever you go, there you are: Mindfulness meditation in everyday life.* New York: Hyperion.

Kabat-Zinn, J., Lipworth, L., & Burney, R. (1985). The clinical use of mindfulness meditation for the self-regulation of chronic pain. *Journal of Behavioral Medicine, 8*, 163–190.

Kabat-Zinn, J., Massion, M. D., Kristeller, J., Peterson, L. G., Fletcher, K. E., Pbert, L., et al. (1992). Effectiveness of a meditation-based stress reduction program in the treatment of anxiety disorders. *American Journal of Psychiatry, 149*, 936–943.

Lawrence, R. C., Helmick, C. G., Arnett, F. C., Deyo, R. A., Felson, D. T., Giannini, E. H., et al. (1998). Estimates of the prevalence of arthritis and selected musculoskeletal disorders in the United States. *Arthritis and Rheumatism, 41*, 778–799.

Mather, M., Canli, T., English, T., Whitfield, S., Wais, P., Ochsner, K. G., et al. (2004). Amygdala responses to emotionally valenced stimuli in older and younger adults. *Psychological Science, 15*, 259–263.

McCrae, R. R., & Costa, P. T., Jr. (1999). A five-factor theory of personality. In L. Pervin & O. P. John (Eds.), *Handbook of personality* (2nd ed., pp. 139–153). New York: Guilford Press.

Melzak, R., & Wall, P. D. (1965). Pain mechanisms: A new theory. *Science, 150*, 971–979.

Moskowitz, J. T. (2003). Positive affect predicts lower risk of AIDS mortality. *Psychosomatic Medicine, 65*, 620–626.

Mroczek, D. K., & Kolarz, C. M. (1998). The effect of age on positive and negative affect: A developmental perspective on happiness. *Journal of Personality and Social Psychology, 75*, 1333–1349.

Nicassio, P. M., & Greenberg, M. A. (2001). The effectiveness of cognitive-behavioral and psychoeducational interventions in the management of arthritis. In M. H. Weisman, M. Weinblatt, & J. Louie (Eds.), *Treatment of rheumatic diseases* (2nd ed., pp. 147–161). Orlando, FL: Saunders.

Ong, A. D., Bergeman, C. S., Bisconti, T. L., & Wallace, K. A. (in press). The contours of resilience and the complexity of emotions in later life. *Journal of Personality and Social Psychology.*

Ostir, G. V., Ottenbacher, K. J., & Markides, K. S. (2004). Onset of frailty in older adults and the protective role of positive affect. *Psychology and Aging, 19*, 402–408.

Pennebaker, J. W., & Stone, L. D. (2004). Translating traumatic experiences into language: Implications for child abuse and long-term health. In L. J. Koenig, L. S.

Doll, A. O'Leary, & W. Pequegnat (Eds.), *From child sexual abuse to adult sexual risk: Trauma, revictimization, and intervention* (pp. 201–216). Washington, DC: American Psychological Association.

Pruchno, R. A., & Meeks, S. (2004). Health-related stress, affect and depressive symptoms experienced by caregiving mothers of adults with a developmental disability. *Psychology and Aging, 19*, 394–401.

Reich, J. W., Zautra, A. J., & Davis, M. (2003). Dimensions of affect relationships: Models and their integrative implications. *Review of General Psychology, 7*, 66–83.

Reich, J. W., Zautra, A. J., & Potter, P. T. (2001). Cognitive structure and the independence of positive and negative affect. *Journal of Social and Clinical Psychology, 20*, 99–115.

Robinson-Whelen, S., Cheongtag, K., MacCallum, R. C., & Kiecolt-Glaser, J. K. (1997). Distinguishing optimism from pessimism in older adults: Is it more important to be optimistic or not to be pessimistic? *Journal of Personality and Social Psychology, 73*, 1345–1353.

Salovey, P., & Mayer, J. D. (1990). Emotional intelligence. *Imagination, Cognition and Personality, 9*(3), 185–211.

Salovey, P., Rothman, A. J., Detweiler, J. B., & Steward, W. T. (2000). Emotional states and physical health. *American Psychologist, 55*, 110–121.

Salovey, P., Stroud, L. R., Woolery, A., & Epel, E. S. (2002). Perceived emotional intelligence, stress reactivity, and symptom reports: Further explorations using the trait meta-mood scale. *Psychology and Health, 17*, 611–627.

Segal, Z. V., Williams, J. M. G., & Teasdale, J. D. (2002). *Mindfulness-based cognitive therapy for depression*. New York: Guilford Press.

Srivastava, S., John, O. P., Gosling, S. D., & Potter, J. (2003). Development of personality in early and middle adulthood: Set like plaster or persistent change? *Journal of Personality and Social Psychology, 84*, 1041–1053.

Teasdale, J. D., Moore, R. G., Hayhurst, H., Pope, M., Williams, S., & Segal, Z. V. (2002). Metacognitive awareness and prevention of relapse in depression: Empirical evidence. *Journal of Consulting and Clinical Psychology, 70*, 275–287.

Teasdale, J. D., Segal, Z. V., & Williams, M. G. (1995). How does cognitive therapy prevent depressive relapse and why should attentional control (mindfulness training) help? *Behaviour Research and Therapy, 33*, 25–39.

Wijeratne, C., Shome, S., Hickie, I., & Koschera, A. (2001). An age-based comparison of chronic pain clinic patients. *International Journal of Geriatric Psychiatry, 16*, 477–483.

Zautra, A. J. (2003). *Emotions, stress, and health*. New York: Oxford University Press.

Zautra, A. J., Affleck, G., Tennen, H., Reich, J. W., & Davis, M. C. (2005). Dynamic approaches to emotions and stress in everyday life: Bolger and Zuckerman reloaded with positive as well as negative affects. *Journal of Personality, 73*, 1–28.

Zautra, A. J., Berkhof, J., & Nicolson, N. A. (2002). Changes in affect interrelations as a function of stressful events. *Cognition and Emotion, 16*(2), 309–318.

Zautra, A. J., Fasman, R., Reich, J. W., Harakas, P., Johnson, L. M., Olmsted, M. E., et al. (2005). Fibromyalgia: Evidence for deficits in positive affect regulation. *Psychosomatic Medicine, 67*, 147–155.

Zautra, A. J., Johnson, L. M., & Davis, M. C. (2005). Positive affect as a source of resilience for women in chronic pain. *Journal of Consulting and Clinical Psychology*, 73 212–220.

Zautra, A. J., Reich, J. W., Davis, M. C., Potter, P. T., & Nicolson, N. A. (2000). The role of stressful events in the relationship between positive and negative affects: Evidence from field and experimental studies. *Journal of Personality*, 68, 927–951.

Zautra, A., Smith, B., Affleck, G., & Tennen, H. (2001). Examinations of chronic pain and affect relationships: Applications of a dynamic model of affect. *Journal of Consulting and Clinical Psychology*, 69, 786–795.

# CHAPTER 14

# Optimizing Social Relationships as a Resource for Health and Well-Being in Later Life

KAREN S. ROOK, SHAHRZAD MAVANDADI,
DARA H. SORKIN, *and* LAURA A. ZETTEL

Social relationships influence health and well-being throughout the lifespan, with effects evident for multiple dimensions of health. At the most basic level, involvement in satisfying social relationships has been shown to predict mortality after adjusting for biomedical (e.g., cholesterol levels, hypertension) and behavioral (e.g., smoking, diet) risk factors (see reviews by Cohen, 2004; Seeman, 2000). Social support has been linked to decreased risks for cardiovascular disease, cancer mortality, and functional decline (Seeman & McEwen, 1996; Uchino, Cacioppo, & Kiecolt-Glaser, 1996). Such associations are impressive in size, as evidenced by the fact that relationship variables predict mortality and morbidity nearly as well as do conventional risk factors, such as smoking (House, Umberson, & Landis, 1988).

Social relationships also contribute to emotional well-being and quality of life. For example, close relationships influence positive affect by serving as a source of enjoyable social interaction and companionship (Rook, 1994). Research on subjective well-being confirms, moreover, that having close relationships is a reliable and powerful predictor of happiness and life satisfaction (Diener & Seligman, 2004).

Supportive relationships play an important role as well in facilitating adaptation to life stress, including physical disability and illness. Given that the onset or progression of disability is often accompanied by distress and

267

difficulties such as pain, progressive declines, energy loss, and changes in self-concept, the need for others and the value of supportive relationships may increase during this time (Seeman, 2000). A lack of social support, for example, has been found to contribute to worse health outcomes among individuals with chronic illness, with especially detrimental effects on the physical functioning of chronically ill older adults (Sherbourne, Meredith, Rogers, & Ware, 1992).

Some of the beneficial physical and psychological effects of social relationships in later life are believed to stem from a proactive role that older adults play in regulating their relationships. Theorists have suggested that older adults play an active role in managing their social relationships, seeking to invest their time in emotionally rewarding relationships and to avoid or minimize their involvement in unrewarding or aversive relationships (Carstensen, Issacowitz, & Charles, 1999; Lang, 2001). In this sense, older adults may be regarded as actively involved in efforts to shape their social environment, by cultivating and benefiting from the strengths of their most supportive social network relationships.

Yet it is not always possible for older adults to manage their social relationships so that interactions with others are consistently rewarding. Some older adults are entangled in problematic social relationships from which disengagement is difficult (Krause & Rook, 2003). Others who enjoy largely harmonious social relationships for an extended period of time may experience life events that threaten these relationships. Declining health or mobility, for example, can disrupt established patterns of interaction with social network members. Experiences such as widowhood and residential relocation can lead to the loss of important social relationships, creating adaptational challenges. Thus, in some contexts, older adults' social network ties may be characterized by limitations or tensions that erode, rather than enhance, their health and well-being. A fertile direction for future research, and the goal of this chapter, is to consider how older adults seek to manage their social worlds to maximize positive interactions with others, prevent negative interactions, and to meet their social needs in the wake of relationship losses.

Aging is often accompanied by physical decline; we begin, therefore, by illustrating the role social relationships may play in disability onset and progression in later life. We then consider how older adults seek to regulate their social relationships to maximize positive interactions, to minimize negative interactions, and to adapt to relationship losses. Three perspectives on the processes of relationship regulation are examined. The first perspective emphasizes older adults' selective engagement with other people as a means of limiting their social contacts to those that are most supportive and emotionally rewarding. The second perspective emphasizes older adults' efforts to prevent or resolve tensions and disagreements that arise in their relationships with social network members. A third perspective emphasizes older adults' efforts to derive support and companionship from alternative sources following the loss or disruption of important social relationships. We conclude by suggesting directions for further research on the nature and effectiveness of older adults' efforts to optimize their social relationships.

## BENEFICIAL AND DETRIMENTAL EFFECTS OF SOCIAL RELATIONSHIPS IN THE CONTEXT OF PHYSICAL DISABILITY

Physical disability leads to difficulties in the performance of activities needed for daily living and is highly associated with health and well-being, leading researchers to be interested in identifying psychosocial factors that may influence the onset and developmental course of impairment and subsequent disability. One factor that has been studied extensively is the nature of individuals' social network relationships. Research has documented both beneficial and detrimental effects of social relationships on disability onset and progression in later life.

### Beneficial Effects of Social Relationships

Research has documented that structural (e.g., network size) and functional (e.g., perceived adequacy) aspects of social support are related to a reduced risk of developing disability in later life. For example, a longitudinal study of community-dwelling older adults revealed that greater baseline social network involvement was related to a significantly lower risk of future impairments in the ability to carry out activities of daily living (ADLs; Mendes de Leon et al., 1999). In a study of initially disability-free, community-dwelling older adults, having more close social network relationships predicted a lower incidence of disability 2 years later (Seeman, Bruce, & McAvay, 1996). Confirming the importance of close social ties, Strawbridge, Cohen, Shema, and Kaplan (1996) found that older adults who reported such ties at a baseline assessment were 82% less likely to develop disability at a 6-year follow-up than were older adults who lacked such ties.

Social relationships have been linked not only to the onset but also to the progression of disability in later life. In an early study demonstrating this latter association, both more frequent and more satisfying emotional support predicted fewer declines in older adults' physical functioning over a 2-year period (Seeman et al., 1995). Structural, but not functional, aspects of social networks predicted physical functioning in another study (Unger, McAvay, Bruce, Berkman, & Seeman, 1999). Older adults who reported more social ties at baseline evidenced fewer declines in functioning 7 years later. The effects were stronger, however, for individuals who had lower levels of baseline physical performance, suggesting that the effects of social ties may vary as a function of the severity of the disability. In a study spanning 9 years, Mendes de Leon, Glass, and Berkman (2003) found that more socially engaged older adults (i.e., who participated in a greater number of social and productive activities) at baseline reported less subsequent disability.

Additional research has focused on the potential role of social support in predicting recovery from disability, because older adults with physical impairments can experience periods of partial or complete recovery, as well as periods of stability in their level of functioning over time. Glass, Matchar, Belyea, and Feussner (1993), for example, followed surviving stroke patients for 6 months in a prospective study of the impact of social support on physical recovery. Patients with greater perceived social support experienced faster and more extensive recovery of ADLs following a stroke. In fact, among patients who had more severe strokes, those with the greatest social support scored 65% higher on ADL measures than did those with the least social support. Similarly, in a study examining physical recovery following hospitalization for one of three medical conditions (hip fracture, stroke, or myocardial infarction), greater perceived adequacy of instrumental support assessed shortly after admission to the hospital was associated with greater recovery of ADLs 6 months postadmission (Wilcox, Kasl, & Berkman, 1994). Such studies illustrate the beneficial effects of social support on recovery from disability, as well as disability onset and progression.

## Detrimental Effects of Social Relationships

The research we have just reviewed suggests that aspects of older adults' involvement with members of their social networks often exhibit positive associations with physical functioning. Yet social network members' actions are not always positive and may instead include criticism, neglect, demands, and other insensitive or inconsiderate behaviors that detract from health and well-being (Rook, 1998).

Moreover, network members' very efforts to be supportive sometimes backfire, resulting in worse, rather than better, health outcomes (Coyne, Wortman, & Lehman, 1988). For example, among individuals with an illness, increased support from family and friends, and preferential treatment (e.g., more attention and concern directed toward the individual after disease onset) predict greater manifestations of disability (e.g., Seeman et al., 1996).

The receipt of instrumental support (i.e., receiving help with self-care and other tasks) has been implicated in several studies as contributing to disability onset and progression among originally high-functioning older adults (e.g., Mendes de Leon, Gold, Glass, Kaplan, & George, 2001). In one study of community-dwelling older adults, more frequent receipt of instrumental support predicted an increased risk of new disability onset, as well as recurrent ADL disability 2 years later (Seeman et al., 1996). Similar results emerged in a study of over 1,300 initially nondisabled older adults: High levels of instrumental support predicted an increased risk of functional decline in men, but not women (Avlund, Lund, Holstein, & Due, 2004).

Although such findings appear counterintuitive, a number of explanations have been offered to account for them. First, social learning theorists have suggested that behavioral manifestations of disability may be positively reinforced by supportive responses from network members; thus, the two processes become mutually reinforcing over time (Turk, Kerns, & Rosenberg, 1992). The individual with a disability may come to realize that adopting the "sick role" is rewarding, and secondary gain in the form of preferential treatment from network members may be enough to perpetuate symptoms of disability (Baltes, 1996).

Second, a loved one's disability sometimes causes network members to act in counterproductive and overprotective ways (Coyne et al., 1988). Such support can foster dependency, leading to reduced participation in physical activities that would help to prevent physical decline. Overprotective support also may erode one's confidence in being able to care for oneself and to engage in productive activities, thereby threatening feelings of autonomy, independence, and overall well-being (Coyne et al., 1988; Seeman et al., 1996).

The receipt of instrumental support, in particular, has been shown to be threatening to self-esteem and emotional well-being (Newsom, 1999) and may act as a recurring reminder of one's inability to perform tasks independently (Martire, Stephens, Druley, & Wojno, 2002; Oxman, Freeman, Manheimer, & Stukel, 1994). Such feelings of dependency have in turn been shown to elicit a greater frequency of negative interactions with support providers, leading to more negative affect and distress (Boerner, Reinhardt, Raykov, & Horowitz, 2004). Also damaging is the potential for declines in self-efficacy and personal competence to thwart involvement in activities that would help to sustain physical health (Baltes & Wahl, 1992), resulting in further declines and greater disability.

It is clear, then, that relationships with others do not guarantee that an individual will experience health-related benefits. Not only can people receive, in a sense, too much social support, but also not all relationships may be supportive. Rather, some social relationships may be sources of acute or chronic stress. Indeed, research that has examined both interpersonal and noninterpersonal stressors has found that stressors of an interpersonal nature are often more distressing than other kinds of stressors (Bolger, DeLongis, Kessler, & Schilling, 1989).

Experiencing negative exchanges in one's social relationships, not surprisingly, has been linked to adverse psychological and physical health outcomes. Although the majority of research examining the physical health effects of negative social interactions has examined either short-term reactions in laboratory settings or effects on cardiovascular, neuroendocrine, and immunological functioning (see review by Seeman & McEwen, 1996), a few studies have focused on disability as an outcome. For example, older adults' negative interactions with social network members were shown in a prospective study to predict greater functional impairment, with the effects being more pronounced among those with less education (Krause & Shaw, 2002). Complementing such findings regarding the role of negative social exchanges and physical disability is a fairly large literature documenting adverse effects of such exchanges on mental health and psychological well-being (see reviews by Rook, 1998; Finch, Okun, Pool, & Ruehlman, 1999). Moreover, the prospective designs of a growing number of studies in this literature increase confidence in the causal direction of the associations reported.

In light of the empirical evidence indicating that both positive and negative aspects of older adults' social relationships affect disability, as well as other physical and psychological health outcomes, it becomes important to understand how older adults attempt to regulate their relationships to maximize positive interactions with others and minimize negative interactions. An emerging literature, discussed below, is beginning to address this issue.

## OLDER ADULTS' STRATEGIES FOR OPTIMIZING THEIR SOCIAL RELATIONSHIPS

On balance, positive experiences with social network members occur far more often than do negative experiences (Rook, 1998), and this is particularly true as people age (Carstensen et al., 1999). Moreover, satisfaction with social network relationships tends to be high in later life (Settersten, 2002), and levels of loneliness tend to be lower in this life stage than in earlier life stages, although loneliness rises in advanced old age (Perlman, 1988).

Such findings are striking in view of evidence that social networks become smaller (Lang & Carstensen, 1994), and interaction with network members becomes less frequent as people grow older (Carstensen et al., 1999). These findings raise the question of how older adults manage their social relationships to maximize support and companionship, and to minimize relationship tensions and difficulties, thereby optimizing their relationships as a resource for physical health and psychological well-being. We draw upon existing theory and research to compare three different perspectives on this question. These perspectives emphasize older adults' (1) selective engagement with social network members to maximize positive experiences, (2) their efforts to prevent or resolve problems that do occur with social network members, and (3) their efforts to compensate for the loss or disruption of important social network relationships by seeking alternative sources of support and companionship.

## Engaging Selectively with Social Network Members

An age-related contraction of social network size is a robust finding that has been documented since the 1950s and 1960s (Cumming & Henry, 1961). Early interpretations portrayed such contraction as reflecting either older adults' disengagement from social involvements to facilitate the developmental task of coming to grips with the approaching end of life (Cumming & Henry, 1961) or, alternatively, societal rejection of older adults (Maddox, 1964). More recently, socioemotional selectivity theory has offered an alternative interpretation that attributes the declining rate of social interaction to an age-related increase in the selectivity of social involvement, so that interaction occurs primarily with social network members who offer the greatest emotional rewards (Carstensen et al., 1999).

According to socioemotional selectivity theory (Carstensen et al., 1999), the underlying motivations for social interaction change as people age, with social interaction as a means of acquiring information about the world or solidifying one's self-concept becoming less important over time. By later life, a substantial store of information about the world has already been amassed and other, nonsocial means of acquiring information have been mastered. Similarly, the self-concept tends to have solidified by later life, reducing the motivation to interact with others as a means of learning about oneself through social comparisons. Instead, emotional goals assume greater importance as a motivation for social contact. The opportunity for emotionally meaningful interaction with others becomes more important than other social goals and, according to the theory, leads older people to prefer to engage selectively with emotionally rewarding interaction partners. Such partners tend to be those with whom close, long-term bonds exist (Carstensen et al., 1999).

These developmental shifts in the basic motivations for social contact are hypothesized to lead older adults to exhibit a narrower range of preferred interaction partners, with partners who offer the greatest potential to assist in the regulation of affective states preferred over others. The amount of social contact also declines as it becomes focused on fewer partners and fewer categories of interaction (those most relevant to emotional goals). Continuity of contact is maintained over time with a select subset of social network members, and psychological well-being is enhanced through involvement with emotionally rewarding interaction partners.

Substantial empirical evidence supports the propositions of socioemotional selectivity theory (see reviews by Carstensen et al., 1999; Lockenhoff & Carstensen, 2004). Research suggests that prospective social interaction is construed in terms of the social goals emphasized by socioemotional selectivity theory, that the emotional dimensions of social interaction have greater salience to older adults, and that older adults prefer familiar inter-action partners over unfamiliar partners because familiar partners offer more emotional rewards (Frederickson & Carstensen, 1990). Moreover, as predicted by the theory, declines in social network size with advancing age tend to be limited to peripheral social ties; neither the number of close rela-tionships nor the level of satisfaction with social network members exhibit age-related declines (Fung, Carstensen, & Lutz, 1999; Lang & Carstensen, 1994).

The extensively documented age-related declines in social network size and in the frequency of social interaction thus appear to result from a pro-cess of selective investment in social ties that offer the greatest emotional rewards (Carstensen et al., 1999). Selective engagement in close network relationships allows older adults' social interactions to provide an arena for experiencing positive affect. From this perspective, age-related declines in social activity do not represent threats to health and well-being; instead, they reflect older adults' proactive regulation of their social lives in a man-ner that preserves their health and well-being.

The changing circumstances in later life, however, can create chal-lenges and impose limits on selectivity as a strategy for the regulation of social relationships. Chronic illness and disability can erode established patterns of social activity, leading to involuntary, rather than voluntary, re-ductions in contact. Consistent with this idea, deteriorating health has emerged as the strongest predictor of declines in older adults' friendship in-volvement in longitudinal studies (e.g., Johnson & Troll, 1992). Chronic conditions often require long-term support from network members, creat-ing the conditions for conflict and the resurrection of dormant resentments (Johnson & Catalano, 1983). The potential for conflict increases when more distant family members (e.g., nieces, nephews) are called upon to take over the support functions previously performed by others (Johnson & Catalano, 1983). Disengaging from such support providers can prove diffi-cult, even when the receipt of support carries psychological costs.

Apart from relationships that may deteriorate in the context of serious illness, some social relationships can be persistently stressful over a period of many year but, nonetheless, difficult to avoid or terminate. For example, proximity or kinship may cause some stressful relationships to persevere, such as unpleasant or demanding relationships with neighbors or extended kin. Krause and Rook (2003), in a longitudinal study, found that a measure of older adults' negative interactions with social network members exhib-ited a high degree of stability over a 6-year period. Research needs to exam-ine, therefore, not only selective engagement as a strategy for experiencing positive social interactions in later life but also older adults' strategies for dealing with negative social interactions when they do occur.

## Responding to Negative Exchanges with Social Network Members

Despite evidence documenting the harmful effects of negative exchanges with social network members, relatively little research has examined how people respond to such exchanges (Rook, Sorkin, & Zettel, 2004). The coping literature has focused primarily on how people cope with stressors that are not interpersonal in nature, such as life-threatening illness or financial stress. The theoretical perspectives that have guided investigations of coping may, nonetheless, be useful in examining how older adults seek to cope with negative exchanges with members of their social networks.

Coping researchers have distinguished between two basic kinds of coping: problem-focused coping (externally directed responses aimed at changing the stressful situation itself) and emotion-focused coping (internally directed responses aimed at managing the negative emotions generated by the stressful event; Lazarus & Folkman, 1984). This distinction has been incorporated in the small body of research that has begun to examine how people cope with negative social exchanges (e.g., Birditt & Fingerman, 2005). Examples of problem-focused forms of coping emphasized in this literature include compromise (efforts to achieve with the interaction partner a mutually satisfactory resolution of the problem), assertion or confrontation (efforts to change the interaction partner's behavior), and support seeking (solicitation of advice or support from others about the problem). Examples of emotion-focused forms of coping with negative social exchanges include cognitive distancing (efforts to keep from thinking about the interpersonal problem, or to minimize its significance), emotional restraint or self-control (efforts to keep one's feelings about the problem to oneself), and self-blame (efforts to accept responsibility for the problem).

Forgiveness also has begun to receive attention as an additional emotion-focused coping strategy, with most research to date conducted with younger and middle-aged adults. "Forgiveness" refers to an internal process of releasing anger or other negative feelings toward a person who is believed to have engaged in some form of transgression, with a resulting decline in the motivation to avoid the person or to seek revenge (Fincham, Beach, & Davila, 2004). Evidence has linked forgiveness to less retaliatory behavior and more conciliatory behavior among married couples (Fincham et al., 2004). Nevertheless, Jones, Moore, Schratter, and Negel (2000) have cautioned that "forgiving is not the same as forgetting" (p. 249). In their research, nearly one-third of participants who had experienced a betrayal reported that they had forgiven the betrayer, but further examination revealed that their forgiveness often was qualified and resentments persisted.

When trying to understand the effectiveness of particular coping responses, coping theorists often have assumed that coping efforts are directed toward one of two goals: the resolution of the problem or the reduction of emotional distress (Lazarus & Folkman, 1984). In general, existing research suggests that problem-focused coping responses are more reliably linked to reduced emotional distress and greater problem resolution than are emotion-focused coping responses, when the stressor is perceived as being controllable (Aldwin, 1999). Furthermore, emotion-focused strategies, such as self-blame and avoidant coping, appear to be particularly maladaptive, having been linked to increased psychological distress (Penley, Tomaka, & Wiebe, 2002). The extent to which similar associations would be evident in older adults' efforts to deal with negative social exchanges is not yet known.

In the interpersonal domain, a third goal, the goal of preserving good will in the social relationship, has unique importance. This goal sometimes may be more important than the goal of reducing one's own distress and may lead to a different set of coping responses (Rook et al., 2004).

Although coping goals may not always be subject to conscious deliberation, evidence suggests that individuals can reflect upon and identify such goals if prompted. For example, Sorkin and Rook (in press) asked older adults to report the primary goal they had in mind when responding to a recently experienced, negative exchange with a social network member. Participants' responses revealed that preserving good will in the relationship was reported most often as the primary coping goal, followed by reducing one's own distress, and, last, by inducing the other person to change his or her behavior. Coping responses to interpersonal problems, accordingly, may differ as a function of people's coping goals. For example, an older adult whose primary goal is to prevent a recurrence of the problem may be motivated to confront or to seek a compromise with the network member. An older person whose primary goal is to maintain harmony in the relationship, in contrast, may forgo even broaching the problem with the other person as a means of avoiding tensions. Older adults do appear to be sensitive to the risks involved in raising interpersonal problems for discussion (Fingerman, 1998), causing some problems to remain submerged.

Consideration of the goals that older adults pursue as they seek to deal with interpersonal problems has implications for evaluating the effectiveness of their coping efforts. A common barometer of coping effectiveness is the extent to which coping efforts reduce the emotional distress caused by a stressor (Coyne & Racioppo, 2000). Yet some coping goals may be pursued at the expense of reducing emotional distress. In the interpersonal context, for example, an older person whose paramount goal is to maintain harmony in an important relationship may engage in coping responses directed toward attaining this goal, even if doing so causes emotional distress to linger. For example, the individual might refrain from expressing feelings of anger to avoid tensions in the relationship. Such emotional inhibition may serve the immediate objective of maintaining harmony in the relationship, but it may do little to reduce emotional distress.

Despite the fact that emotional distress may linger, people nevertheless appraise such coping responses as successful if they achieve a primary goal (e.g., maintaining or restoring good will in a relationship). From this perspective, coping strategies identified in the literature as being ineffective might prove to be effective when evaluated with reference to personal coping goals. To test this possibility, Sorkin and Rook (in press) evaluated older adults' coping effectiveness by assessing not only the intensity and duration of emotional distress aroused by a recent negative social exchange, but also by assessing participants' perceptions of how successful or unsuccessful they had been in achieving their primary coping goal. In general, the coping responses that predicted less emotional distress were not associated with greater perceived success in achieving participant's paramount coping goal. Such findings underscore the idea that not all coping efforts are motivated by the desire to manage one's own distress; some coping efforts are undertaken in pursuit of other goals, even at the expense of forgoing distress reduction. Evaluating coping effectiveness through multiple lenses will continue to be important in future research.

More generally, researchers only recently have begun to examine how older adults respond to the conflicts and disappointments that arise in their social relationships. A great deal more remains to be learned about this aspect of older adults' efforts to regulate their social relationships, and, specifically, to limit the health-related toll of negative exchanges with others.

## Compensating for the Loss or Disruption of Social Network Relationships

We have thus far focused on forms of relationship regulation in later adulthood that reflect older adults' efforts to engage selectively with emotionally rewarding network members or to grapple with intermittent or chronic strains in their relationships with network members. In this section, we consider a third form of relationship regulation that occurs in response to the loss of a close relationship or the disruption of established patterns of interaction within a close relationship. Relationship losses arise from such events as the death or residential relocation of important members of one's social network. Relationship disruptions occur when deteriorating health or other life circumstances limit a social network member's ability to participate in established patterns of interaction. Such losses and disruptions detract from well-being in later life and often require older adults to seek support and companionship from alternative sources.

Both the toll and the adaptive challenges presented by relationship losses are illustrated by research on conjugal bereavement. Widowhood is a common experience in later life, with nearly two-thirds of women and one-fifth of men likely to be widowed by their mid-70s (U.S. Bureau of the Census, 2000). Moreover, widowhood involves not only the loss of the spouse but often also the loss of other relationships. Contacts with in-laws and couples with whom the widowed person once socialized often dwindle (Lamme, Dykstra, & Broese van Groenou, 1996). It is not surprising, therefore, that the loss of a spouse poses a threat to the physical and psychological health of the bereaved. The death of a spouse is associated with not only immediate declines in health but also more enduring vulnerabilities. The lifespan of widows and widowers, for example, is significantly shorter than that of married individuals (see review by Stroebe & Stroebe, 1987). Depression and loneliness levels are often high among the recently bereaved as well (Lund, Caserta, & Diamond, 1993; but see Bonanno et al., 2002).

The loss of the spouse is not the only relationship loss that people may expect to face as they age. The deaths of relatives and friends are distressingly common experiences. In one study, 25% of older adults reported having experienced the death of a friend in the preceding year (Aldwin, 1990). This figure increases among the old-old, with 59% of men and 42% of women over the age of 85 reporting the death of a close friend in the past year in one study (Johnson & Troll, 1992). In this context, too, older adults are at risk for adverse psychological and physical health effects.

Research provides indications, however, that bereaved individuals experience at least some rebounding of well-being after a period of time. For example, although the depression rates of widows tend to be significantly higher than those of the general population immediately following the spouse's death, these initially inflated rates return to normal levels for most widows after about 2 years (Shuchter & Zisook, 1993). Social network members may play a role in this recovery process, possibly by assuming some of the social support functions that were previously performed by the spouse.

Antonucci (1985) has described social network substitution as a natural response to the loss of social ties and the resulting tendency for people to add new members to their social networks. Research suggests that older adults who have experienced the loss of a major relationship do appear to engage in several different forms of social network substitution (Zettel & Rook, 2004), including establishing new ties (Morgan, Carder, & Neal, 1997), rekindling dormant ties (Cicirelli, 1995), and modifying their pattern of interaction and exchange with existing members of their social network (Connidis & Davies, 1992). For example, in one study (Lamme et al., 1996), widowed older adults were asked whether they had engaged in explicit efforts to "obtain, maintain, or intensify contact" with other people following the death of their spouse. More than 25% of participants reported establishing a new social relationship after their spouse's death. Of those who reported having made deliberate attempts to create or intensify a social tie, 44% were successful. Such figures suggest that older adults do actively seek to reconstitute their social lives as a means of compensating for relationship losses.

Simply establishing a substitute social relationship following a major loss, however, does not ensure that the substitute relationship will restore psychological well-being effectively, thus compensating for the lost relationship (Rook et al., 2004). "Substitution," which refers to the extent to which people derive support from alternative social ties, needs to be distinguished from "compensation," which refers to the extent to which these alternative social ties enhance well-being (Zettel & Rook, 2004). This distinction is sometimes blurred in studies of either process, in which substitute ties simply have been assumed to compensate for lost ties (Zettel & Rook, 2004). Because substitution and compensation are conceptually related but distinct processes, it is possible for an individual to establish substitute ties without actually deriving significant psychological or health-related benefits from them.

This conclusion was suggested by recent research demonstrating that widowed older women often form substitute relationships but do not necessarily derive compensatory benefits from these relationships (Zettel & Rook, 2004). In fact, greater substitution was related to worse, rather than better, psychological health over a 1-year period. Such findings suggest that social support obtained from substitute ties may be inherently different from the support previously obtained from the spouse. For example, the support and companionship derived from alternative sources may seem to be less natural, inconsistently available, or even grudgingly delivered, resulting in a negative impact on psychological well-being. Thus, substitute social ties may not impart the same psychological benefits as the social tie that has been lost.

This discussion is not meant to imply that spouses or other significant social partners can easily, or perhaps ever truly, be replaced by other social ties. Many aspects of long-term, intimate relationships (e.g., shared experiences and memories, idiosyncratic and treasured patterns of interaction) cannot easily be replicated or replaced. Yet people do attempt to find alternative sources of support and companionship following the loss or disruption of a close relationship (e.g., Morgan et al., 1997). How well these efforts succeed in restoring or preserving physical and emotional health remains an important question for future research.

## CONCLUSION

Social relationships serve as a source of uplifting and disheartening experiences. We sought to highlight the health-related effects of both kinds of interpersonal experiences. Given that social relationships can both bolster and drain emotional well-being, we examined research on three classes of strategies that older adults might pursue to maximize positive experiences, minimize negative experiences, and adapt to the loss or disruption of close relationships.

We first considered older adults' efforts to structure their social network to spend time with rewarding interaction partners. According to socioemotional selectivity theory, social networks and rates of social interaction decrease as people age, but these decreases are neither random nor involuntary, and instead reflect selective engagement with close, emotionally gratifying social network members. Thus, by choosing to interact with a subset of their closest network members, older adults enhance the quality of their interpersonal experiences and, in turn, their psychological well-being.

Selective engagement with rewarding interaction partners is not always possible, however, and unpleasant or stressful interactions with network members sometimes cannot be avoided. This led us to consider how older adults might seek to respond to interpersonal difficulties with members of their social networks. When negative interactions occur, the manner in which older adults respond is likely to have implications for their own emotional well-being and sense of coping efficacy, as well as for the relationship itself. Persistently stressful social relationships are strongly implicated in depression in later life (Krause & Rook, 2003), and depression is linked to negative physical health outcomes (e.g., Ormel, Rijsdijk, Sullivan, van Sonderen, & Kempen, 2002). Such evidence underscores the importance of efforts to understand how well older adults' coping efforts mitigate the health-related toll of conflict and tensions with social network members.

Finally, we sought to examine older adults' efforts to respond to the loss or disruption of important social relationships. Given that bereavement is associated with declines in mental and physical health, older adults' ability to identify alternative sources of support and companionship may play an important role in sustaining their psychological and physical health. Our discussion emphasized, however, that beneficial effects of alternative sources of social support cannot simply be assumed and, instead, must be evaluated. Further research is needed to understand the conditions under which compensatory benefits of substitute social ties actually emerge.

A variety of questions come to the fore in thinking about research that will extend our current understanding of older adults' strategies for protecting and strengthening their social relationships. For instance, to what extent are such strategies conscious and subject to planful actions? When do members of older adults' social networks, rather than older adults themselves, seek to intervene to enhance the older person's social ties in some way? Do self-initiated versus other-initiated strategies of relationship regulation have different outcomes? What roles do age and prior experience play in these efforts? For example, do developmental shifts in problem-solving skills or the capacity to regulate emotions lead older adults to respond to relationship conflicts and stressors differently than do younger or middle-aged adults? Research on everyday problem solving (Blanchard-Fields, Stein, & Watson, 2004) and on marital interaction during conflicts (Levenson, Carstensen, & Gottman, 1994) suggests that important age differences may exist, but extensions of this work to the broader interpersonal domain remain scarce. What are the physical and emotional health consequences of success versus failure in efforts to regulate social relationships in later life? Finally, how are older adults' efforts to optimize their social relationships influenced by constraints and opportunities that exist in the social environment (cf. Heckhausen & Schulz, 1995)? Pursuing such questions in future research will help to shed light on how older adults seek to preserve and enhance an important resource for physical and psychological health—their social relationships.

## REFERENCES

Aldwin, C. M. (1990). The Elders Life Stress Inventory (ELSI): Egocentric and nonegocentric stress. In M. A. P. Stephens, S. E. Hobfoll, J. H. Crowther, & D. L. Tennenbaum (Eds.), *Stress and coping in late-life families* (pp. 49–69). New York: Hemisphere.

Aldwin, C. M. (1999). *Stress, coping, and development: An integrative approach.* New York: Guilford Press.

Antonucci, T. C. (1985). Personal characteristics, social networks, and social behavior. In R. H. Binstock & E. Shanas (Eds.), *Handbook of aging and the social sciences* (2nd ed., pp. 94–128). New York: Van Nostrand Reinhold.

Avlund, K., Lund, R., Holstein, B. E., & Due, P. (2004). Social relations as determinant of onset of disability in aging. *Archives of Gerontology and Geriatrics, 38,* 85–99.

Baltes, M. M. (1996). *The many faces of dependency in old age.* New York: Cambridge University Press.

Baltes, M. M., & Wahl, H. W. (1992). The dependency–support script in institutions: Generalization to community settings. *Psychology and Aging, 7,* 409–418.

Birditt, K. S., & Fingerman, K. L. (2005). Do we get better at picking our battles?: Age group differences in descriptions of behavioral reactions to interpersonal problems. *Journals of Gerontology: Psychological Sciences and Social Sciences, Series B, 60,* P121–P128.

Blanchard-Fields, F., Stein, R., & Watson, T. L. (2004). Age differences in emotion-regulation strategies in handling everyday problems. *Journals of Gerontology: Psychological Sciences and Social Sciences, Series B, 59,* P261–P269.

Boerner, K., Reinhardt, J. P., Raykov, T., & Horowitz, A. (2004). Stability and change in social negativity in later life: Reducing received while maintaining initiated negativity. *Journals of Gerontology: Psychological Sciences and Social Sciences, Series B, 59,* S230–S237.

Bolger, N., DeLongis, A., Kessler, R. C., & Schilling, E. A. (1989). Effects of daily stress on negative mood. *Journal of Personality and Social Psychology, 57,* 808–818.

Bonanno, G. A., Wortman, C. B., Lehman, D. R., Tweed, R. G., Haring, M., Sonnega, J., et al. (2002). Resilience to loss and chronic grief: A prospective study from pre-loss to 18 months post-loss. *Journal of Personality and Social Psychology, 83,* 1150–1164.

Carstensen, L. L., Isaacowitz, D. M., & Charles, S. T. (1999). Taking time seriously: A theory of socioemotional selectivity. *American Psychologist, 54,* 165–181.

Cicirelli, V. G. (1995). *Sibling relationships across the life span.* New York: Plenum Press.

Cohen, S. (2004). Social relationships and health. *American Psychologist, 59,* 676–684.

Connidis, I. A., & Davies, L. (1992). Confidants and companions: Choices in later life. *Journal of Gerontology, 47,* S115–S122.

Coyne, J. C., & Racioppo, M. W. (2000). Never the twain shall meet?: Closing the gap between coping research and clinical intervention research. *American Psychologist, 55,* 655–664.

Coyne, J. C., Wortman, C. B., & Lehman, D. R. (1988). The other side of support: Emotional overinvolvement and miscarried helping. In B. H. Gottlieb (Ed.), *Marshalling social support: Formats, processes, and effects* (pp. 305–330). Newbury Park, CA: Sage.

Cumming, E., & Henry, W. E. (1961). *Growing old: The process of disengagement.* New York: Basic Books.

Diener, E., & Seligman, M. E. P. (2004). Beyond money: Toward an economy of well-being. *Psychological Science in the Public Interest, 5,* 1–31.

Finch, J. F., Okun, M. A., Pool, G. J., & Ruehlman, L. S. (1999). A comparison of the influence of conflictual and supportive social interactions on psychological distress. *Journal of Personality, 67,* 581–621.

Fincham, F. D., Beach, S. R. H., & Davila, J. (2004). Forgiveness and conflict resolution in marriage. *Journal of Family Psychology, 18,* 72–81.

Fingerman, K. L. (1998). Tight lips?: Aging mothers' and adult daughters' responses to interpersonal tensions in their relationships. *Personal Relationships, 5,* 121–138.

Frederickson, B. L., & Carstensen, L. L. (1990). Choosing social partners: How old age and anticipated endings make people more selective. *Psychology and Aging, 5,* 335–347.

Fung, H. H., Carstensen, L. L., & Lutz, A. M. (1999). Influence of time on social preferences: Implications for life-span development. *Psychology and Aging, 14,* 595–604.

Glass, T. A., Matchar, D. B., Belyea, M., & Feussner, J. R. (1993). Impact of social support on outcome in first stroke. *Stroke, 24,* 64–70.

Heckhausen, J., & Schulz, R. (1995). A life-span theory of control. *Psychological Review, 102,* 284–304.

House, J. S., Umberson, D., & Landis, K. (1988). Structures and processes of social support. *Annual Review of Sociology, 14,* 293–318.

Johnson, C. L., & Catalano, D. J. (1983). A longitudinal study of family supports to impaired elderly. *Gerontologist, 23,* 612–625.

Johnson, C. L., & Troll, L. (1992). Family functioning in late late life. *Journals of Gerontology: Psychological Sciences and Social Sciences, Series B, 47,* S66–S72.

Jones, W. H., Moore, D. S., Schrater, A., & Negel, L. A. (2000). Interpersonal transgressions and betrayals. In R. M. Kowalski (Ed.), *Behaving badly* (pp. 233–256). Washington, DC: American Psychological Association.

Krause, N., & Rook, K. S. (2003). Negative interaction in late life: Issues in the stability and generalizability of conflict across relationships. *Journals of Gerontology: Psychological Sciences and Social Sciences, Series B, 58*, P88–P99.

Krause, N., & Shaw, B. A. (2002). Negative interaction and changes in functional disability during late life. *Journal of Social and Personal Relationships, 19*, 339–359.

Lamme, S., Dykstra, P. A., & Broese van Groenou, M. I. (1996). Rebuilding the network: New relationships in widowhood. *Personal Relationships, 3*, 337–349.

Lang, F. R. (2001). Regulation of social relationships in later adulthood. *Journals of Gerontology: Psychological Sciences and Social Sciences, Series B, 56*, P321–P326.

Lang, F. R., & Carstensen, L. L. (1994). Close emotional relationships in late life: Further support for proactive aging in the social domain. *Psychology and Aging, 9*, 315–324.

Lazarus, R. S., & Folkman, S. (1984). *Stress, appraisal, and coping.* New York: Springer.

Levenson, R. W., Carstensen, L. L., & Gottman, J. M. (1994). Influence of age and gender on affect, physiology, and their interrelations: A study of long-term marriages. *Journal of Personality and Social Psychology, 67*, 56–68.

Lockenhoff, C. E., & Carstensen, L. L. (2004). Socioemotional selectivity theory, aging, and health: The increasingly delicate balance between regulating emotions and making tough choices. *Journal of Personality, 72*, 1395–1424.

Lund, D. A., Caserta, M. S., & Diamond, M. R. (1993). The course of spousal bereavement. In M. S. Stroebe, W. Stroebe, & R. O. Hansson (Eds.), *Handbook of bereavement: Theory, research, and intervention* (pp. 240–254). Cambridge, UK: Cambridge University Press.

Maddox, G. L. (1964). Disengagement theory: A critical evaluation. *Gerontologist, 4*, 80–82.

Martire, L. M., Stephens, M. A. P., Druley, J. A., & Wojno, W. C. (2002). Negative reactions to received spousal care: Predictors and consequences of miscarried support. *Health Psychology, 21*, 167–176.

Mendes de Leon, C. F., Glass, T. A., Beckett, L. A., Seeman, T. E., Evans, D. A., & Berkman, L. F. (1999). Social networks and disability transitions across eight intervals of yearly data in the New Haven EPSES. *Journals of Gerontology: Psychological Sciences and Social Sciences, Series B, 54*, S162–S172.

Mendes de Leon, C. F., Glass, T. A., & Berkman, L. F. (2003). Social engagement and disability in a community population of older adults: The New Haven EPESE. *American Journal of Epidemiology, 157*, 633–642.

Mendes de Leon, C. F., Gold, D. T., Glass, T. A., Kaplan, L., & George, L. K. (2001). Disability as a function of social networks and support in elderly African Americans and whites: the Duke EPESE 1986–1992. *Journals of Gerontology: Psychological Sciences and Social Sciences, Series B, 56*, P179–P190.

Morgan, D. L., Carder, P. C., & Neal, M. B. (1997). Are some relationships more useful than others?: The value of similar others in the networks of recent widows. *Journal of Social and Personal Relationships, 14*, 745–759.

Newsom, J. T. (1999). Another side to caregiving: Negative reactions to being helped. *Current Directions in Psychological Science, 8,* 183–187.

Ormel, J., Rijsdijk, F. V., Sullivan, M., van Sonderen, E., & Kempen, G. (2002). Temporal and reciprocal relationship between IADL/ADL disability and depressive symptoms in late life. *Journals of Gerontology, Psychological Sciences and Social Sciences, Series B, 57,* P338–P347.

Oxman, T. E., Freeman, D. H., Manheimer, E. D., & Stukel, T. (1994). Social support and depression after cardiac surgery in elderly patients. *American Journal of Geriatric Psychiatry, 2,* 309–323.

Perlman, D. (1988). Loneliness: A life-span family perspective. In R. M. Milardo (Ed.), *Families and social networks.: New perspectives on family* (pp. 190–220). Thousand Oaks, CA: Sage.

Penley, J. A., Tomaka, J., & Wiebe, J. S. (2002). The association of coping to physical and psychological health outcomes: A meta-analytic review. *Journal of Behavioral Medicine, 25,* 551–603.

Rook, K. S. (1994). Assessing the health-related dimensions of older adults' social relationships. In M. P. Lawton & J. Teresi (Eds.), *Annual review of gerontology and geriatrics* (Vol. 14, pp. 142–181). New York: Springer.

Rook, K. S. (1998). Investigating the positive and negative sides of personal relationships: Through a lens darkly? In B. H. Spitzberg & W. R. Cupach (Eds.), *The dark side of close relationships* (pp. 369–393). Mahwah, NJ: Erlbaum.

Rook, K. S., Sorkin, D. H., & Zettel, L. A. (2004). Stress in social relationships: Coping and adaptation across the life span. In F. Lang & K. Fingerman (Eds.), *Growing together: Personal relationships across the lifespan* (pp. 210–239). New York: Cambridge University Press.

Seeman, T. E. (2000). Health promoting effects of friends and family on health outcomes in older adults. *American Journal of Health Promotion, 14,* 362–370.

Seeman, T. E., Berkman, L. F., Charpentier, P. A., Blazer, D. G., Albert, M. S., & Tinetti, M. E. (1995). Behavioral and psychosocial predictors of physical performance: MacArthur Studies of Successful Aging. *Journals of Gerontology: Biological Sciences and Medical Sciences, Series A, 50,* M177–M183.

Seeman, T. E., Bruce, M. L., & McAvay, G. J. (1996). Social network characteristics and onset of ADL disability: MacArthur Studies of Successful Aging. *Journals of Gerontology: Psychological Sciences and Social Sciences, Series B, 51,* S191–S200.

Seeman, T. E., & McEwen, B. S. (1996). Impact of social environment characteristics on neuroendocrine regulation. *Psychosomatic Medicine, 58,* 459–471.

Settersten, R. A., Jr. (2002). Challenges of the third age: Meaning and purpose in later life. In R. S. Weiss & S. A. Bass (Eds.), *Challenges of the third age: Meaning and purpose in later life* (pp. 55–79). London: Oxford University Press.

Sherbourne, C. D., Meredith, L. S., Rogers, W., & Ware, J. E. (1992). Social support and stressful life events: Age differences in their effects on health-related quality of life among the chronically ill. *Quality of Life Research, 1,* 235–246.

Shuchter, S. R., & Zisook, S. (1993). The course of normal grief. In M. S. Stroebe, W. Stroebe, & R. O. Hansson (Eds.), *Handbook of bereavement: Theory, research, and intervention* (pp. 23–43). Cambridge, UK: Cambridge University Press.

Sorkin, D. H., & Rook, K. S. (in press). Dealing with negative social exchanges in later life: Coping responses, goals, and effectiveness. *Psychology and Aging.*

Strawbridge, W. J., Cohen, R. D., Shema, S. J., & Kaplan, G. A. (1996). Successful aging: Predictors and associated activities. *American Journal of Epidemiology, 144,* 135–141.

Stroebe, W., & Stroebe, M. S. (1987). *Bereavement and health: The psychological and physical consequences of partner loss.* Cambridge, UK: Cambridge University Press.

Turk, D. C., Kerns, R. D., & Rosenberg, R. (1992). Effects of marital interaction on chronic pain and disability: Examining the down side of social support. *Rehabilitation Psychology, 37,* 259–274.

Uchino, B. N., Cacioppo, J. T., & Kiecolt-Glaser, J. K. (1996). The relationship between social support and physiological processes: A review with emphasis on underlying mechanisms and implications for health. *Psychological Bulletin, 119,* 488–531.

Unger, J. B., McAvay, G., Bruce, M. L., Berkman, L., & Seeman, T. (1999). Variation in the impact of social network characteristics on physical functioning in elderly persons: MacArthur Studies of Successful Aging. *Journals of Gerontology: Psychological Sciences and Social Sciences, Series B, 54,* S245–S251.

U. S. Bureau of the Census, Current Population Survey. (2000). *America's families and living arrangements: Population characteristics.* Retrieved on September 9, 2003, from www.census.gov/prod/2001pubs/p20–537.pdf.

Wilcox, V. L., Kasl, S. V., & Berkman, L. F. (1994). Social support and physical disability in older people after hospitalization: A prospective study. *Health Psychology, 13,* 170–179.

Zettel, L. A., & Rook, K. S. (2004). Substitution and compensation in the social networks of older widowed women. *Psychology and Aging, 19,* 433–443.

# CHAPTER 15

# Issues of Diversity
# in Health Psychology and Aging

BARBARA W. K. YEE
*and* DAVID A. CHIRIBOGA

In a landmark book entitled *Unequal Treatment* (Smedley, Stith, & Nelson, 2003), the Institute of Medicine showed that cultural and social contexts play an important role in health disparities beyond the influence of socioeconomic status. Biological and genetic differences across groups may be involved, but causal inferences about these differences must be treated with care (Anderson & Nickerson, 2005). One result is that race is now treated more as a social construct when considering differences in health and functioning. Gender differences also represent a mixture of social–cultural and biological imperatives.

Disparities in the physical and mental health of ethnic minorities and women have been acknowledged, although disparities among older groups have only recently come to the attention of researchers (Glass, 2003; U.S. Department of Health and Human services, 2001; Whitfield, 2004). A key marker was the Congressionally mandated National Institutes of Health (NIH) Revitalization Act of 1993, following which NIH created guidelines for the inclusion of minorities and women in research projects (NIH, 1994). Without the specific decision to incorporate gender and ethnic diversity into sampling frames, we appeared destined to base an empirical literature of human health on samples of the nondiverse. Only now are investigators making progress in testing whether empirical findings based on advantaged populations generalize to other populations, such as older adults, females, and ethnic/minority or poor people. The continuing need for targeted funding is exemplified by the fact that from 2000 to 2003, only

3% of the NIH budget was devoted to understanding sex/gender differences (Simon et al., 2005).

In the following sections we discuss key constructs, why they are relevant, and how health psychologists might create more cultural- and gender-responsive research. This chapter focuses on aging, race, ethnicity, and culture, then discusses gender issues. The chapter concludes with a highlight of research opportunities in health psychology, diversity, and aging.

## WHY RACE, ETHNICITY, AND CULTURE?

Ambiguities cloud the empirical literature on health disparities. We have already noted that race is now considered more a social than a biological construct. As another example of ambiguity, consider the definition of "minority group"—a key definition in studying disparities—offered by the NIH (2004): "A minority group is a readily identifiable subset of the U.S. population that is distinguishable by racial, ethnic, and/or cultural heritage" (pp. 6–7). Because of their ambiguity, Bhopal (1997, p. 1751) has called investigations using terms such as "minority group" or "race" "black box epidemiology."

### Culture, Labeling, and Labeling Theory

Despite numerous definitional problems, the terms used still help us to frame the issues surrounding diversity and health disparities. Culture and ethnicity represent additional examples. "Culture" can be defined as a pattern of traditions, values, beliefs, norms, and attitudes that are transmitted across generations (e.g., Kroeber & Kluckhohn, 1952; Sternberg, 2004). "Ethnicity" refers to self-identity and membership in a group manifesting specific cultural patterns (Bhopal, 1997). Used inappropriately, ethnic and racial/minority labels can lead to simplistic interpretations, confusion, and even conflict. Are African-born individuals living in the United States equivalent in culture and ethnicity to African Americans? Cubans living in Florida may view themselves as members of the more generic "white" group. Although a recent national poll indicated that 65% preferred the term "Hispanic," there is regional variation, and some people are strongly opposed to being called "Hispanic" (Granado, 2003). Such controversies simply highlight the complexities of ethnic labeling.

Whereas a group label may be a convenience in communication, it can inadvertently suggest homogeneity, facilitate negative stereotypes, and not infrequently facilitate the expression of derogatives and prejudice. Negative stereotyping may be subtle but have destructive consequences. Minority groups can be portrayed as economically disadvantaged and less educated, criminally minded, or fanatically religious, thus yielding stereotypical responses toward all ethnic group members. Unfortunately, being pulled over for a DWB (driving while black) is not a rare event for African American males of all ages. More importantly, society's lowered expectations and stereotyping of certain minorities may produce performance that is consistent with these expectancies (Steel, 1997). As described in social labeling theory (e.g., Scheff, 1974), if society comes to view one as a failure, there is a greater chance that a person will eventually accept that label. Bengtson and Kuypers (1986) adapted social labeling theory to aging and noted that the downward spiral of negativity could be reversed through interventions providing opportunities for success in activities associated with a more positive self-image.

The multiple jeopardy and cumulative disadvantage hypotheses suggested that minorities and women are more likely to enter later life with a history of financial and educational disadvantages, and poorer access to physical and mental health care. Both hypotheses may lead to overgeneralization, because not all members of minority groups, or women, enter later life with a history of disadvantage. The multiple jeopardy hypothesis (i.e., being old, minority, and female) spoke to the cumulative disadvantages that accrued over a lifetime, such as lack of education and employment, leading to reduced access to physical and mental health services (Dowd & Bengtson, 1978).

A recent cumulative disadvantage hypothesis states that the impact of disadvantages faced by ethnic minorities and women increase over time (Whitfield, 2004). Evidence supporting this idea can be found in annual Medicare expenditures for older blacks, who average over $2,000 more than non-Hispanic whites (Federal Interagency Forum on Aging-Related Statistics, 2004). As a result, older minorities may arrive at later life bearing the burden of greater health problems and a lifelong pattern of service underutilization, even when covered by Medicare services (Williams & Rucker, 2000)

## Putting Theory and Research to Practice

Social labeling theory and historical disadvantage hypotheses underscore the point that physical and mental health disparities are not solely the result of genetic differences, but have significant psychosocial and behavioral components. Granted, the genetic component of adult-onset diabetes, for example, modifiable lifestyle factors, and nutrition and exercise still play an important role. Because certain minority groups, such as Mexican Americans, are more likely to engage in behaviors associated with greater risk of diabetes, effective intervention programs that target these groups are clearly in order.

On a more general note, the *Diagnostic and Statistical Manual of Mental Disorders* (American Psychiatric Association, 1994) now recognizes the existence of culture-specific constellations of behaviors with adverse consequences. Such behaviors are labeled "culture-bound syndromes." Readers may be familiar with the concepts of *amok* (a murderous frenzy followed by apathy), *koro* (perceived genital retraction), or *dhat* (anxiety about semen loss). Guarnaccia and Rogler (1999) have noted that the increasing diversity in America, coupled with DSM-IV recognition of the importance of culture, generates a need for research to understand these culturally linked syndromes in the context of assimilation and acculturation. Such syndromes may be more evident in older immigrants to America than in American-born (or higher) generation of ethnic minorities.

## The Scope of the Problem

The diversity of the U.S. population poses challenges to the health psychologist. In 2003, 83% of persons age 65 and older were non-Hispanic whites, approximately 8% were black, and 3% were Asian (single race); older Hispanics of any race accounted for about 6% of the older population (Federal Interagency Forum on Aging-Related Statistics, 2004). By 2050, the percentage of older, non-Hispanic whites drops to 61%, percentage of blacks increase to 12%, Asians to 8%, and Hispanics of any race, to 18%. Thus, the Hispanic older adults will increase the most: from slightly over 2 million in 2003 to 15 million by 2050. For health psychologists interested in developing interventions, it is critical to note that older Hispanics, as a group, are the least educated: Only 36% had attained a high school degree compared to 76% of non-Hispanic whites, 70% of Asians, and 52% of blacks.

In the context of these demographics, current health disparities in nearly all disease states are both striking and widely documented. High mortality and poor morbidity rates for African Americans in virtually all domains exceed those of non-Hispanic white populations (Smedley et al., 2003). For the Hispanic population, there are marked variations in incidence and prevalence of disease states and associated mortality rates (e.g., Vega & Amaro, 1994). Some years ago Markides and Coreil (1986) identified what they called an "epidemiologic paradox," in which Hispanics were found to have a significantly lower mortality rate than would be anticipated on the basis of sociodemographics; although partially attributable to return migration after retirement, this paradox has more recently been substantiated for most foreign-born Hispanics (Palloni & Arias, 2004) and immigrant Asian elderly (Hummer, Benjamins, & Rogers, 2004). Of concern is the rise of chronic diseases and negative health outcomes associated with the acculturation of immigrant populations (Jasso, Massey, Rosenzweig & Smith, 2004).

Less researched are the disparities in mental health (e.g., U.S. Department of Health and Human Services, 2001). In seeking to understand the causes underlying such disparities, researchers and practitioners alike should keep in mind the multiplicity of factors potentially at work. A number of factors at the individual and social level that have consequences for physical and mental health problems and treatment (see discussion by Alvidrez, Azocar, & Miranda, 1996) are presented below.

## Immigration

In 2002, approximately 40% of Hispanics, the largest ethnic/minority group in the United States, were foreign born. Of these, over one-half had immigrated to America between 1990 and 2002 (U.S. Bureau of the Census, 2003). Similarly, disproportionately large numbers of Asian elders (65.4%) other than the Japanese are foreign born. Typically, immigrants are less likely to be 65 and older when they arrive, which helps to explain why the proportion of Asian and Hispanic elders is still low relative to that of non-Hispanic whites and even blacks. However, the growth rate of both Asians and Hispanic elders is significantly greater (U.S. Bureau of the Census, 2003).

## The Fragmented Family

One consequence of immigration to the United States is that older family members, and members of the extended family, may be left behind. Another source of fragmentation may arise over time as younger members of the family acculturate to the host culture, whereas older members continue to hold to traditional expectations of support that are unmet.

## Posttraumatic Stress Disorder

Refugees who have involuntarily left their homelands during war or political conflict have experienced great losses, including their social networks (Alvidrez et al., 1996). Greater trauma has been experienced by refugees from Central America and from Southeast Asia. In nearly all instances, older refugees have been most affected (Handelman & Yeo, 1996; Knight, 2000; Tran, 1991; Yee, 1997). The resulting trauma continues to affect quality of life decades later, because it has not been adequately addressed by health professionals.

## Acculturation

Generally those who are more educated and hold higher paying jobs experience fewer problems in adaptation (e.g., Moyerman & Forman, 1992). Controlling for socioeconomic status does not eliminate the differences. Among older Mexican Americans, for example, those with less acculturation report more symptoms of depression, even among second-generation individuals (e.g., Chiriboga, Black, Aranda, & Markides, 2002).

## Gatekeepers

To the extent that older family members have difficulty speaking English, they may rely on gatekeepers, people who interface in situations that range from everything transportation services to shopping at the grocery store, to utilizing the health care system. Undocumented aliens are also more likely to rely on gatekeepers, or on informal and uncredentialed service providers, regardless of language barriers.

## Health Insurance

As noted earlier, ethnic/minority groups are more likely to have lacked insurance when of working age. This is in large part a consequence of lower average incomes and greater likelihood that employers did not cover health insurance. In later life, their lower incomes and often poorer health status make it more difficult for them to afford medications, despite having national health insurance (e.g., Klein, Turvey, & Wallace, 2004). These problems are more likely to be the case for older immigrants, especially the undocumented ones.

## Generational Effects

Although immigrants face a number of challenges, each successive generation faces new sets of challenges. Second-generation minorities usually have high levels of acculturation and assimilation, unless they live in ethnic minority enclaves, such as a classic "Chinatown" or in a *barrio* near the Mexican border, where the majority of residents speak Chinese, Spanish, and so forth. First- and second-generation immigrant families may face barriers imposed by members of the host culture, but for Hispanics in the United States, these barriers may be blurred (Alba, 2005). The third generation is most likely to first attain full assimilation (Alba, 2002). On the other hand, while awareness of one's cultural heritage and preference for ancestral language decreases with each successive generation, loyalty to one's ethnic group remains relatively stable (e.g., Keefe & Padilla, 1987).

## Education and Income

Ethnic/minority groups as a rule have less education and lower incomes than non-Hispanic whites (Federal Interagency Forum on Aging-Related Statistics, 2004; U.S. Bureau of the Census, 2003). Although education and income affect health and health care utilization, ethnic minority status generally exerts an independent effect. Health beliefs, values, dietary patterns, familiarity with the health care system, language barriers, citizenship status, a history of oppression or discrimination, and other factors all influence health.

## Health Beliefs

Depending on circumstances such as country of origin, generation within the United States, and neighborhood context, members of ethnic minority groups may hold health beliefs that differ from those of the host culture (Guarnaccia & Rogler, 1999). Vaillant (2003) points out at least six models of mental health, and that members of different cultural groups—and therapists—may differ in what model they use when identifying good or bad mental health.

## Stigma

Cultural groups may vary in the degree to which mental illness is stigmatized in their native lands. Stigmatization of mental illness, can in turn lead to avoidance of seeking treatment (Major & O'Brien, 2005).

## Communication

When a client or research participant does not speak English, the potential communication problem is clear. However, even in the absence of an obvious problem, communication issues may exist. Older patients from any group may have difficulty hearing, a problem that may be compounded when English is a second language. The words used by the health professional or researcher may be difficult for the client to understand—and the client may be hesitant to mention this fact. These communication problems may lead health professionals to treat minority clients differently than their more mainstream clients. For example, one study of 458 white and black patients (mean age = 50) who met with over 60 different physicians revealed that physicians were more demanding and authoritative with their black patients, and exhibited more negative affect (Johnson, Roter, Powe, & Cooper, 2004). In turn, a lack of respect or perception of unfair treatment by ethnic minority clients has been associated with reduced compliance and follow-up.

## Cultural Competence in Practice

The preceding section dealt with topics about which practitioners and researchers should have some knowledge—what is often referred to as "cultural competence." Contrary to some interpretations, competence is not simply about language. Cultural competence is a construct that deals generally and most simply with a practitioner's knowledge about a group and his or her appropriate use of clinical skills (e.g., Sue, Arredondo, & McDavis, 1992). One of the more complete operational definitions of "cultural competence" was developed by the U.S. Department of Health and Human Services, Office of Minority Health (2001): The set of 14 standards that apply to the provision of "culturally and linguistically appropriate services" (CLAS) consist of four mandates required of all recipients of federal services, nine recommended guidelines, and one general recommendation.

For example, the first mandated standard states, "Health care organizations must offer and provide language assistance services, including staff and interpreter services, at no cost to each patient/consumer with limited English proficiency at all points of contact, in a timely manner during all hours of operation" (Office of Minority Health, 2001, p. 10). One solution to the demand posed by this particular standard is for local and regional intervention programs to form partnerships with community-based programs that serve the needs of the various ethnic/minority populations. These community partners can assist in the identification of individuals in need. To facilitate such activities, intervention specialists can develop training programs for community partners.

## Access and Appropriateness

Older minority individuals are more likely to be diagnosed at a later stage of illness than are non-Hispanic whites, and are less likely to obtain adequate medical care. These problems are actually more pronounced among younger minorities, since they are the least likely to have health insurance (with certain exceptions, Medicare becomes available at age 65). However, as noted earlier, a personal history of underutilization may create its own barriers to access, even when economic considerations are removed. Underutilization is enhanced by language barriers and, for some, undocumented or "illegal" status in this country.

Although it may be impractical to tailor interventions for every ethnic/minority group, health psychologists and others have been successful when the intervention team has understood the needs and behaviors of the target population. Campbell et al. (2004) designed a colorectal cancer prevention program specifically for older African Americans that significantly improved both diet and exercise. Similarly, a recent U.S. Food and Drug Administration (FDA) trial has demonstrated the efficacy of a new drug for congestive heart failure (CHF), BiDil, that is particularly effective with African Americans (Taylor et al., 2004). In both instances, the interventions work because the researchers understand the target population: understanding how one relates to African American churchgoers in the one case, and that African Americans with CHF are more likely to have a deficiency in nitric oxide, a substance involved in heart health, in the other.

## Cultural Competence in Research

Many of the CLAS clinical guidelines are also appropriate to research. There are a host of additional concerns and issues, some of which have been documented by the National Research Council (Van Ploeg & Perrin, 2004). Here we provide more detail on several issues of particular relevance to health psychologists studying older adults. Overall, there seems to be agreement that consideration of cultural issues not only helps to ensure compliance with local and federal research guidelines but also helps in identifying research gaps (e.g., Beiser, 2003).

### Recruitment

Access is a problem not only for the ethnic/minority group member seeking help but also for health psychologists and others who seek to include ethnic/minority subjects in their studies (Gauthier & Clarke, 1999). Some barriers to access stem from a community's past exposure to research. Historically, there are many instances of researchers coming to a community and conducting a study that is insensitive to the perceptions and behaviors of residents, or simply using the data for scientific publications, without any attempt to give back to the community. Distrust of research involving health issues is not uncommon. In the African American community, older adults may be particularly distrustful of health-related research due to instances such as the infamous Tuskegee Syphilis Study (Jones, 1993). Similarly, Manson, Garroutte, Goins, and Henderson (2004) report that because of a past history of flawed research activities conducted on their populations, a number of American Indian and Alaska Native communities have implemented programs that control access by outside researchers. In one case cited by Manson et al. (2004), research preparation for a study of community elders included institutional review board (IRB) reviews by eight different programs and 13 months of negotiations.

The greater effort often required to conduct research with ethnic/minority populations demonstrates both the impact of past experiences with outside researchers and the urgent need for researchers to be sensitive to the needs of the minority communities they study. Failure to understand the community or population being studied can lead to systematic biases in recruitment and, subsequently, in results. This is particularly true when studying older adult minorities, who are often markedly fewer in number and require special efforts. As an example of potential biases, Conroy and Heer (2003) report that because homeless Hispanic men may not live in the same areas as non-Hispanic whites and blacks, they are often overlooked in studies of the homeless. Cabral et al. (2003) found that middle-aged and older blacks recruited by random digit dialing (RDD) were more likely to manifest risk factors for lung cancer than those who were recruited through community-based efforts, such as working with religious organizations. However, the RDD approach took more than 18 times longer per subject recruited than did the community-based methods.

## Instrumentation

Recruitment is not the only challenge facing researchers working with minority communities. Instrumentation can pose a threat to generalizability. The problem may be reduced when the study or intervention is qualitative or case-focused, reflecting what linguists and anthropologists (e.g., Triandis, McCusker, Betacourt, Iwao, Leung, Salazar, et al., 1993) have called the "emic" approach to data collection. Studies that follow the emic tradition are devoted to understanding a particular people rather than attempting to generalize across cultures.

The contrasting "etic" approach attempts to use a standard battery of instruments or questions across groups or cultures. Several potential problems can be anticipated with an etic approach, centering on what is called the "cultural equivalence" of an instrument (e.g., Matias-Carrelo et al., 2003). Sternberg (2004) lists four scenarios with broad relevance: (1) The nature of the phenomenon under study is sufficiently similar across cultures that it allows use of the same measure; (2) the nature of the phenomenon differs across cultures, but existing instruments are adequate; (3) the nature of the phenomenon is the same, but instruments should differ because the meaning of the items differ and interpretations may therefore be erroneous; and (4) the nature of the phenomenon is so different from culture to culture that different measures are required.

What Sternberg's scenarios point out is that even with adequate, culturally appropriate translations and content, problems may remain with instrumentation. A particular concern is whether the structure of responses is the same across groups of interest. Anyone familiar with cross-cultural applications of the Center for Epidemiologic Studies—Depression Scale (CES-D; Radloff, 1977) knows that factor analyses of this instrument yield a wide range of solutions. The differences in structure may be meaningful. Jang, Kim, and Chiriboga (2005) have found that Korean American older adults with higher or lower scores on acculturation vary significantly in the factor structure of the CES-D, which suggests that more traditional Korean older adults experience symptoms differently than do more assimilated individuals. On the other hand, structural differences for this instrument are not universal. Analyses of blacks have been found to yield structures very similar to those of white groups (e.g., Nguyen, Kitner-Tiolo, Evans, & Zonderman, 2004). Generally, both researchers and practitioners would be well-advised to examine not only the adequacy of translations and similarity of factorial structure across cultures of interest but also the concurrent and predictive validity of instruments within the cultures.

## WHY GENDER?

As illustrated earlier, culture, ethnicity, and race are important sources of diversity in the later years. Other important sources of variability during the second half of life are sex and gender. Like culture, ethnicity, and race, the influences of sex and gender reflect far more than biological, physiological, and genetic factors: The influence of the lifelong sociocultural context plays an important role in what it means to be an older man or woman.

Gender research has had a long tradition in health psychology and the behavioral sciences in general. Stewart and McDermott (2004) highlighted two important research themes in the study of gender in psychology. The first theme highlights differentials in power relationships traditionally attached to gender. These power differentials drive the nature and outcomes of resource access throughout the lifespan and social relationships in families, communities, and society. For instance, these power relationships may color the relationships between spouses, within families, and between patients and their physicians in ways that reflect societal expectations. Gender roles with prescribed societal expectations are socialized in specific ways by generation and culture.

The second theme relates to improving our understanding of how the social status of men and women contributes to and shapes personality characteristics such as social identity and behavior throughout the lifespan. Gender identify and its behavioral ramifications are developed, solidified, and modified as a result of personal experiences and feedback from the social environment.

Only in the last decade have the studies of biological, genetic, and physiological underpinnings of sex differences developed into a mature science. There are now some reasonable genetic, physiological, and biological tools with which to measure and account for these influences in our explanatory models of aging.

At the same time, we have not made significant research progress regarding how the environmental, developmental, and psychosocial contexts interact with the biological underpinnings over the lifespan to produce gender effects in later life. The overarching themes for research on women's health at NIH largely focus upon the biological and genetic sciences, as outlined by the *Agenda for Research in Women's Health for the 21st Century* (USDHHS, 1999a) and the Institute of Medicine report, *Exploring the Biological Contributions to Human Health: Does Sex Matter?* (Wizemann & Pardue, 2001). These reports acknowledge that more gender-related behavioral and social science research is needed, yet federal research initiatives have not materialized.

A major stumbling block is the lack of multifactorial and multidisciplinary frameworks to guide gender-related research after the reproductive phase of the life cycle and in the context of biological and sociocultural factors. For instance, according to theorists Wood and Eagly (2002), who examined the behavior of men and women in the context of social roles and biological imperatives before and during the reproductive phase of the life cycle across cultures and societies, older members of the culture have supportive roles in the rearing of children, whereas parents attend to basic needs for subsistence. This perspective is not unusual: There is an absence of theoretical frameworks and empirical research related to gender development in the second half of life.

## Gender, Aging, and Health Psychology

Health psychology has played a key role in shaping the empirical research on the relationships among the brain, cognitions, and health (Ray, 2004); health disparities (Anderson, Castro, Kilty, Schneiderman & Yee, 1995); and coping, stress, and aging (Aldwin & Park, 2004). To explain more fully complex human behavior and its resulting health outcomes, psychological research must examine how important sources of diversity, such as gender differences, mediate and moderate health and quality of life in late life (Anderson, Bulatao, & Cohen, 2004; Yali & Revenson, 2004). Much of the research typically focuses on processes within a specific sex or gender, or may not purposefully examine gender in its research design or analysis.

The NIH expends a significant share of its budget on disease-specific research and health care initiatives focused on cardiovascular disease, cancer, HIV/AIDS, immunizations, and diabetes. Historically, these initiatives have done little to address cross-cutting issues such as the influence of gender, or underlying contributing factors such as poverty, lack of health access, and discriminatory barriers. Health psychology can make significant research contributions to understanding psychological, social, and behavioral mechanisms that have directly and indirectly contributed to diseases and resulting health outcomes. The following paragraphs provide examples of how health psychology has made, or might make major inroads in reducing health disparities during later life.

### Heart Disease and Gender

There is a critical need to examine the influence of gender upon heart disease in the later years. Heart disease is the number one killer of older women (for Asian American women, cancer is the number one killer). Women are at high risk after menopause, are underdiagnosed, and often are unaware of this issue, because the public believes heart disease to be a "man's disease" (Marcuccio, Loving, Bennett, & Hayes, 2003; Shulman et al., 1999). This mistaken belief is a barrier to appropriate heart disease interventions for women during perimenopause and menopause (Travis, 2005). Even after being diagnosed, older women are less likely than men to receive gold standard, gender-appropriate treatment. Health psychologists can investigate behavioral and social issues related to higher risk of heart disease among poor and minority populations.

## Cancer and Gender

Cancer is the number two killer of women, with lung cancer as the leading subcategory. Women may be more vulnerable than men to the carcinogenic effects of smoking (Patel, Bach, & Kris, 2004), with possible tumor promotion by estrogen. Not only are women more susceptible to lung cancer from smoking themselves, but they may also reap greater negative health consequences, such as increased risk of cervical, breast, and lung cancer, from passive smoking exposures (Trimble et al., 2005). Health education and smoking cessation interventions appear to more effectively reduce smoking among men than among women. More competent and responsive interventions need to be developed to decrease smoking among women.

## Sex, Gender, and Physiological Differences

Much research indicates women's vulnerability to physical pain and a greater incidence of painful disorders in women. An important question is, what aspects of pain perception and emotional/behavioral reactions result from gender and sociocontextual variables such as stress exposure over the lifespan? Some investigators suggest that women are more sensitive to pain during the menstrual cycle and become vigilant to other pain sensations over the lifespan (Wizeman & Pardue, 2001). Women are more likely than men to use a wide variety of therapies for pain in response to their higher incidence of painful disorders and heightened sensitivity to pain. Social and behavioral causal factors related to pain experiences have yet to be identified. An important question is whether female pain sensitivity, established earlier in the lifecycle, is later modified in the absence of female hormones during and after menopause. Attention to the protective factors, such as positive affect (Zautra, Johnson, & Davis, 2005) or religion (Park, Chapter 16, this volume), can be a source of resilience for women with chronic pain.

The increased attention to sex and gender differences in energy metabolism, body composition, and obesity may ultimately reveal significant environmental and sociocultural factors. Although differences in body composition are mediated by sex hormones, these differences tend to diminish after puberty. With menopause, there is an increase in the amount of body fat and its deposition in the abdominal region of the body. Health psychologists have been involved in the clinical and behavioral management of weight loss and physical activity, and more attention should be directed at middle-aged and premenopausal women.

A promising area of research that explores gender and sex differences in neurobiology uses improved technology developed in the last decade (Cahill, 2005). Although the debate about sex differences in functional organization of the brain for language, reading, or other specific cognitive processes continues, there appear to be specific sex differences in phonological processing, with brain activation in the left inferior frontal gyrus among men, and in the left and right inferior frontal gyri among women (Shaywitz et al., 1995). Other research has found that sex differences in language processing may occur between as well as within hemispheres of the brain (Baxter et al., 2003). These sex differences suggest that memory and language interventions after a stroke may need to be modified by gender.

### Alcohol, Health Outcomes, and Gender

Women are at higher health risk from not only smoking but also alcohol. Dose–response studies of alcohol consumption indicate that women have a higher risk of liver cirrhosis and brain disorders earlier in their drinking careers and at half the dose required for men (U.S. Department of Health and Human Services, 1999b). Alcohol may protect bone density but increase the risk of early tumor promotion (Gapstur, Potter, Sellers, & Folson, 1992). Thus, alcohol within a narrow dose range may provide protection for one health condition, while being a risk factor for another. Such findings suggest the need for gender-targeted interventions, because the negative consequences of some risky behaviors (e.g., smoking, alcohol consumption, unprotected sex) for women may be far more serious than for men.

### Gender, Risk, and Protective Health Mechanisms

The study of how social environments interact with the biology and genetics of aging may advance our understanding of protective health mechanisms and pathways to health or illness (Ryff & Singer, 2003). For instance, in the Midlife Development in the United States Study (Ryff, Singer, Wing, & Love, 2001), adults ages 25–74 who reported better health also reported more positive social/relational experiences. Longitudinal research has shown high allostatic load to be a important predictor of cardiovascular disease, decline in cognitive and physical functioning, and death over a 7-year period (Karlamangla, Singer, McEwen, Rowe, & Seeman, 2002; Seeman, Rowe, McEwen, & Singer, 2001). The Wisconsin Longitudinal Study (Ryff et al., 2001) found that a positive social environment in childhood and adulthood served as protective factors in midlife. The effect was significant for both genders, but it was far more dramatic for men than for women. This research suggests that a positive social environment in the first half of life is heath protective to a greater degree for men than for women.

Seeman, Singer, Rygg, Love, and Levy-Storms (2002) found a gender difference in the impact of the social environment upon middle-aged and older adults. Among the younger cohort, 58–59 years of age, positive social relationships over the lifespan were related to lower allostatic load for both men and women. Older men, 70–79 years of age, who were more socially integrated and had frequent emotional/social supports, had lower allostatic loads than those lacking these socially protective factors. No significant associations were seen for older women. These age and gender differences in how social relationships and environments impact health must be explored to untangle and identify important predictors of the social environment that have significant health implications for older women.

Whereas cortisol response to challenge was significantly stronger for older women (Otte et al., 2005), aerobic fitness counteracted these high cortisol responses and greater systolic blood pressure in older women (Traustadóttir, Bosch, & Matt, 2005). The implication is that significant lifestyle changes, such as improved physical fitness, could dramatically improve health outcomes among elderly women.

## Emotions, Aging, and Gender

Emotions are an important mediator between stressors and health outcomes. Both culture and gender expectations shape how people express emotions, respond to life's challenges, and devise problem-solving strategies. For example, responses to stress by females may be closer to the "tend-and-befriend" than the "fight-or-flight" reaction (Taylor et al., 2000). One of the suggested biological links of the "tend-and-befriend" responses to stress is oxytocin, a female reproductive hormone. An empirical question is whether these stress response behaviors are lessened or absent after menopause. Research must determine whether this female response to stress, facilitated by oxytocin, is maintained by lifelong habitual patterns or diminished when these biological underpinnings are absent.

Psychosocial studies on how emotions mediate and regulate stressors and their impact on health outcomes has led to some of the more fruitful developments in the last decade. According to Carstensen, Fung, and Charles (2003), a lifetime of experience allows older people to regulate their emotions more effectively than do younger people. Ong and Bergemen (2004) suggested that resilient elders are better than younger people at differentiating their positive and negative emotions, and have higher emotional complexity. Resilient elderly adults are also more likely to possess dispositions such as openness to experience, mindfulness, and emotional intelligence. Middle-aged adults use more proactive emotion regulation strategies than do older adults, and older adults use more passive emotion regulation than middle-aged adults in highly emotional situations (Blanchard-Fields, Stein, & Watson, 2004). In highly emotional situations, adaptive emotional strategies may vary by life stage. Culture has also been demonstrated to influence emotional expression and display rules for emotions (Matsumoto, Yoo, Hirayama, & Petrova, 2005). Overall, emotional regulation serves an integrative function among self-regulation, positive and negative affect, and dyadic processes, topics worthy of intense study during the later years (Diamond & Aspinwall, 2003).

## Health Beliefs

An important area of investigation is the role of health beliefs, attitudes, and knowledge, and their relationships to lifestyle behaviors. A substantial body of literature suggests that there may be a universal gender difference, with women having greater health knowledge and better lifestyle habits than men; however, the level of knowledge and lifestyle behaviors may vary across age, socioeconomic, and ethnic populations. For example, Beier and Ackerman (2003) found that older people may have greater health knowledge except in the mental health domain; their knowledge does not necessarily translate into better behavioral health lifestyle practices. Investigators found that older Vietnamese had greater knowledge about health but poorer lifestyle behaviors than younger Vietnamese (Yee, Nguyen, & Ha, 2003). In the same study, Vietnamese women had greater health knowledge and better lifestyle habits than Vietnamese men. Studies indicate that level of health knowledge regarding chronic diseases may be significantly improved among immigrant elders.

Even in national prevention programs such as WISEWOMAN (Will, Farris, Sanders, Stockmyer, & Finkelstein, 2004) or the Study of Women's Health across the Nation (SWAN), little attention has been paid to the needs of high risk and underserved populations such as Hmong, Cambodian, or Pacific Islander women. Most national surveys of older individuals exclude non-English-speaking aged populations that are often at greatest risk for poor health outcomes due to the lack of health care information and access.

## Health Behaviors, Aging, and Gender

Another fruitful area of investigation is an examination of the relationship between use of complementary and alternative medicine (CAM), help-seeking patterns, and delay of timely access to medical care. It has been estimated that 33% of women and 24% of men use CAM, with usage highest among those ages 35–54 (Berman & Straus, 2004). The most commonly used CAM modalities were prayer (14%), herbal medicine (10%), and chiropractic therapies (8%; Ni, Simile, & Hardy, 2002). Health psychologists can take a major role in investigation and developing instruments/measurements of expectation or placebo effects; patients' hopes; the influence of emotional states, risk perceptions, motivations; and other self-healing processes that may facilitate healing or promote help seeking on a timely basis, when therapies are most effective. Health service access, decision-making strategies for use of CAM or traditional health care, medication compliance, and disclosure relative to CAM (Piette, Heisler, & Wanger, 2004) can be fruitful areas of investigations.

## Gender Differences in Access to Care, Treatment Efficacy, and Outcomes

Gender appears to make a difference in access to care, treatment efficacy, and its resulting health outcomes. A major socioeconomic barrier, the high rate of poverty among older women (12% in comparison to 7.7% for men), is most problematic among minority older women (10.1% for non-Hispanic whites alone, 27.4% for blacks alone, 9.6% for Asians alone, and 23% for Hispanics; Federal Interagency Forum on Aging-Related Statistics, 2004). Lifelong health risks that accumulate over the life cycle, with increasing chronic and acute health episodes causing significant health crises, are not easily remedied by access to Medicare in late life.

Although Medicare helps to minimize the erosion of health access for many older women, it does not provide services to noncitizen older adults, and access to Medicaid services varies by state. Sexism, racism, and ageism put older, minority females at greater risk for not receiving preventive care and gold standard treatment for their health conditions (Shulman et al., 1999).

An area that has received increased attention is preventable adverse events such as medical errors and the iatrogenic effects of pharmacological therapeutic agents or CAMs (Kohn, Corrigan, & Donaldson, 2000). Although many medical errors are preventable, elders are at higher risk because of the potential for medication error as the number of drugs and the complexity of regimen increases. Sex, age, and ethnic differences in body composition (e.g., body fat and weight), metabolism (e.g., gastric emptying, cytochrome P450 that modulates oxidative metabolism of drugs in the liver), and excretion (e.g., kidney functioning) are especially likely to put older women and some minority populations at higher risk for adverse medication events. Antihistamines (terfenadine), antibiotics (erythromycin) and antiarrhythmic drugs, for example, can produce lethal cardiac rhythm, and the risk is far greater in females than males. According to Wizemann and Pardue (2001), sex differences may be more problematic with drugs that have narrow dose safety rather than wide therapeutic ranges. These types of sex differences imply that older females must either comply more closely with the prescribed treatment regimen or suffer more severe, health damaging consequences than older men or younger people.

Hewitt, Herdman, and Holland (2004) found that psychosocial interventions such as imagery, relaxation, and hypnosis are effective in reducing negative psychiatric symptoms and improving quality of life among individuals with early and metastatic breast cancer. They suggested that behavioral and psychosocial interventions should be offered as a routine aspect of medical care to improve quality of life during the later years. To accomplish this goal, psychosocial interventions must achieve parity in medical care reimbursement as a health policy issue. Cuff and Vanselow (2004) noted that there are compelling reasons for all physicians to possess basic knowledge and skills of the behavioral sciences; however, there is an equally compelling need for greater medical reimbursement for treatment by behavioral intervention specialists. As important, equal partnerships, and multidisciplinary treatment and research teams, would significantly enhance and improve care to reduce health disparities found in later life.

## BEYOND RACE, CULTURE, AND GENDER: SETTING AN AGENDA FOR THE FUTURE

As illustrated earlier in this chapter, health psychologists can make major contributions in reducing health disparities by conducting basic and applied research on ethnic minority and gender issues in gerontology. The task is a challenging one: Research progress in addressing disparities from a health psychology perspective has been insufficient, as has attention to the contextual variables that mediate disparities in health and behavior (Yali & Revenson, 2004). The topic of discrimination provides an example. Important social–environmental and contextual issues that arise from a history of discrimination produce behavioral and health outcomes (e.g., Jones, 1993). For instance, chronic stress and ongoing discrimination, social exclusion, and negative stereotyping may produce both social pain (MacDonald & Leary, 2005) and negative health outcomes, such as subclinical carotid artery disease (Troxel, Matthews, Bromberger, & Sutton-Tyrrell, 2003).

Other instances of the damaging effect of discrimination and social exclusion include impaired self-regulation (Baumeister, DeWall, Ciarocco, & Twenge, 2005), patronizing environments that produce decrements in female performance in masculine domains (Vescio, Gervais, Snyder, & Hoover, 2005), or backlash against people who exhibit counterstereotypical behaviors (Rudman & Fairchild, 2004). The damaging effects of discrimination and social exclusion deserve further attention, with a focus on proximal and distal relationships to health outcomes. The damaging effects of discrimination experienced during childhood or early adulthood, for example, may influence health outcomes in later life.

Another promising research area is the roles of trust and stigmatization to explain individuals' lack of research participation or disclosure, delay in seeking health care, or underutilization of health care services for the older adult population. In an important area related to trust, gender differences in self-disclosure (Dindia & Allen, 1992), self-disclosure has been shown to be diminished when the patient does not trust the health professional. Patients who do not trust their health care professional may not reveal that they are taking CAMs, or engaging in risky behaviors. Ethnicity or gender mismatches with health professionals may result in patients' dropping out prior to therapy completion, noncompliance with a prescribed treatment regimen, or failure to show up for a return checkup. After a trusting relationship has been established, ethnic or gender match may not matter.

A relatively understudied topic in health psychology is the impact of acculturation on future generations of older adults, such as baby boomers and children or grandchildren of immigrants. The immigrant health paradox has puzzled researchers; given the educational and economic circumstances of immigrants, both their birth outcomes and chronic disease outcomes are often better than those of Americans or more acculturated generations (Hernandez, 1999).

Investigators have attributed this immigrant health paradox to selective migration (e.g., only healthier migrants are able to survive long journeys) and the fact that sicker or retired immigrants may return to the country of origin (the so-called "salmon effect") and/or have better lifestyle habits (e.g., not smoking, having a plant-based diet, or being more physically active). Systematic data errors may contribute to this immigrant health paradox (e.g., missing data, the wrong ethnic identifier recorded at death, errors due to small sample size). We need to investigate this immigrant health paradox systematically and more carefully.

Investigation into the impact of health literacy and utilization of health information and health-promoting behavioral changes in late life may be a fruitful area of research (Institute of Medicine, 2003). Health literacy is influenced by educational level and cultural or familial upbringing (tools and conceptual health knowledge), exposure to health information (oral and print literacy, English language skills), underlying health beliefs, and lifestyle practices. A growing literature suggests that many cultural and health literacy factors influence breast and cervical cancer screening among Latinas (Buki, Borrayo, Feigal, & Carrillo, 2004) and Vietnamese women (Yee et al., 2003). Major contributions may be made by health psychologists in health literacy, cultural and gender competence in health measurement, and research methodologies.

A fruitful area of investigation must target the underlying gender, culture, and ethnic differences in risky behavior (Yee et al., 1995) and in risk perceptions and risk management during the second half of life. Optimistic risk perceptions create barriers to health screening ("It won't happen to me"), and pessimistic risk perceptions lead to overscreening and unnecessary health expenditures (Quillin, Fries, McClish, deParedes, & Bodurtha, 2004).

As we gather more research on gender, culture, and ethnicity, we need to pay close attention to those research areas in which the dose–response across genders or ethnic groups may differ from that found among middle-class, young, or white populations. We also need to become increasingly attentive to the notion that relationships among mainstream populations may not generalize to the poor, or across genders and ethnic groups. According to Smedley and Smedley (2005), there is much broader empirical support for health differences due to environmental inequities than for biological differences related to race or ethnicity. Still, there remains an ongoing legacy of racism that systematically influences health over the lifespan. For example, Farmer and Ferraro (2005) found that the positive relationship between education and morbidity among white Americans over a 20-year period was not found among black Americans. In other words, even with increased educational attainment, the health outcomes (e.g., morbidity and self-reported health) for middle-class blacks remained poor relative to their white counterparts. Perhaps large differences in negative emotions, such as those resulting from discrimination or sexism, may account for these health disparities in late life. Another example is the finding that with equivalent doses of smoking or alcohol, females may be at higher risk than males for negative health outcomes.

National research policy must incorporate a strategy to target high-risk but understudied and smaller populations. Funding for oversampling of gender and ethnically diverse groups should be dramatically increased to fill data gaps in large national surveys and longitudinal studies of aging. As a nation, we need this basic information to formulate effective national health policies to reduce health disparities.

In conclusion, an important theme throughout this chapter is that gender and ethnicity/cultural characteristics are proxy variables for important underlying life experiences and biological–environmental interactions that contribute to health disparities. As such, exclusive use of these demographics as explanatory variables oversimplifies the relationships between moderating/ mediating variables, and health and quality of life. Critical to future research in health psychology and aging is a better understanding of the cognitive, social, and behavioral changes at multiple levels of analysis. The simultaneous study of risk and protective factors holds promise to advance our understanding of how diverse social contexts and life experiences produce health disparities in late life.

# REFERENCES

Aldwin, C. M., & Park, C. L. (2004). Coping and physical health outcomes: An overview. *Psychology and Health, 19,* 277–281.

Alba, R. (2002). Only English by the third generation?: Mother-tongue loss and preservation among the grandchildren of contemporary immigrants. *Demography, 39,* 467–484.

Alba, R. (2005). Bright versus blurred boundaries: Second generation assimilation and exclusion in France, Germany, and the United States. *Ethnic and Racial Studies, 28*(1), 20–49.

Alvidrez, J., Azocar, F., & Miranda, J. (1996). Demystifying the concept of ethnicity for psychotherapy researchers. *Journal of Consulting and Clinical Psychology, 64*(5), 903–908.

American Psychiatric Association. (1994). *Diagnostic and statistical manual of mental disorders* (4th ed.). Washington, DC: Author.

Anderson, N. B., Bulatao, R. A., & Cohen, B. (Eds.). (2004). *Critical perspectives on racial and ethnic differences in health in late life.* Washington, DC: National Research Council, National Academies Press.

Anderson, N. B., Castro, F. G., Kilty, M. F., Schneiderman, N., & Yee, B. W. K. (Eds.). (1995). Behavioral and sociocultural perspectives on ethnicity and health [Special issue]. *Health Psychology, 14,* 589–653.

Anderson, N. B., & Nickerson, K. J. (2005). Genes, race, and psychology in the genome era [Special issue]. *American Psychologist, 6*(1).

Baumeister, R. F., DeWall, C. N., Ciarocco, N. J., & Twenge, J. M. (2005). Social exclusion impairs self-regulation. *Journal of Personality and Social Psychology, 88,* 589–604.

Baxter, L. C., Saykin, A. J., Flashman, L. A., Johnson, S. C., Guerin, S. J., Babcock, D. R., et al. (2003). Sex differences in semantic language processing: A functional MRI study. *Brain and Language, 84,* 264–272.

Beier, M. E., & Ackerman, P. L. (2003). Determinants of health knowledge: An investigation of age, gender, abilities, personality, and interests. *Journal of Personality and Social Psychology, 84,* 439–448.

Beiser, M. (2003). Why should researchers care about culture? *Canadian Journal of Psychiatry, 48*(3), 154–160.

Bengtson, V. L., & Kuypers, J. A. (1986). The family support cycle: Psycho-social issues in the aging family. In J. M. A. Munnichs, P. Mussen, & E. Olbrich (Eds.), *Life-span and change in a gerontological perspective* (pp. 61–77). New York: Academic Press.

Berman, J. D., & Straus, S. E. (2004). Implementing a research agenda for complementary and alternative medicine. *Annual Review of Medicine, 55,* 239–254.

Bhopal, R. (1997). Is research into ethnicity and health racist, unsound, or important science? *British Medical Journal, 314,* 1751–1756.

Blanchard-Fields, F., Stein, R., & Watson, T. L. (2004). Age differences in emotion-regulation strategies in handling everyday problems. *Journals of Gerontology: Psychological Sciences and Social Sciences, Series B, 59,* 261–269.

Buki, L. P., Borrayo, E. A., Feigal, B. M., & Carrillo, I. Y. (2004). Are all Latinas the same?: Perceived breast cancer screening barriers and facilitative conditions. *Psychology of Women Quarterly, 28,* 400–411.

Cabral, D. N., Napoles-Springer, A. M., Milke, R., McMillan, A., Sison, J. D., Wrensch, M. R., et al. (2003). Population- and community-based recruitment of African Americans and Latinos: The San Francisco Bay Area Lung Cancer Study. *American Journal of Epidemiology, 158,* 272–279.

Cahill, L. (2005). His brain, her brain. *Scientific American, 292,* 40–47.

Campbell, M. K., James, A., Hudson, M. A., Carr, C., Jackson, E., Oates, V., Demissie, S., et al. (2004). Improving multiple behaviors for colorectal cancer prevention among African American church members. *Health Psychology, 23,* 492–502.

Carstensen, L. L., Fung, H. H., & Charles, S. T. (2003). Socioemotional selectivity theory and the regulation of emotion in the second half of life. *Motivation and Emotion, 27,* 103–123.

Chiriboga, D. A., Black, S. A., Aranda, M., & Markides, K. (2002). Stress and depressive symptoms among Mexican American elderly. *Journals of Gerontology: Psychological Sciences and Social Sciences, Series B, 57,* 559–568.

Conroy, S. J., & Heer, D. M. (2003). Hidden Hispanic homelessness in Los Angeles: The "Latino paradox" revisited. *Hispanic Journal of Behavioral Sciences, 25*(4), 530–538.

Cuff, P. A., & Vanselow, N. A. (Eds.). (2004). *Improving medical education: Enhancing the behavioral and social science content of medical school curricula* (Committee on Behavioral and Social Sciences in Medical School Curricula and Board on Neuroscience and Behavioral Health). Washington, DC: National Academies Press.

Diamond, L. M., & Aspinwall, L. G. (2003). Emotion regulation across the life span: An integrative perspective emphasizing self-regulation, positive affect, and dyadic processes. *Motivation and Emotion, 27,* 125–156.

Dindia, K., & Allen, M. (1992). Sex differences in self-disclosure: A meta-analysis. *Psychological Bulletin, 112,* 106–124.

Dowd, J. J., & Bengtson, V. L. (1978). Aging in minority populations: An examination of the double jeopardy hypothesis. *Journal of Gerontology, 33*(3), 427–443.

Farmer, M. M., & Ferraro, K. F. (2005). Are racial disparities in health conditional on socioeconomic status? *Social Science and Medicine, 60,* 191–204.

Federal Interagency Forum on Aging-Related Statistics. (2004). *Older Americans 2004: Key indicators of well-being.* Washington, DC: U.S. Government Printing Office.

Gapstur, S. M., Potter, J. D., Sellers, T. A., & Folson, A. R. (1992). Increased risk of breast cancer with alcohol consumption in postmenopausal women. *American Journal of Epidemiology, 136,* 1221–1231.

Gauthier, M. A., & Clarke, W. P. (1999). Gaining and sustaining minority participation in longitudinal research projects. *Alzheimer's Disease and Associated Disorders, 13*(Suppl. 1), S29–S33.

Glass, T. A. (Ed.). (2003). *Health inequalities: Lifecourse approaches.* Bristol, UK: Policy Press.

Granado, C. (2003). "Hispanic" vs. "Latino." *Diversity Currents, 4*(4), 1, 6–7. Accessed on December 9, 2004, from www.hispaniconline.com/res&res/polls/hisp_vs_lat.html.

Guarnaccia, P. J., & Rogler, L. H. (1999). Research on culture-bound syndromes. *American Journal of Psychiatry, 156*(9), 13322–13327.

Handelman, L., & Yeo, G. (1996). Using explanatory models to understand chronic symptoms of Cambodian refugees. *Family Medicine, 28*(4), 271–276.

Hernandez, D. J. (Ed.). (1999). *Children of immigrants: Health, adjustment, and public assistance* (Committee on the Health and Adjustment of Immigrant Children and Families, National Research Council and Institute of Medicine). Washington, DC: National Academy Press.

Hewitt, M., Herdman, R., & Holland, J. (Eds.). (2004). *Meeting the needs of women with breast cancer* (National Cancer Policy Board, Institute of Medicine and National Research Council). Washington, DC: National Academy Press.

Hummer, R. A., Benjamins, M. R., & Rogers, R. G. (2004). Racial and ethnic disparities in health and mortality among the U.S. elderly population. In N. B. Anderson, R. A. Bulatao, & B. Cohen (Eds.), *Critical perspectives on racial and ethnic differences in health in late life* (pp. 53–94). Washington, DC: National Research Council and National Academies Press.

Institute of Medicine. (2003). *Health literacy: A prescription to end confusion.* Washington, DC: National Academies Press.

Jang, Y., Kim, G., & Chiriboga, D. A. (2005). Acculturation and manifestation of depressive symptoms among Korean American older adults. *Journal of Aging and Mental Health, 9*, 500–507.

Jasso, G., Massey, D. S., Rosenzweig, M. R., & Smith, J. P. (2004). Immigrant health: Selectivity and acculturation. In N. B. Anderson, R. A. Bulatao, & B. Cohen (Eds.), *Critical perspectives on racial and ethnic differences in health in late life* (pp. 53–94). Washington, DC: National Research Council and National Academy Press.

Johnson, R. L., Roter, D., Powe, N. R., & Cooper, L. A. (2004). Patient race/ethnicity and quality of patient–physician communication during medical visits. *American Journal of Public Health, 94*(12), 2084–2090.

Jones, J. H. (1993). *Bad blood: The Tuskegee syphilis experiment.* New York: Free Press.

Karlamangla, A., Singer, B. H., McEwen, B., Rowe, J., & Seeman, T. E. (2002). Allostatic load as a predictor of functional decline. *Journal of Clinical Epidemiology, 55*, 699–710.

Keefe, S. M., & Padilla, A. M. (1987). *Chicano ethnicity.* Albuquerque: University of New Mexico Press.

Klein, D., Turvey, C., & Wallace, R. (2004). Elders who delay medication because of cost: Health insurance, demographic, health, and financial correlates. *Gerontologist, 44*(6), 779–787.

Knight, L.-A. (2000). Humanitarian crises and old age: Guidelines for best practice. *Age and Ageing, 29*, 293–295.

Kohn, L. T., Corrigan, J. M., & Donaldson, M. S. (Eds.). (2000). *To err is human: Building a safer health system.* Washington, DC: Institute of Medicine, National Academies Press.

Kroeber, A. L., & Kluckhohn, C. (1952). *Culture: A critical review of concepts and definitions.* Cambridge, MA: Peabody Museum.

MacDonald, G., & Leary, M. R. (2005). Why does social exclusion hurt?: The relationship between social and physical pain. *Psychological Bulletin, 131,* 202–223.

Major, B., & O'Brien, L .T. (2005). The social psychology of stigma. *Annual Review of Psychology, 56,* 393–421.

Manson, S. M., Garroutte, E., Goins, R. T., & Henderson, P. N. (2004). Access, relevance, and control in the research process. *Journal of Aging and Health, 16*(Suppl. 5), 58S–77S.

Marcuccio, E., Loving, N., Bennett, S. K., & Hayes, S. N. (2003). A survey of attitudes and experiences of women with heart disease. *Women's Health Issues, 13,* 23–31.

Markides K. S., & Coreil J. (1986). The health of Hispanics in the southwestern United States: An epidemiologic paradox. *Public Health Reports, 101,* 253–265.

Matias-Carrelo, L. E., Chavez, L. M., Negron, G., Canino, G., Aguilar-Gaxiola, S., & Hoppe, S. (2003). The Spanish translation and cultural adaptation of five mental health outcome measures. *Culture, Medicine and Psychiatry, 27*(3), 291–313.

Matsumoto, D., Yoo, S. H., Hirayama, S., & Petrova, G. (2005). Development and validation of a measure of display rule knowledge: The Display Rule Assessment Inventory. *Emotion, 5,* 23–40.

Moyerman, D. R., & Forman, B. D. (1992). Acculturation and adjustment: A meta-analytic study. *Hispanic Journal of Behavioral Sciences, 14*(2), 163–200.

National Institutes of Health. (1994). Guidelines on the inclusion of women and minorities as subjects in clinical research. *Federal Register, 59,* 14508–14513.

National Institute of Health. (2004). NIH policy and guidelines on the inclusion of women and minorities as subjects in clinical research—amended, October 2001 (pp. 1–11). Last updated on August 10, 2004. Retrieved on December 26, 2004, from grants.nih.gov/grants/funding/women_min/guidelines_amended_10_2001.htm.

Nguyen, H. T., Kitner-Triolo, M., Evans, M. K., & Zonderman, A. B. (2004). Factorial invariance of the CES-D in low socioeconomic status African Americans as compared with a nationally representative sample. *Psychiatry Research, 126*(2), 177–187.

Ni, H., Simile, C., & Hardy, A. M. (2002). Utilization of complementary and alternative medicine by United States adults: Results from the 1999 National Health Interview Survey. *Medical Care, 40,* 353–358.

Ong, A. D., & Bergemen, C. S. (2004). The complexity of emotions in later life. *Journals of Gerontology: Psychological Sciences and Social Sciences, Series B, 59,* 117–122.

Office of Minority Health. (2001). National standards for culturally and linguistically appropriate services in health care. Washington, DC: U.S. Department of Health and Human Services. Retrieved October 2004 from www.omhrc.gov/omh/programs/2pgprograms/finalreport.pdf.

Otte, C., Hart, S., Neylan, T. C., Marmar, C. R., Yaffe, K., & Mohr, D. C. (2005). A meta-analysis of cortisol response to challenge in human aging: Importance of gender. *Psychoneuroendocrinology, 30,* 80–91.

Palloni, A., & Arias, E. (2004). Paradox lost: Explaining the Hispanic adult mortality advantage. *Demography, 41*(3), 385–415.

Patel, J. D., Bach, P. B., & Kris, M. G. (2004). Lung cancer in U.S. women: A contemporary epidemic. *Journal of the American Medical Association, 291,* 1763–1768.

Piette, J. D., Heisler, M., & Wanger, T. H. (2004). Cost related medication underuse: Do patients with chronic illnesses tell their doctors? *Archives of Internal Medicine, 164,* 1749–1755.

Quillin, J. M., Fries, E., McClish, D., deParedes, E. S., & Bodurtha, J. (2004). Gail model risk assessment and risk perceptions. *Journal of Behavioral Medicine, 27,* 205–214.

Radloff, L. S. (1977). The CES-D scale: A self-report depression scale for research in the general population. *Applied Psychological Measurement, 1,* 385–401.

Ray, O. (2004). How the mind hurts and heals the body. *American Psychologist, 59,* 29–40.

Rudman, L. A., & Fairchild, K. (2004). Reactions to counterstereotypic behavior: The role of backlash in cultural stereotype maintenance. *Journal of Personality and Social Psychology, 87,* 157–176.

Ryff, C. D., & Singer, B. H. (2003). Flourishing under fire: Resilience as a prototype of challenged thriving. In C. L. M. Keyes & J. Haidt (Eds.), *Flourishing: Positive psychology and the life well-lived* (pp. 15–36). Washington, DC: American Psychological Association.

Ryff, C. D., Singer, B. H., Wing, E., & Love, G. D. (2001). Elective affinities and uninvited agonies: Mapping emotion with significant others onto health. In C. D. Ryff & B. H. Singer (Eds.), *Emotion, social relationships and health* (pp. 133–175). New York: Oxford University Press.

Scheff, T. J. (1974). The labeling theory of mental illness. *American Sociological Review, 39,* 444–452.

Seeman, T. E., Rowe, J. W., McEwen, B. S., & Singer, B. H. (2001). Allostatic load as a marker of cumulative biological risk: MacArthur Studies of Successful Aging. *Proceedings of the National Academy of Sciences of the United States of America, 98,* 4770–4775.

Seeman, T. E., Singer, B. H., Ryff, C. D., Love, G. D., & Levy-Storms, L. (2002). Social relationships, gender, and allostatic load across two age cohorts. *Psychosomatic Medicine, 64,* 395–406.

Shaywitz, B. A., Shaywitz, S. E., Pugh, K. R., Constable, R. T., Skudlarski, P., Fulbright, R. K., et al. (1995). Sex differences in the functional organization of the brain for language. *Nature, 373,* 607–609.

Shulman, K. A., Berlin, J. A., Harless, W., Kerner, J. F., Sistrunk, S., Gersh, B. J., et al. (1999). The effect of race and sex on physicians' recommendations for cardiac catheterization. *New England Journal of Medicine, 340,* 618–626.

Simon, V. R., Hai, T., Williams, S. K., Adams, E., Ricchetti, K., & Marts, S. A. (May, 2005). National Institutes of Health: Intramural and extramural support for research on sex differences, 2000–2003. (Scientific Report Series: Understanding the biology of sex differences). *Society for Women's Health Research,* 1–11.

Smedley, A., & Smedley, B. D. (2005). Race as biology is fiction, racism as a social problem is real: Anthropological and historical perspectives on the social construction of race. *American Psychologist, 60,* 16–26.

Smedley, B. D., Stith, A. Y., & Nelson, A. R. (Eds.). (2003). *Unequal treatment: Confronting racial and ethnic disparities in health care.* Washington, DC: National Academies Press.

Steele, C. M. (1997). A threat in the air: How stereotypes shape intellectual identity and performance. *American Psychologist, 52,* 613–629.

Sternberg, R. J. (2004). Culture and intelligence. *American Psychologist, 59*(5), 325–338.

Steward, A. J., & McDermott, C. (2004). Gender in psychology. *Annual Review of Psychology, 55,* 519–544.

Sue, D. W., Arredondo, P., & McDavis, R. J. (1992). Multicultural counseling competencies and standards: A call to the profession. *Journal of Counseling and Development, 70,* 477–486.

Taylor, A. L., Ziesche, S., Yancy, C., Carson, P., D'Agostino, R., Jr., Ferdinand, K., et al. (2004). Combination of isosorbide dinitrate and hydralazine in blacks with heart failure. *New England Journal of Medicine, 351*(20), 2049–2057.

Taylor, S. E., Klein, L. C., Lewis, B. P., Gruenewald, T. L., Gurung, R. A. R., & Updegraff, J. A. (2000). Biobehavioral responses to stress in females: Tend-and-befriend, not fight-or-flight. *Psychological Review, 107,* 411–429.

Tran, T. V. (1991). Family living arrangements and social adjustment among three ethnic groups of elderly Indochinese refugees. *International Journal of Aging and Human Development, 32*(2), 91–102.

Traustadóttir, T., Bosch, P. R., & Matt, K. S. (2005). *Psychoneuroendocrinology, 30,* 392–402.

Travis, C. B. (2005). 2004 Carolyn Sherif Award Address: Heart disease and gender inequity. *Psychology of Women Quarterly, 29,* 15–23.

Triandis, H. C., McCusker, C., Betancourt, H., Iwao, S., Leung, K., Salazar, J. M., et al. (1993). An etic–emic analysis of individualism and collectivism. *Journal of Cross-Cultural Psychology 24,* 366–383.

Trimble, C. L., Genkinger, J. M., Burke A. E., Hoffman S. C., Helzlsouer K. J., Diener-West M., et al. (2005). Active and passive cigarette smoking and the risk of cervical neoplasia. *Obstetrics and Gynecology, 105,* 174–181.

Troxel,W. M., Matthews, K. A., Bromberger, J. T., & Sutton-Tyrrell, K. (2003). Chronic stress burden, discrimination, and subclinical carotid artery disease in African American and Caucasian Women. *Health Psychology, 22,* 300–309.

U.S. Bureau of the Census. (2003). *Statistical abstract of the United States.* Washington, DC: Author.

U.S. Department of Health and Human Services. (1999a). *Agenda for research in women's health for the 21st century: A report of the Task Force on the NIH Women's Health Research Agenda for the 21st century: Vol. 1. Executive summary NIH Publication No. 99–4385).* Bethesda, MD: Author.

U.S. Department of Health and Human Services. (1999b). *Agenda for research in women's health for the 21st Century: A report of the Task Force on the NIH Women's Health Research Agenda for the 21st century: Vol. 2. NIH Publication No. 99–4386).* Bethesda, MD: Author.

U.S. Department of Health and Human Services. (2001). *Mental Health: Culture, race and ethnicity—A supplement to mental health: A report of the Surgeon General* (NIH Publication No. SMA01-3613). Rockville, MD: U.S. Department of Health and Human Services, Substance Abuse and Mental Health Services Administration, Center for Mental Health Services, National Institutes of Health, National Institute of Mental Health.

Vaillant, G. E. (2003). Mental health. *American Journal of Psychiatry, 160*(8), 1373–1384.

Van Ploeg, M., & Perrin, E. (Eds.). (2004). *Eliminating health disparities: Measurement and data needs.* Washington, DC: National Academies Press.

Vega, W. A., & Amaro, H. (1994). Latino outlook: Good health, uncertain progress. *Annual Review of Public Health, 15,* 39–67.

Vescio, T. K., Gervais, S. J., Snyder, M., & Hoover, A. (2005). Power and the creation of patronizing environments: The stereotype-based behaviors of the powerful and their effects on female performance in masculine domains. *Journal of Personality and Social Psychology, 88,* 658–672.

Whitfield, K. E. (Ed.). (2004). *Closing the gap: Improving the health of minority elders in the new millenium.* Washington, DC: Gerontological Society of America.

Will, J. C., Farris, R. P., Sanders, C. G., Stockmyer, C. K., & Finkelstein, E. A. (2004). Health promotion intervention for disadvantaged women: Overview of the WISEWOMAN projects. *Journal of Women's Health, 13,* 484–502.

Williams, D., & Rucker, T. D. (2000). Understanding and addressing racial disparities in health care. *Health Care Financing Review, 21*(4), 75–90.

Wizemann, R. M., & Pardue, M. L. (2001). *Exploring the biological contributions to human health: Does sex matter?* Washington, DC: National Academies Press.

Wood, W., & Eagly, A. H. (2002). A cross-cultural analysis of the behavior of women and men: Implications for the origins of sex differences. *Psychological Bulletin, 128,* 699–727.

Yali, A. M., & Revenson, T. A. (2004). How changes in population demographics will impact health psychology: Incorporating a broader notion of cultural competence into the field. *Health Psychology, 23,* 147–155.

Yee, B. W. K., Nguyen, H. T., & Ha, M. (2003). Chronic disease, health beliefs and lifestyle practices among Vietnamese adults: Influence of gender and age. *Women and Therapy, 26*(1), 111–127.

Yee, B. W. K. (1997). The social and cultural context of adaptive aging among Southeast Asian elders. In J. Sokolovsky (Ed.), *The cultural context of aging* (2nd ed., pp. 293–303). New York: Greenwood.

Yee, B. W. K., Castro, F., Hammond, R., John, R., Wyatt, G., & Yung, B. (1995). Risk taking and abusive behaviors among ethnic minority individuals. *Health Psychology, 14*(7), 622–631.

Zautra, A. J., Johnson, L. M., & Davis, M. C. (2005). Positive affect as a source of resilience for women in chronic pain. *Journal of Consulting and Clinical Psychology, 73,* 212–220.

# CHAPTER 16

# Religious and Spiritual Issues
# in Health and Aging

## CRYSTAL L. PARK

Recent research has focused on the relationships between religiousness and spirituality and health, and many of these reports indicate primarily protective effects: Researchers have found links between various dimensions of religiousness and spirituality, and lower rates of cancer, heart disease, alcoholism, and mental illness, as well as lower blood pressure, higher health-related quality of life, and higher levels of positive health behaviors. It has been suggested that religious and spiritual resources may become more salient and more closely linked to health in older adults as health problems increase and other resources diminish. This chapter examines the issues relevant to religious and spiritual factors in the health of older adults, including evidence regarding whether the links appear to grow stronger with age.

## THE IMPORTANCE OF RELIGION AND
## SPIRITUALITY IN THE LIVES OF AMERICANS

Religion is highly prevalent in the United States and exerts a strong influence on both the social institutions and the personal lives of most Americans (Koenig, 2000). Nationwide polls repeatedly reflect Americans' strongly held beliefs and widely held practices. For example, Gallup polls show that 96% of Americans believe in God or a universal spirit, 90% pray, 85% say religion is very or fairly important to them, and 41% attend church or synagogue weekly or more often (Gallup Organization, 2004). In recent years, researchers have begun to investigate in earnest how religion and spiritual-ity may intersect with health. For example, studies have examined how reli-gious beliefs and practices are related to physical and mental health, as well as health-related lifestyle habits and decisions that people make about seek-ing health care.

Furthermore, it has been noted that religion is commonly used as a way to cope with stress caused by health problems, and studies indicate that it is very commonly used to cope with serious medical illnesses (Aldwin, in press); for example, participants in one study of ill older adults in the southeastern United States reported that religious faith was their most important resource for dealing with their illness (Koenig, George, & Siegler, 1998). It should be noted that the vast majority of the research gen-erated on these topics has been conducted in the United States. In recent years, some efforts have been made to examine issues of religiousness and spirituality and health outside the United States (e.g., Goldbourt, Yaari, & Medalie, 1993), but to date such studies are few and far between.

## CONCEPTUALIZING AND MEASURING RELIGION AND SPIRITUALITY

Within the past 10 years, scholars in the psychology of religion have been actively struggling to define, both conceptually and operationally, the con-structs of religion and spirituality (Miller & Thoresen, 2003). This discus-sion has taken place in the context of changing meanings of these words in U.S. culture, as well as in the scientific community. In the past, "religion" was considered to be the mainstream term, encompassing structural aspects such as ritual, service attendance, and doctrine, as well as the more internal aspects such as transcendence and meaning, whereas "spirituality" was not a widely used term. In recent years, however, a curious polarity has devel-oped, wherein both researchers and the general public increasingly use the term "spirituality" to denote efforts toward a variety of sacred goals, meaning, and transcendence, whereas the term "religion" is often relegated to denoting the structural and institutional aspects (see Zinnbauer & Pargament, 2005).

In introducing a special section of *American Psychologist* on religion, spirituality, and health, Miller and Thoresen (2003) noted that there is cur-rently a great deal of overlap in the meanings of the terms "religion" and "spirituality", particularly as used in the health literature. They therefore used the convention "R/S" to refer to the general construct of religion and spirituality, noting that little research has examined spirituality separate from religion in the context of health. Because of the lack of differentiation in the vast majority of literature reviewed herein, this chapter uses the same convention.

In addition to the energy being put into definitional issues, an important advance in the study of the psychology of religion in the past few decades has been the widespread acceptance of the notion that R/S can only be accurately characterized as a multidimensional construct (Idler et al., 2003). These dimensions include religious denomination or affiliation; attendance at services; fundamentalism; private religious practices, such as prayer, meditation, and reading of religious materials; religious coping; religious motivation (e.g., intrinsic and extrinsic religiousness); religious and spiritual well-being; daily spiritual experiences of the transcendent; and theodicies and beliefs (e.g., beliefs in the afterlife and views of suffering).

This recognition of the need to measure multiple dimensions of R/S has resulted in an expanding universe of measures. Several authors have advocated focusing on and working with existing measures (Hill, 2005), but in the years since Hill and Hood (1999) compiled and reviewed 125 extant scales, new measures have continued to proliferate. One important development was the Fetzer/National Institute on Aging (NIA) initiative, a working group formed in 1997 to examine the literature on R/S and health, and to develop a measure of the dimensions most important to assess vis-à-vis health. This effort resulted in the Brief Multidimensional Measure of Religiousness/Spirituality (BMMR/S; Fetzer Institute/NIA Working Group, 1999), which examines the domains of organizational religiousness, private religious practices, daily spiritual experiences, meaning, values, beliefs, forgiveness, religious/spiritual coping, religious support, religious/spiritual history, commitment, and religious preference. This new measure has demonstrated promising psychometrics and utility (e.g., Idler et al., 2003).

The increased awareness of the need to capture multiple dimensions of R/S, along with the arsenal of available measures, creates opportunities for researchers to examine with much greater sophistication the roles of various aspects of R/S on health, and future publications will likely reflect this. However, to date, most of the literature has used more simplistic measurement approaches. For example, most articles on R/S and health have defined "religion" as denomination or attendance at church/services. Whereas these studies lay the foundation for future research to understand relations between R/S and health, they are limited in what they can reveal. For example, denomination may indicate some important information regarding an individual's religiousness or spirituality but may also be related to socioeconomic status, education, ethnicity, and other potentially confounding factors.

## R/S AND HEALTH: GENERAL FINDINGS

Early research on religion and health concerned the differential prevalence of various diseases across denominations (e.g., Phillips, Kuzma, Beeson, &

Lotz, 1980) and church or service attendance (e.g., Comstock & Partridge, 1972). Although these relationships were known for many years, the numbers of studies published on R/S and health increased dramatically beginning around 1990 (Mills, 2002), and research examining religious and spiritual factors in health has since burgeoned (for reviews, see Powell, Shahabi, & Thoresen, 2003; Thoresen & Harris, 2002; Koenig, McCullough, & Larson, 2001).

The strongest findings, emerging from a number of large-scale epidemiological studies, are that more frequent service attendance is related to lower mortality rates (McCullough, Hoyt, Larson, Koenig, & Thoresen, 2000; Thoresen & Harris, 2002). Even controlling for a variety of potential covariates, such as baseline health, social support, and health behaviors, attendance remains strongly and prospectively related to lower mortality (e.g., Oman, Kurata, Strawbridge, & Cohen, 2002). In addition to mortality, R/S (again, primarily reflected in attendance) is associated with lower rates of a variety of illnesses, including alcoholism, cardiovascular disease, hypertension, and myocardial infarction (Miller & Thoresen, 2003).

Aside from service attendance, little research has focused on dimensions of R/S and health (Thoresen & Harris, 2002). Of those studies conducted using measures other than attendance and examining health outcomes other than mortality, the findings are mixed (Powell et al., 2003). Some studies that examined religious coping with illness, for example, found that it was related to better recovery, but a number of other studies yielded null findings (see Powell et al., 2003, for a review). Still, many of these studies are difficult to interpret given the various ways in which both R/S and health outcomes have been defined, as well as a number of methodological problems (e.g., selective samples, limited power).

## ISSUES OF R/S IN AGING AND HEALTH

The above-mentioned findings indicate that R/S is moderately strongly related to various aspects of health in general population studies and specific groups such as cardiac patients. In addition to these general effects on health, many writers have suggested that R/S may be particularly important in the lives and health of older individuals (e.g., Thorson, 2000). R/S is hypothesized to be more important to health in older adults because of the higher levels of both religiousness and health problems that occur at later ages.

Levels of religiousness, variously measured, are typically higher in older people than in younger people (e.g., Pargament, 1997). For example, 73% of adults age 65 and older say religion is "very important" to them, with lower numbers for younger groups: 65% of 50- to 64-year-olds, 59%

of 30- to 49-year-olds, and 48% of 18- to 29-year-olds say that religion is "very important" to them. Similarly, 46% of people over age 50 report having attended religious services in the past 7 days, compared with 40% of those ages 30–49 and 30% of those ages 18–29 (Gallup Organization, 2004). There is evidence that spirituality also increases as people age (e.g., Wink & Dillon, 2002).

These higher levels of R/S in older individuals, at least to some extent, appear to be a cohort effect (Koenig, Kvale, & Ferrel, 1988). Furthermore, to the extent that R/S has salutary effects on health or is related to factors that do so (e.g., health habits, marital status), the higher levels of R/S observed among older adults may also reflect survival effects, in that those with lower R/S die earlier (Oman et al., 2002) However, recent longitudinal data on multiple cohorts provide some evidence that, regardless of cohort, people become more religious or spiritual as they age (Argue, Johnson, & White, 1999; see Krause, 2006, for a review), although not everyone experiences such increases (Ingersoll-Dayton, Krause, & Morgan, 2002).

Not only does R/S appear to increase with age but so also does the prevalence of acute and chronic illness, and functional disabilities. In addition, older adults are more likely to encounter life-threatening illnesses and to be facing the end of their lives, as well as other stressors that may impact their health, such as spousal bereavement (Krause, 1998; Gall, 2003). All of these conditions provide opportunities for R/S to exert more influence. Recognizing the increased health problems of older adults, a number of recent studies have focused on the issue of whether R/S influences health in older populations, and if so, how.

## Studies of Religion and Health in the Context of Adult Development and Aging

Although many studies included in the previously cited reviews included older individuals in their samples, studies that have focused on older adults in particular, or on health issues that primarily affect them (e.g., cardiac surgery) provide more direct evidence regarding the relevance of R/S in the health of older individuals. In this section, the findings of studies that specifically focus on the health of older individuals are summarized by categories of health outcome, followed by a discussion of the problems that arise in interpreting these findings.

### Subjective Health

Subjective health has been shown to be a predictor of mortality, as well as an important aspect of health and well-being (Idler & Kasl, 1991). Reviewing the literature on religion and subjective health (typically assessed as a single item), conducted primarily in general population studies, Musick (1996) concluded that attendance and religious practices were positively related to subjective health, although not all studies showed this relationship. Two of the studies reviewed by Musick focused on samples of older adults: One found that religious attendance was related to subjective health, but only for African Americans (Boyer, 1981–1982), and the other found that attendance was positively related to subjective health (Broyles & Drenovsky, 1992). More recent studies produced more mixed results. A study of the relation of spiritual well-being and subjective health in members of a community-dwelling sample, most of whom were over 80, found that spiritual well-being, as well as its components of existential and religious well-being, are all related to perceived health (Wotherspoon, 2000), whereas another study found no relation between religious service attendance and subjective health (Idler & Kasl, 1991). Musick (1996) noted, however, that cross-sectional studies such as these cannot rule out the reverse causality (i.e., that those who were more positive about their health may have become more religious or attended services more frequently).

In a prospective study of black and white older adults, private religious activities such as prayer and Bible reading were related to positive changes in subjective health only for blacks, and public religious activity (attendance) was positively related to subjective health for whites and blacks, but the effect disappeared when functional health status was included (Musick, 1996). However, another prospective study of community-dwelling older adults found that affiliation, attendance, and degree of religiousness were unrelated to self-rated health 14 years later (Atchley, 1997). In their review, Musick, Traphagan, Koenig, and Larson (2000) concluded, "Although there is some evidence that religious activity, especially in terms of service attendance, is related to self-rated health, we cannot definitively conclude that this is the case. More work must be done on the subject using prospective data to examine the influence of health on changes in self-ratings of health" (pp. 76–77). It appears that this conclusion remains true.

## Specific Diseases

Little is known about how dimensions of religion influence the incidence of specific diseases in older adults. In general, a large body of literature has documented that people of certain denominations have lower rates of certain diseases. For example, cancer and cancer-related mortality is lower in Seventh-Day Adventists than in the general population (see Musick et al., 2000). However, little research has addressed the issue of whether other dimensions of R/S (e.g., frequency of public or private religious activity) within these denominations have similar effects on disease incidence (Musick et al., 2000).

## Recovery from Illness/Surgery

Studies of religion and recovery from illness or surgery are rare, and very little of that research has focused on older adults. In their review of evidence linking R/S and health, Powell et al. (2003) concluded, "In general, there have been consistent failures to support the hypothesis that religion or spirituality improves recovery from acute illness" (p. 46).

One recent study examined the role of religion and recovery in a sample of heart surgery patients with a mean age of 65 years. "Religiousness," defined as beliefs, attendance, and prayer, was assessed prior to surgery. Several interesting findings emerged: Those with stronger religious beliefs had fewer surgical complications and shorter hospital stays, but attendance at religious services predicted longer hospital stays and was unrelated to complications. However, prayer was not related to recovery. Finally, the effects of beliefs and attendance were both stronger for women than for men (Contrada, Goyal, et al., 2004).

## Physical Functioning/Disability

Some studies suggest that religious attendance is related to higher levels of functioning and less disability in older adults. For example, a series of longitudinal studies of community-dwelling older adults found a prospective relationship between attendance and lowered risk for future disability, an effect that was particularly strong for the subgroup that was disabled at baseline (Idler & Kasl, 1997). When the findings were adjusted to control for health practices, social ties, and indicators of well-being, the effects were smaller but remained significant. Furthermore, these findings suggested that religious service attendance influenced functional health, but that the reverse was not true.

However, in a longitudinal study of medical rehabilitation patients (mean age of 65) found that public and private religiosity and positive religious coping were unrelated to subsequent recovery (assessed in terms of activities of daily living [ADLs] and mobility) when they controlled for levels of health at admission, depression, social support, and other variables (Fitchett, Rybarczyk, DeMarco, & Nicholas, 1999).

## Mortality

Studies examining mortality have the advantages of an objective outcome and a higher chance of eliminating the possibility of reciprocal causation (Musick et al., 2000). In addition to the epidemiological studies cited earlier, a number of studies that have focused specifically on the influences of R/S (primarily church or service attendance) on mortality rates in older adults have found prospective protective effects even after adjusting for demographic, socioeconomic, and health-related confounds (e.g., Oman & Reed, 1998), although not all found such a positive relation (e.g., Kutner, Lin, Fielding, Brogan, & Hall, 1994; Idler & Kasl, 1992; Powell et al., 2003).

A handful of studies examining other aspects of R/S as predictors of mortality in older adults have generally found that various dimensions, such as depth of religiousness or time spent in prayer or scripture readings, are associated with lower mortality rates (see Powell et al., 2003, for a review). Again, however, not all studies have found such effects. For example, in a sample of aged hemodialysis patients, depth of religiousness and finding strength and comfort in religion were unrelated to mortality (Kutner et al., 1994).

Other studies have found effects of R/S on mortality, but only for a subsample. For example, in a nationwide survey of 819 older adults, religious coping was found to offset the effect of stressors on mortality, but only for stresses in highly valued roles, and only among older adults with less educational attainment (Krause, 1998). A longitudinal study of 3,851 community-dwelling adults ages 64–101 in North Carolina found that, in a 6-year follow-up, nearly one-third of the sample had died. Controlling for social support and health behaviors, lack of private religious activity predicted a 47% greater risk of dying. However, low levels of private religious activity (meditation, prayer, or Bible study) were a significant predictor of mortality only for healthy participants, not for those who were disabled at baseline (Helm, Hays, Flint, Koenig, & Blazer, 2000).

Interestingly, several studies have identified aspects of religion that may adversely affect mortality in older patients who are ill. In a prospective study of 444 inpatients, Pargament, Koenig, Tarakeshwar, and Hahn (2001) found that those who had experienced religious struggle in the hospital, such as feeling punished or abandoned by God, had increased mortality rates of 19–28% at the 2-year follow-up, even after adjusting for a variety of demographic, mental health, and physical health variables. Complementary results were found in a study of older open-heart surgery patients. Examining mortality at 6-months postsurgery, Oxman, Freeman, and Manheimer (1995) found that lack of perceiving strength and comfort from religion was related to increased risk of dying when they controlled for age, previous history of cardiac surgery, and impairment in presurgery ADLs.

## Cognitive Functioning

Few studies have explicitly looked at religion in relation to the outcome of cognitive dysfunction or dementia. An analysis of the longitudinal Established Populations for Epidemiological Studies of the Elderly (EPESE) data of community-dwelling older adults found an inverse association between religious attendance in 1982 and cognitive dysfunction in 1985, but religious attendance measured in 1982 did not predict cognitive dysfunction in 1988 (Van Ness & Kasl, 2003). The authors interpreted the short-term nature of the effect of attendance as at least partially due to differential mortality, in that persons with infrequent attendance and high levels of cognitive dysfunction in 1982 were more likely to die in the follow-up period.

## Immune Functioning

Some research has examined the relation between R/S and immune functioning. In their review, Seeman, Dubin, and Seeman (2003) rated the evidence linking the two as "reasonable." Relative to older adults, the best evidence comes from a longitudinal study of individuals age 65 and over, in which Koenig et al. (1997) found a small but significant predictive relationship between religious attendance and lower levels of plasma interleukin-6 that remained significant after they controlled for other factors such as age, sex, race, education, chronic illnesses, physical functioning, depression, and negative life events. This finding provides some support for the hypothesis that older adults who frequently attend religious services have healthier immune systems (however, these significant effects disappeared when psychosocial factors were entered into the model; see Seeman et al., 2003). A more recent study examining the role of interleukin-6 as a mediator in the relationship between religious attendance and mortality in a community-based sample of older adults found that interleukin-6 mediated the prospective relationship between religious attendance and mortality independently of covariates, including age, sex, health behaviors, chronic illness, social support, and depression (Lutgendorf, Russell, Ullrich, Harris, & Wallace, 2004).

## Cardiovascular Health

Studies have linked R/S (again, primarily assessed as attendance) with a variety of indicators of cardiovascular health in older adults, including cardiovascular-related mortality, stroke, and hypertension (Seeman et al., 2003; Powell et al., 2003).

Cardiovascular-related mortality was examined in prospective analyses of the Alameda County Study, which tracked individuals for 31 years. Findings indicated that religious attendance exerted a protective effect against circulatory mortality (including heart disease and stroke) that was greatly reduced when the authors controlled for a variety of sociodemographic and healthy lifestyle variables; furthermore, the effect was strongest for stroke mortality (Oman et al., 2002).

In a prospective study of stroke incidence, religious attendance was a protective factor; however, when controlled for covariates (age, sex, hypertension, diabetes, physical function, and smoking), religious attendance was no longer predictive (Colantonio, Kasl, & Ostfeld, 1992). Further, prestroke religiousness was not related to recovery from stroke in stroke survivors (Colantonio, Kasl, Ostfeld, & Berkman, 1993).

Regarding blood pressure, Seeman et al. (2003) concluded that "studies of blood pressure present a generally consistent pattern relating greater religious involvement to lower blood pressure and/or lower prevalence of hypertension" (p. 54). Several studies have demonstrated this relationship in older samples. For example, one prospective study of community-dwelling older adults found a protective effect of religious activity on subsequent high blood pressure. Respondents who both attended religious services regularly and prayed or studied the Bible frequently were 40% less likely to have high blood pressure compared to those who engaged in those activities infrequently (Koenig, George, Cohen, et al., 1998).

A longitudinal study of 1,723 older Japanese people who had recently lost a loved one examined several aspects of R/S, including the rarely assessed but likely very important aspect of belief, in relation to blood pressure. They assessed R/S and found that, 2 years later, those who reported having beliefs in a good afterlife were less likely to report hypertension than those who did not have this belief. However, neither religious practices nor religious coping were related to reports of hypertension (Krause et al., 2002).

Adding to the studies on hypertension, Masters, Lensegrav-Benson, Kircher, and Hill (2005; see also Masters, Hill, Kircher, Benson, & Fallon, 2004) examined religiousness and cardiovascular reactivity (CVR). CVR, which refers to cardiovascular changes in response to a stressor (usually blood pressure or heart rate), is believed to be a precursor of, or at least marker for, hypertension (Masters et al., 2005; see Cooper, Katzel, & Waldstein, Chapter 8, this volume). Results of two studies with older adults indicated that individuals classified as intrinsically religious (wherein religion is their master motive) had lower reactivity, particularly for interpersonal (as opposed to cognitive) stressors, compared to those classified as extrinsically religious (wherein religion is seen as a means to other ends, such as support; Masters et al., 2005).

Taken together, it appears that relationships between R/S and cardiovascular health are fairly robust, and that they occur largely, but not entirely, from their joint link with healthy lifestyle factors such as abstinence from smoking, moderation in food and alcohol consumption, and maintenance of appropriate weight (Powell et al., 2003; Oman et al., 2002).

## Ways That R/S Can Influence Health in the Elderly

Given that relations between aspects of R/S and of health seem complex but fairly robust, the compelling question becomes: *How* does R/S influence various aspects of health? Although some studies have examined possible mechanisms, most have not (George, Ellison, & Larson, 2002). There is, however, no lack of speculation regarding these links. This section first discusses the issue of confounds and covariates, then describes some of the major theories regarding how R/S may exert an influence on health.

## The Importance of Controlling for Confounds

As has been amply demonstrated, the correlational findings linking R/S factors and health outcomes are very difficult to interpret, because both R/S factors and health outcomes are related to many other factors that may serve as third variables, confounding the extent of the "true" relationship between them (Miller & Thoresen, 2003). For example, R/S and morbidity are both positively linked to gender, particularly in older groups, so to understand the influence of R/S on morbidity in a particular sample, some studies have controlled for the effects of gender. Similarly, studies that have examined R/S (defined as attendance or involvement) and health outcomes (e.g., mortality) have had to carefully control for an underlying disability or illness factor (McCullough et al., 2000). A wide variety of potential covariates or confounds have been identified and, in the more sophisticated studies, controlled. These covariates include demographic characteristics (e.g., age, gender, race, and ethnicity), socioeconomic status, education, health status, general activity levels, health behaviors and lifestyle, social support, and mental health. Yet, as is discussed in the concluding section, such statistical controls may be a poor substitute for an actual understanding of the causal relations among these variables (Pargament, 2002).

Other potential confounds or third variables, however, may be harder to control for but equally important to consider. For example, personality factors such as conscientiousness may underlie or be related to both R/S factors and health behaviors, or other dimensions relevant to health (e.g., Friedman & Martin, Chapter 9, this volume). Although it has been noted that both religiousness and spirituality overlap with conscientiousness (Piedmont, 2005), it has also been argued that both are personality dimensions distinct from the "Big Five" and unique in and of themselves (Piedmont, 1999, 2005). Further work may be needed to tease apart these issues, but the implications for health are important.

In another important caveat to the approach of statistically controlling for confounds, Miller and Thoresen (2003) noted the importance of distinguishing "true confounds" that are appropriately considered as covariates from variables that may serve as mediators or moderators. In other words, confounds should be assessed and statistically controlled to better understand the independent influence of R/S on a given outcome. However, many variables that are treated as confounds are actually mediators or moderators of the effects of R/S on health. Among potential mediators are the factors of health behaviors and lifestyle, social support, meaning, religious coping, and religious comfort versus struggle and doubt. Rather than simply "controlling for" the influence of these variables, Miller and Thoresen (2003) recommend using path analysis or structural equation models to show both their independent and mediational and moderating relations on R/S.

## Potential Mediators of Effects of R/S on Health

Although it remains to be established how R/S factors are translated into health outcomes (Underwood & Teresi, 2002), the most widely proposed mechanisms include health behaviors and social support. Both mechanisms have received some empirical attention (George et al., 2002). Many other pathways have been proposed as linkages between R/S and health outcomes, but few of these have been examined empirically. Below, theory and evidence bearing on these potential mediators are presented.

*Health Behaviors/Lifestyle.* It has long been supposed that certain types of R/S are related to health behaviors, which might then lead to better health. Different religious traditions prescribe certain behaviors (e.g., marital fidelity) and proscribe others (e.g., eating meat), which, although not directed toward affecting health, may nonetheless promote health and prevent diseases ("denominational effect"; George et al., 2002; Gorsuch, 1988; Koenig et al., 2001). Large-scale epidemiological studies that have controlled for the effects of health behaviors when examining the religious service attendance–mortality link have demonstrated that health behaviors partially mediate the effects of attendance on mortality. For example, one study found that, over 28 years, frequency of service attendance was related to subsequent exercise initiation and maintenance, and smoking and drinking cessation or reduction, behaviors related to reduced mortality (Strawbridge, Cohen, Shema, & Kaplan, 1997).

In addition to service attendance, other aspects of R/S beyond denomination may also be associated with better health behaviors. For example, a study of older adults in North Carolina found that both attendance and prayer were related to lower rates of cigarette smoking (Koenig, George, Cohen, et al., 1998). However, time spent watching religious television or listening to religious radio programming was related to higher rates of smoking.

There is some evidence that R/S factors are related to compliance with treatment among those with existing health problems. For example, in the previously cited study of R/S and blood pressure, in those participants who had been told they had high blood pressure, extent of patients' religious activity was positively related to taking their blood pressure medication (Koenig, George, Cohen, et al., 1998). In another study, elderly women recovering from broken hips, rated by their physical therapists as having better responses to physical therapy, also had higher levels of self-rated religiousness (Pressman, Lyons, Larson, & Strain, 1990).

In addition to health behaviors related to existing conditions, religion may be related to preventive health behaviors. One recent study of a nationally representative sample of older adults found that level of religious importance was positively related to the performance of preventive health care behaviors (i.e., flu shots, cholesterol screening, breast self-exams, mammograms, Pap smears, and prostate screening). Furthermore, those with a denominational affiliation were more likely to use preventive care than were nonaffiliated individuals, an effect particularly strong for those who identified themselves as Jewish (Reindl Benjamins & Brown, 2004).

*Social Support.* Religions typically promote socialization among adherents, and various aspects of religiousness are positively associated with social support (Koenig et al., 2001). Studies that have examined relations between attendance and mortality often covary out the influence of social support, which often weakens the relationship (indicating that social support is an important mediator of R/S effects on health). However, effects are inconsistent; it appears that social support is strongly related to mortality, but it often functions as a predictor rather than as a mediator (i.e., it is not strongly related to R/S factors; George et al., 2002). It is likely that those who do not attend religious services regularly seek out other sources of social support, so that general levels of social support may not drive the R/S–health link documented in many studies. However, it may also be true that aspects of social support that are specific to R/S are qualitatively different from non-R/S-related social support, and may have more potent effects on health (Krause, 2002). For example, R/S-related social support can provide what Krause called "spiritual support"—support given with the intent of explicitly enhancing the religious beliefs, behaviors, and experiences of the recipient. Such social support can reinforce communal beliefs and increase a sense of belongingness and closeness to God.

*Sense of Meaning in Life.* One of the hallmarks of most religions is an integrated system of strivings and worldviews (e.g., Park & Folkman, 1997; Spilka, Hood, Hunsberger, & Gorsuch, 2003), and numerous writers have proposed that a sense of meaning or coherence may be a major pathway of its influence on health (e.g., George et al., 2002). Although the mediational pathway of meaning in the R/S–health link remains to be tested (George et al., 2002), it seems likely that the extent to which religion helps people to have a meaningful life would be related to better physical and psychological well-being.

Although surprisingly little research has examined whether religiousness is related to higher levels of meaning, several studies have demonstrated that religiousness is related to a sense of meaning, particularly in older adults (Ardelt, 2003; Krause, 2002), and especially in older black adults compared to older white adults (Krause, 2002). Although the rest of this mediational link—that purpose in life is related to better health—has rarely been examined (cf. Riley et al., 1998), there is some evidence in the literature that meaning in life may be related to better health. For example, in one study of healing from total knee-replacement surgery in a sample of older people (mean age 67 years), meaning in life was related to better recovery at 6 months, when the authors controlled for initial health, age, gender, and education (Smith & Zautra, 2000).

*Meaning in Stressful Circumstances.* In addition to being related to meaning in life, it has also been proposed that R/S may influence health through its ability to mitigate even the most aversive meanings of stressful events, including illness. Religious beliefs provide options for understanding the meaning of a specific stressful event in more benign ways, including the notions that there is a larger plan, that events are not random, or that personal growth or spiritual purification can arise from struggle. Some individuals may believe that God would not harm them or visit upon them more than they could handle, whereas others may believe that God is trying to communicate something important through the event (Furnham & Brown, 1992; Pargament, 1997).

Specific religious beliefs can lead directly to understandings of particular events. For example, death may be appraised very differently—and bereavement experienced very differently—depending on beliefs about the afterlife (Benore & Park, 2004). The earlier study of bereaved Japanese elders (Krause et al., 2002) illustrates how a particular aspect of religious meaning might influence health by providing a more benign meaning in a highly stressful situation. Such provision of meaning may be even more important for those dealing with their own health problems, such as acute or chronic illness. Interestingly, in a recent study of older adults' adjustment to illness, Gall (2003) found that attributing the illness to God's love was related to poorer physical and social functioning. This study, however, was cross-sectional, and it may be that those who were worse off turned to religious explanations for comfort.

*Religious Coping.* Religious coping describes a wide range of religion-related attempts to manage or deal with one's problems. Religious coping may influence health both in dealing with specific health crises and, more generally, in the extent to which it reduces or buffers the effects of stress. Research has sometimes, but not always (e.g., Alferi, Culver, Carver, Arena, & Antoni, 1999), found that using religion to cope with illness is helpful (see Koenig et al., 2001, for a review). More recent research attempts have included measures of both "positive" and "negative" religious coping

(Pargament, Koenig, & Perez, 2000), which may help to delineate its multiple influences on health. Positive religious coping involves "benevolent religious involvement and the search for significance" (Pargament, 1999, p. 46), whereas negative religious coping involves spiritual discontent and anger in coping with stressors. One study found that negative religious coping had deleterious effects on health, whereas positive religious coping appeared to have beneficial, but weaker, effects on health in a sample of medically ill older adults (Koenig, Pargament, & Nielsen, 1998). In this cited study of medical rehabilitation patients, negative religious coping, particularly anger with God, was significantly related to lower ADL levels at a 1-month follow-up (Fitchett et al., 1999).

*Strength/Comfort versus Struggle/Doubt.* Some researchers have found that the extent to which an individual feels that God provides comfort and strength is related to positive psychological adjustment, whereas the extent to which one feels estranged from God and struggles with his or her faith is related to poorer adjustment (Exline & Rose, 2005). As noted earlier, several studies have linked this aspect of R/S to disability and mortality, and it may be that certain types of religious beliefs or affiliations lead to different levels of strength or comfort and struggle or doubt. Such feelings may then lead to different levels of enactment of health behaviors and, for those who are already dealing with chronic illnesses, may also influence adjustment to physical illness. For example, those who find strength and comfort in their religious or spiritual life may be better able to endure or live with their illness and more likely to comply with treatments. Such conjectures await empirical testing.

*Other Possible Mediators.* In addition to the previously mentioned variables, a number of other pathways have been proposed, although research testing these links remains to be conducted. Some of the promising mediators awaiting examination that may have particular relevance for older individuals include the ongoing experience of positive emotions and the absence of negative emotions, self-esteem, lack of hostility, marital and family stability, hope and optimism, meaningful social roles, helping and volunteerism, and the sense that one's life is sanctioned and supported by God. In addition, it is likely that the well-documented links between R/S and mental health (Koenig et al., 2001) may be pathways through which R/S influences physical health.

## DOES AGE MODERATE THE R/S–HEALTH LINK?

It is widely presumed that R/S factors influence health more as people age—in other words, that age strengthens the R/S–health link. Several competing hypotheses may be advanced. For example, on the one hand, it may be that religion becomes a more potent or salient resource as other resources, such as vitality and social support, are lost (Brandtstädter, Meiniger, & Graeser, 2003; Gall, 2003), thus exerting stronger effects on health as people age or become more ill. It may also be that there is a cumulative effect of R/S on health over a lifetime (e.g., due to health habits), so that effects become stronger with age (George et al., 2002). On the other hand, it may be that as individuals become more frail, some effects of R/S on well-being may be lessened, while others remain constant or become stronger. For example, religious service attendance may be strongly linked to physical functioning, so that attendance may become more strongly related to health with age (e.g., Idler & Kasl, 1997), whereas daily spiritual experiences may be less strongly linked with functioning and therefore less strongly moderated by age.

However, there is very little evidence for moderation (primarily because researchers have not looked!). In spite of many theoretical notions suggesting that R/S may play complex roles, surprisingly little research has addressed the issue of age as a moderator of the R/S–health link. Many of the studies linking religion to health have been conducted with samples of older people, in part because of their higher rates of morbidity and mortality, so there is substantial evidence that R/S factors are related to health in older people. However, most of these studies simply report or control for age rather than examine its potential impact on R/S–health relationships; very few studies have specifically examined age moderation.

Reports from two large-scale studies provide some data on age as a moderator in the religiousness–mortality link. In the Alameda County Study, religious service attendance was related to mortality, but there were also interactions by both age and gender (Oman et al., 2002). Results indicated that service attendance exerted more protective effects for younger than for older men, but more protective effects for older than for younger women. The results were interpreted as possibly due either to the link between maintenance of annual checkups and attendance, or the buffering effect of religion on work stress, both of which might disproportionately benefit younger men.

In a prospective study of a national sample of 3,617 persons age 25 and over in the United States (the Americans Changing Lives Study), frequency of attendance at religious services was inversely related to mortality rates 7½ years later. These analyses controlled for socioeconomic status, health status (functional impairment, chronic health problems, self-rated health), health behaviors (weight, physical activity, drinking, smoking), social integration (network size, confidence, social interaction, meeting attendance, subjective social support), other religious factors (volunteering for church, private religious activity, subjective religiosity), and beliefs (concerning justice, fatalism, rewards in the afterlife). However, the effects of service attendance were stronger among those under age 60 (Musick, House, & Williams, in press).

Virtually no studies have examined age and aspects of R/S other than service attendance. Exceptions are, first, the study of patients recovering from heart surgery (Contrada, Goyal, et al., 2004), cited earlier, in which stronger religious beliefs were associated with shorter lengths of hospital stay for the sample as a whole. Regarding age, these results indicated a trend ($p = .07$) toward a stronger beneficial effect of religious beliefs among older patients. Second, a study of forgiveness in a large representative U.S. sample found that forgiveness of others is more strongly related to self-reported physical health for middle-aged and old-age adults than for young adults (Toussaint, Williams, Musick, & Everson, 2001).

Although these studies offer tantalizing hints of the possible moderating effects of age, no conclusions can be drawn at this point. Instead, much more work is needed that focuses carefully and specifically on the question of moderation. This research needs to assess various aspects of R/S and also attend to the possibly differential influences of race and gender on moderation.

## A CAUTIONARY NOTE

Although much has been written in recent times about the strong connections between R/S and health, not everyone agrees that the evidence is so conclusive. One group of scholars has described the body of literature linking R/S and health as "weak and inconsistent" (Sloan, Bagiella, & Powell, 1999). Some of the inconsistencies found across studies may be due to the fact that different R/S dimensions influence different health dimensions in different populations, accounting for the sometimes spotty or null findings (Idler et al., 2003). Furthermore, many studies of R/S–health links fail to employ adequate statistical controls, thus drawing misleading conclusions (Freedland, 2004). Sloan and Bagiella (2002) have been among the most vocal critics of the rush to judgment regarding positive effects of R/S on health, concluding in their review of R/S–health links that "there is little empirical basis for assertions that religious involvement or activity is associated with beneficial health outcomes" (p. 14).

## CONCLUSIONS

Surveying the vast array of findings from studies that use various methodologies with various populations, Miller and Thoresen (2003, p. 33), concluded that "the evidence is clearly suggestive and, though not definitive or conclusive, is sufficient to warrant further methodologically sound investigation that will clarify health risk or protective effects of spiritual/ religious factors." This statement appears to be a reasonable reflection of the current state of this area of research. Specific to the issues of aging and health, the findings are even more sporadic and tentative, but, again, the evidence seems to suggest that this is a fruitful area in which to proceed. It is clear that much more work is needed to develop theoretical models of the influences of R/S on health, and more research based on these models is needed, using sophisticated measures to tease apart the dimensions of R/S, the confounds, the mediators, the moderators, and the various health-related outcomes. Below are several suggestions for those interested in advancing work in the area of religion and spirituality, health, and aging, followed by a comment on clinical implications.

## Development of Theory

Stepping back from the myriad research findings, it may be observed that this is an area of inquiry in desperate need of theory; that is, many of these studies have been conducted without a strong theoretical framework, and the resultant jumble of findings, many of which are contradictory, present a hazy picture indeed. A thorough conceptual model of the relations between multidimensional constructs of R/S and multiple dimensions of health, with consideration of mediating and moderating factors, is greatly needed. Such a model can take cues from extant research findings but should also draw heavily from broader biopsychosocial models of health.

## Sophisticated Prospective Research

Clearly, the need for more and better research is great. Few studies have addressed whether and how different dimensions of R/S influence the development and course of common disabling health problems such as heart disease and stroke, cancer, and arthritis—problems that increase in prevalence and severity as people age. In addition, many questions remain regarding the mechanisms of effect. Mediators such as social support and health behaviors are only now being examined in this regard, and many others, such as meaning and religious coping, await scrutiny. The issue of moderation is one that, again, has only recently begun to be tapped. To advance the field, research must be derived from and grounded in solid theoretical models.

## Attention to Diversity

As noted earlier, most of the research on R/S and health has been conducted in the United States, and has focused mostly on individuals with Judeo-Christian backgrounds. Very little is known about the R/S–health links for persons with different religious preferences and affiliations within the

United States, and even less is known about those outside the United States. Given that the United States is "famously religious relative to other industrialized countries" (Sherkat & Ellison, 1999, p. 364), it is not clear how relevant the results of current studies are to those living in other parts of the world, or with other religious beliefs, denominations, or spiritual practices.

## Clinical Applications

Although considerable disagreement and uncertainty remain regarding the actual significance of the effects of R/S factors on health, it is in the other half of the endeavor—the potential translation into clinical practice—that the more substantive controversies exist (Mills, 2002). If R/S is indeed relevant to health, what do we then do with this knowledge? Much has been written in recent years about the role of religion in medicine, and the ethical responsibilities and constraints for medical professionals (e.g., Koenig et al., 2001). For example, Koenig et al. addressed the following issues for physicians interested in clinical applications: meeting patients' religious and spiritual needs, taking a religious history, supporting or encouraging religious beliefs, ensuring access to religious resources, respecting visits by clergy, viewing chaplains as part of the health care team, being ready to step in when clergy are unavailable, and using advanced spiritual interventions (e.g., praying with patients) cautiously.

Some writers appear to endorse religiousness as a part of routine health care. For example, in their *American Psychologist* review, Powell et al. (2003) concluded, "When one considers that attending religious services is an inexpensive but widely available resource in the community, this could be a very cost-effective way to maintain the health of elderly people with disability or chronic diseases" (p. 49). However, researchers have acknowledged that patients may neither be religious nor have such interests. Contrada, Idler, et al. (2004) proposed a number of ways that R/S may be useful in the health care of patients, even when direct manipulation is impossible or impractical. For example, assessing aspects of religiousness or spirituality may help to identify patients at high risk. Studies suggest that patients experiencing religious struggle and doubt are at higher risk for negative consequences, which may warrant intervention. Furthermore, for those who identify themselves as religious, it may be possible to use religious involvement as a motivating factor for making or maintaining particular health behaviors (Contrada, Idler, et al., 2004).

## The Promise Ahead

Because religion and spirituality are so central to the lives of so many people, the development of a deeper and more considered understanding of their influences on physical and psychological illness and health may greatly enrich our knowledge base and also lead to the development of more effective prevention and intervention strategies. Significant efforts are needed to develop theoretical models and to conduct theoretically based studies. Such work is subject not only to many of the same challenges as work on other psychosocial factors (e.g., unassessed confounds, third variables) but also to some challenges that are specific to religion and spirituality (e.g., definitional issues, potential ideological biases). In spite of these obstacles, the research to date suggests that religiousness and spirituality may play a unique role in the psychological functioning of human beings, and that this is a promising area to pursue, with much left to be learned.

## REFERENCES

Aldwin, C. M. (in press). *Stress, coping, and human development, second edition.* New York: Guilford Press.

Alferi, S., Culver, J., Carver, C. S., Arena, P., & Antoni, M.H. (1999). Religiosity, religious coping and distress: A prospective study of Catholic and Evangelical Hispanic women in treatment for early stage breast cancer. *Journal of Health Psychology, 4,* 343–356.

Ardelt, M. (2003). Effects of religion and purpose in life on elders' subjective well-being and attitudes toward death. *Journal of Religious Gerontology, 14,* 55–77.

Argue, A., Johnson, D. R., & White, L. K. (1999). Age and religiosity: Evidence from a three-wave panel analysis. *Journal for the Scientific Study of Religion, 38,* 423–435.

Atchley, R. C. (1997). The subjective importance of being religious and its effect on health and morale 14 years later. *Journal of Aging Studies, 11,* 131–141.

Benore, E. R., & Park, C. L. (2004). Religiousness and beliefs in continued attachment after death. *International Journal of the Psychology of Religion, 14,* 1–22.

Boyer, E. (1981–1982). Variations in health perception between black and white elderly. *International Quarterly of Community Health Education, 2,* 157–173.

Broyles, P. A., & Drenovsky, C. K. (1992). Religious attendance and the subjective health of the elderly. *Review of Religious Research, 34,* 152–160.

Brandtstädter, J., Meiniger, C., & Graeser, H. (2003). Handlungs- und Sinnressourcen: Entwicklungsmuster und protektive Effekte [Action resources and meaning resources: Developmental patterns and protective effects]. *Zeitschrift für Entwicklungspsychologie und Paedagogische Psychologie, 35,* 49–58.

Colantonio, A., Kasl, S. V., & Ostfeld, A. M. (1992). Depressive symptoms and other psychosocial factors as predictors of stroke in the elderly. *American Journal of Epidemiology, 136,* 884–889.

Colantonio, A., Kasl, S. V., & Ostfeld, A. M., & Berkman, L. F. (1993). Psychosocial predictors of stroke outcomes in an elderly population. *Journal of Gerontology, 4,* S261–S268.

Comstock, G. W., & Partridge, K. (1972). Church attendance and health. *Journal of Chronic Disease, 25,* 665–672.

Contrada, R. J., Goyal, T. M., Caher, C., Rafalson, L. L., & Krause, T. J. (2004).

Psychosocial factors in outcomes of heart surgery: The impact of religious involvement and depressive symptoms. *Health Psychology, 23,* 227–238.

Contrada, R. J., Idler, E., Goyal, T. M., Caher, C., Rafalson, L. L., & Krause, T. J. (2004). Why not find out whether religious beliefs predict surgical outcomes?: If they do, why not find out why?: Reply to Freedland (2004). *Health Psychology, 23,* 243–246.

Exline, J. J., & Rose, E. (2005). Religious and spiritual struggles. In R. F. Paloutzian & C. L. Park (Eds.), *Handbook of the psychology of religion and spirituality* (pp. 315–330). New York: Guilford Press.

Fetzer Institute/National Institute on Aging Working Group (1999). *Multidimensional measurement of religiousness/spirituality for use in health research* [A report of a national working group supported by the Fetzer Institute and the National Institute on Aging]. Kalamazoo, MI: John E. Fetzer Institute.

Fitchett, G., Rybarczyk, B. D., DeMarco, G. A., & Nicholas, J. J. (1999). The role of religion in medical rehabilitation outcomes: A longitudinal study. *Rehabilitation Psychology, 44,* 333–353.

Freedland, K. E. (2004). Religious beliefs shorten hospital stays?: Psychology works in mysterious ways: Comment on Contrada et al. (2004). *Health Psychology, 23,* 239–242.

Furnham, A., & Brown, L. B. (1992). Theodicy: A neglected aspect of the psychology of religion *International Journal for the Psychology of Religion, 2,* 37–45.

Gall, T. L. (2003). Religious and spiritual attributions in older adults' adjustment to illness. *Journal of Psychology and Christianity, 22,* 210–222.

The Gallup Organization. (2004). *Focus on religion.* Retrieved December 15, 2006, from www.gallup.com/poll/focus/sr040302.asp.

George, L., Ellison, C., & Larson, D. (2002). Explaining the relationships between religious involvement and health. *Psychological Inquiry, 13,* 190–200.

Goldbourt, U., Yaari, S., & Medalie, J. H. (1993). Factors predictive of long-term coronary heart disease mortality among 10,059 male Israeli civil servants and municipal employees: A 23-year mortality follow-up in the Israeli Ischemic Heart Disease Study. *Cardiology, 82,* 100–121.

Gorsuch, R. L. (1988). Psychology of religion. *Annual Review of Psychology, 39,* 201–221.

Helm, H., Hays, J. C., Flint, E., Koenig, H. G., & Blazer, D. G. (2000). Effects of private religious activity on mortality of elderly disabled and nondisabled adults. *Journals of Gerontology: Biological Sciences and Medical Sciences, Series A, 55,* M400–M405.

Hill, P. C. (2005). Measurement issues. In R. F. Paloutzian & C. L. Park (Eds.), *Handbook of the psychology of religion and spirituality* (pp. 43–61). New York: Guilford Press.

Hill, P. C., & Hood, R. W., Jr. (1999). *Measures of religiosity.* Birmingham, AL: Religious Education Press.

Idler, E., & Kasl, S. V. (1991). Health perceptions and survival: Do global evaluations of health status really predict mortality? *Journal of Gerontology, 46,* S55–S65.

Idler, E. L., & Kasl, S. (1992). Religion, disability, depression, and the timing of death. *American Journal of Sociology, 97,* 1052–1079.

Idler, E. L., & Kasl, S. V. (1997). Religion among disabled and nondisabled persons: II. Attendance at religious services as a predictor of the course of disability. *Journal of Gerontology: Psychological Sciences and Social Sciences, Series B, 52,* S306–S316.

Idler, E. L., Musick, M. A., Ellison, C. G., George, L. K., Krause, N., Ory, M. G., et al. (2003). Measuring multiple dimensions of religion and spirituality for health research. *Research on Aging, 25,* 327–365.

Ingersoll-Dayton, B., Krause, N., & Morgan, D. (2002). Religious trajectories and transitions over the life course. *International Journal of Aging and Human Development, 55,* 51–70.

Koenig, H. G. (2000). Religion, well-being, and health in the elderly: The scientific evidence for an association. In J. A. Thorson (Ed.), *Perspectives on spiritual well-being and aging* (pp. 84–97). Springfield, IL: Thomas.

Koenig, H. G., Cohen, H. J., George, L. K., Hays, J. C., Larson, D. B., & Blazer, D. G. (1997). Attendance at religious services, interleukin-6, and other biological parameters of immune function in older adults. *International Journal of Psychiatry and Medicine, 27,* 233–250.

Koenig, H. G., George, L. K., Cohen, H. J., Hays, J. C., Larson, D., & Blazer, D. G. (1998). The relationship between religious activities and cigarette smoking in older adults. *Journals of Gerontology: Biological Sciences and Medical Sciences, Series A, 53,* M426–M434.

Koenig, H. G., George, L. K., & Siegler, I. (1998). The use of religion and other emotion-regulating coping strategies among older adults. *Gerontologist, 38,* 303–310.

Koenig, H. G., Kvale, J. N., & Ferrel, C. (1988). Religion and well-being in later life. *Gerontologist, 28,* 18–28.

Koenig, H. G., McCullough, M. E., & Larson, D. B. (2001). *Handbook of religion and health.* New York: Oxford University Press.

Koenig, H. G., Pargament, K. I., & Nielsen, J. (1998). Religious coping and health status in medically ill hospitalized older adults. *Journal of Nervous and Mental Disease, 186,* 513–521.

Krause, N. (2006). Religion and health in later life. In J. E. Birren & K. W. Shail (Eds.), *Handbook of the psychology of aging, sixth edition* (pp. 500–518). Burlington, MA: Academic Press.

Krause, N. (1998). Stressors in highly valued roles, religious coping, and mortality. *Psychology and Aging, 13,* 242–255.

Krause, N. (2002). Church-based social support and health in old age: Exploring variations by race. *Journals of Gerontology: Psychological Sciences and Social Sciences, Series B, 57,* S332–S347.

Krause, N., Liang, J., Shaw, B. A., Sugisawa, H., Kim, H., & Sugihara, Y. (2002). Religion, death of a loved one, and hypertension among older adults in Japan. *Journals of Gerontology: Psychological Sciences and Social Sciences, Series B, 57,* S96–S107.

Kutner, N. G., Lin, L. S., Fielding, B., Brogan, D., & Hall, W. D. (1994). Continued survival of older hemodialysis: Investigation of psychosocial predictors. *American Journal of Kidney Diseases, 24,* 42–49.

Lutgendorf, S. K., Russell, D., Ullrich, P., Harris, T. B., & Wallace, R. (2004). Religious participation, interleukin-6, and mortality in older adults. *Health Psychology, 3,* 465–475.

Masters, K. S., Hill, R. D., Kircher, J. C., Benson, T. L. L., & Fallon, J. A. (2004). Religious orientation, aging, and blood pressure reactivity to interpersonal and cognitive stressors. *Annals of Behavioral Medicine, 228,* 171–178.

Masters, K. S., Lensegrar-Benson, T. L., Kirchere, J. C., & Hill, R. D. (2005). Effects of religious orientation and gender on cardiovascular reactivity among older adults. *Research on Aging, 27,* 221–240.

McCullough, M. E., Hoyt, W. T., Larson, D. B., Koenig, H. G., & Thoresen, C. (2000). Religious involvement and mortality: A meta-analytic review. *Health Psychology, 19,* 211–222.

Miller, W. R., & Thoresen, C. E. (2003). Spirituality, religion, and health: An emerging research field. *American Psychologist, 58,* 24–35.

Mills, P. J. (2002). Spirituality, religiousness, and health: From research to clinical practice. *Annals of Behavioral Medicine, 24,* 1–2.

Musick, M. A. (1996). Religion and subjective health among black and white elders. *Journal of Health and Social Behavior, 37,* 221–237.

Musick, M. A., House, J. S., & Williams, D. R. (2004). Attendance at religious services and mortality in a national sample. *Journal of Health and Social Behavior, 25,* 198–213.

Musick, M. A., Traphagan, J. W., Koenig, H. G., & Larson, D. B. (2000). Spirituality in physical health and aging. *Journal of Adult Development, 7,* 73–86.

Oman, D., Kurata, J. H., Strawbridge, W. J., & Cohen, R. D. (2002). Religious attendance and cause of death over 31 years. *International Journal of Psychiatry in Medicine, 32,* 69–89.

Oman, D., & Reed, D. (1998). Religion and mortality among the community-dwelling elderly. *American Journal of Public Health, 87,* 1469–1475.

Oxman, T. E., Freeman, D. H., Jr., & Manheimer, E. D. (1995). Lack of social participation or religious strength and comfort as risk factors for death after cardiac surgery in the elderly. *Psychosomatic Medicine, 57,* 5–15.

Pargament, K. I. (1997). *The psychology of religion and coping: Theory, research, practice.* New York: Guilford Press.

Pargament, K. I. (1999). Religious/spiritual coping. In Multidimensional measurement of religiousness/spirituality for use in health research (pp. 43–56). Kalamazoo, MI: Fetzer Foundation.

Pargament, K. I. (2002). Is religion nothing but . . . ?: Explaining religion versus explaining religion away. *Psychological Inquiry, 13,* 239–244.

Pargament, K. I., Koenig, H. G., & Perez, L. 2000. The many methods of religious coping: Development and initial validation of the RCOPE. *Journal of Clinical Psychology, 56,* 519–543.

Pargament, K. I., Koenig, H. G., Tarakeshwar, N., & Hahn, J. (2001). Religious struggle as a predictor of mortality among medically ill elderly patients: A 2-year longitudinal study. *Archives of Internal Medicine, 61,* 1881–1885.

Park, C. L., & Folkman, S. (1997). Meaning in the context of stress and coping. *General Review of Psychology, 1,* 115–144.

Phillips, R. L., Kuzma, J. W., Beeson, W. L., & Lotz, T. (1980). Influence of selection versus lifestyle on risk of fatal cancer and cardiovascular disease among Seventh-Day Adventists. *American Journal of Epidemiology, 112,* 296–314.

Piedmont, R. L. (1999). Does spirituality represent the sixth factor of personality?:

Spiritual transcendence and the five-factor model. *Journal of Personality, 67,* 985–1023.

Piedmont, R. L. (2005). The role of personality in uderstanding religious and spiritual constructs. In R. F. Paloutzian & C. L. Park (Eds.), *Handbook of the psychology of religion and spirituality* (pp. 253–273). New York: Guilford Press.

Powell, L. H., Shahabi, L., & Thoresen, C. E. (2003). Religion and spirituality: Linkages to physical health. *American Psychologist, 58,* 36–52.

Pressman, M. A., Lyons, J. S., Larson, D. B., & Strain, J. J. (1990). Religious belief, depression, and ambulation status in elderly women with broken hips. *American Journal of Psychiatry, 147,* 758–760.

Reindl Benjamins, M., & Brown, C. (2004). Religion and preventative health care utilization among the elderly. *Social Science and Medicine, 58,* 109–118.

Riley, B. B., Perna, R., Tate, D. G., Forchheimer, M., Anderson, C., & Luera, G. (1998). Types of spiritual well-being among persons with chronic illness: Their relation to various forms of quality of life. *Archives of Physical Medicine and Rehabilitation, 79,* 258–264.

Seeman, T. E., Dubin, L. F., & Seeman, M. (2003). Religiosity/spirituality and health: Critical review of the evidence for biological pathways. *American Psychologist, 58,* 53–63.

Sherkat, D. E., & Ellison, C. G. (1999). Recent developments and current controversies in the sociology of religion. *Annual Review of Sociology, 25,* 363–394.

Sloan, R. P., & Bagiella, E. (2002). Claims about religious involvement and health outcomes. *Annals of Behavioral Medicine, 24,* 14–21.

Sloan, R. P., Bagiella, E., & Powell, T. (1999). Religion, spirituality, and medicine. *Lancet, 353,* 664–667.

Smith, B. W., & Zautra, A. J. (2000). Purpose in life and coping with knee-replacement surgery. *Occupational Therapy Journal of Research, 20,* 96S–99S.

Spilka, B., Hood, R.W., Jr., Hunsberger, B., & Gorsuch, R. (2003). *The psychology of religion: An empirical approach* (3rd ed.). New York: Guilford Press.

Strawbridge, W. J., Cohen, R. D., Shema, S. J., & Kaplan, G. A. (1997). Frequent attendance at religious services and mortality over 28 years. *American Journal of Public Health, 87,* 957–961.

Thoresen, C. E., & Harris, A. H. S. (2002). Spirituality and health: What's the evidence and what's needed? *Annals of Behavioral Medicine, 24,* 3–13.

Thorson, J. A. (Ed.). (2000). *Perspectives on spiritual well-being and aging.* Springfield, IL: Thomas.

Toussaint, L. L., Williams, D. R., Musick, M. A., & Everson, S. A. (2001). Forgiveness and health: Age differences in a U.S. probability sample. *Journal of Adult Development, 8,* 249–257.

Underwood, L. G., & Teresi, J. A. (2002). The Daily Spiritual Experience Scale: Development, theoretical description, reliability, exploratory factor analysis, and preliminary construct validity using health-related data. *Annals of Behavioral Medicine, 24,* 22–33.

Van Ness, P. H., & Kasl, S. V. (2003). Religion and cognitive dysfunction in an elderly cohort. *Journals of Gerontology: Psychological Sciences and Social Sciences, Series B, 56,* S21–S29.

Wink, P., & Dillon, M. (2002). Spiritual development across the adult life course: Findings from a longitudinal study. *Journal of Adult Development, 9,* 79–94.

Wotherspoon, C. M. (2000). The relationship between spiritual well-being and health in later life. In J. A. Thorson (Ed.), *Perspectives on spiritual well-being and aging* (pp. 69–83). Springfield, IL: Thomas.

Zinnbauer, B., & Pargament, K. I. (2005). Religiousness and spirituality. In R. F. Paloutzian & C. L. Park (Eds.), *Handbook of the psychology of religion and spirituality* (pp. 21–42). New York: Guilford Press.

# PART IV

# CLINICAL ISSUES

# CHAPTER 17

# Self-Regulation of Health Threats, Affect, and the Self

## Lessons from Older Adults

HOWARD LEVENTHAL, RACHEL FORSTER,
and ELAINE LEVENTHAL

During an annual physical examination, Mr. X, a 70-year-old male academic, reported being awakened on a regular basis at about 2 A.M., feeling physically stressed. The stress caused him to "toss about" in bed. Sometimes whatever it was—and it was a vague set of sensations—seemed to be more prominent on the left side of his body. Taking 500 mg of acetaminophen or ibuprofen helped. There was no palpable evidence of change on physical examination. The doctor recommended that Mr. X continue using the "pain medication" when needed.

Two years later, Mr. X was seen again by his primary care physician because of severe pain in the left side of his neck and left upper back. At times he could find no way of making himself comfortable; he said he could not imagine having to live for 20 or more years with such pain. The 20-year time frame fit his life expectancy, because his parents had lived into their late 80s, and he had no life-threatening illnesses. The pain was disrupting sleep and made it impossible for Mr. X to use the computer. He had been "living with" this condition for at least a month when he finally decided he had to do something about it.

Mr. X's visits with his primary care physician and his subsequent visits to specialists and physical therapists will provide a concrete illustration of the themes comprising the main body of our chapter. These themes are (1) quality of care and its significance for older persons; (2) the common-sense psychology underlying the everyday management of chronic illness threats;

(3) constructing common-sense representations of illness, including process and content; and (4) effects of age-related physical and psychological changes on the processes involved in the common-sense management of health threats and emotional stress. Although each of these topics could make a separate chapter, considering them together sharpens our view of the relationships among them and compensates for the necessary omission of numerous details relevant to each.

## AGING AND QUALITY OF CARE

### Are Chronic Conditions Treated Successfully?

Although typical chronic illnesses develop over a lifetime, most begin to intrude on functioning in the 6th decade of life, with disruption increasing in the 7th and 8th decades. The typical 70-year-old is likely to report three to five chronic illnesses. Older adults also comprise the bulk of patients in hospital and the greatest use of the health care system, generate the highest cost of health care, and suffer the most when medical care is suboptimal (Institute of Medicine, 1999).

Although in-hospital deaths are well advertised as part of the quality picture, they are probably less of a problem than the deficits in the out-of-hospital management of chronic illnesses such as diabetes, hypertension, congestive heart failure, and arthritis. Management for each of these conditions requires the patient's active participation in his or her care. Indeed, as expert geriatric physicians tell their patients, "I can diagnose your condition and suggest a path for its management, but treatment takes place at home, and you and your spouse are the ones who have to do it. We need to discuss an action plan for treatment that will fit into your life situation." Unfortunately, words such as these and the shared decision making and planning they suggest are likely all too rare in clinical practice, because less than 50% of hypertensives, diabetics, and asthmatics have their conditions adequately controlled (e.g., Wang et al., 2004). The medical care system often fails to respond to and monitor the self-management processes involved in chronic illness management, a situation labeled "clinical inertia" (Phillips et al., 2001).

### Access to Care and Care Seeking

Access to care and timely seeking of care are necessary conditions for quality. Delay in care seeking due to cultural, social, and personal beliefs about the health care system and interpretations of somatic changes can compromise quality and threaten the patient's function and life. Failure to seek care for acute onset of serious conditions such as myocardial infarction (Bunde & Martin, 2006) or bowel obstruction can result in severe complications, such as infection spreading throughout the body. Episodes of bowel obstruction are common among elderly patients, and are likely understood by laypersons as an age-related disease as opposed to episodes related to an underlying, chronic condition (Bickell, Rojas, Anderson, & Leventhal, 2004). Indeed, at any age, patients tend to see illnesses as episodic and acute, and not as permanent conditions of their bodies. The acute perception is adaptive when it matches biological reality, and maladaptive when it does not. That outlook affected Mr. X.

At his 2-year "follow-up" visit, Mr. X reported that he had had severe pain for over 1½ months. He did not call sooner because he thought the pain might go away by itself, and it was not specific and probably not important. But it seemed to get worse rather than better, and Mr. X's wife finally urged him either to see his doctor or to stop complaining.

Consistent with empirical findings, Mr. X's symptoms were necessary for patient-motivated health care visits (as opposed to annually scheduled and other doctor- or work-scheduled visits), but they were not sufficient. The duration, novelty, and severity (in apparent order of importance) were critical motivators (Mora, Robitaille, Leventhal, Swigar, & Leventhal, 2002). Symptoms lacking these properties may be insufficient to motivate care seeking. It is likely that Mr. X would have used health care more quickly if he had had chest pain rather than upper back pain, and if the chest pain were experienced with a history of cardiovascular disease (Bunde & Martin, 2006; Evangelista, Dracup, & Doering, 2000). In addition, Mr. X's pathway to the doctor included both social pressure and the pressure of pain.

The perception of quality was also involved in Mr. X's delay; he did not believe that quality care was available for his symptoms. Indeed, he initially appraised his symptoms as neither serious (not life threatening) nor treatable and felt that an effective treatment was highly unlikely. He also did not want to bother his physician with symptoms that might be perceived as "psychological" rather than physical. But as the symptoms persisted, disrupted daily function, and failed to follow a familiar pattern, Mr. X stopped trying to evaluate what was causing his problem, and moved from an extended period of appraisal delay to illness, a period during which he regarded himself as living with an illness whose origin and label was unknown (Safer, Tharps, Jackson, & Leventhal, 1979).

## THE COMMON SENSE OF EVERYDAY SELF-MANAGEMENT OF CHRONIC ILLNESS THREATS

Mr. X's care-seeking behaviors illustrate how social influence and personal history interact to form a psychological rationale for care seeking; his wife's urging succeeded because ongoing interpretation of his somatic changes led him to worry that they might be serious. His actions also illustrate the interrelationship between self-management behavior and quality of care.

Mr. X's symptoms—the tingling in his arm, the neck pain, and the distress in the region of the left hip—were beginning to coalesce into the representation of a possibly serious spinal problem! He had read Reynolds Price's description of the discovery of a spinal tumor and some of Price's experiences and his own overlapped. The symptoms and the heuristics he used and questions he raised in interpreting their meaning added a potential threat to the underlying uncertainty. The heuristics involved in this process of translating somatic events into an illness representation have been the focus of the research described in this section.

## A Model of the Processes Involved in Deciding One Is Sick and Needs Care

Given that symptoms precede but are not sufficient to motivate care seeking, multiple studies have been conducted to identify the variables that affect the magnitude of the relationship of symptoms to care seeking. We have labeled these factors "heuristics," the simple rules of thumb that either automatically or with deliberate thought affect decisions as to whether one or more symptoms merit medical care. Of course, people seek care for unbearably severe symptoms regardless of their suspicions of their meaning.

### Heuristics Are Used When the Nonconscious Enters Consciousness

Damasio's (1999) model of the mind posits a sharp boundary between homeostatic mechanisms and consciousness. This picture is only partially true. When we feel sick, which is not equivalent to being sick, we are conscious of usually invisible homeostatic processes, because they deviate from normal function. Feeling sick includes physical symptoms that may be fairly specific, such as aches, pains that may be dull or sharp and specific or vague in location, feeling bloated and hearing noises in the gut, and vague feelings (e.g., fatigue, exhaustion, and tension) often accompanied by emotional distress. Conscious experiences of somatic problems lack the detail, however, of the underlying, dysregulated biological system. A severe pulmonary or intestinal inflammation can generate fever, fatigue, localized pain, abdominal bloating, constipation, and diarrhea. Consciousness will not, however, have a picture of the type, quantity, or exact location of the infectious agent, nor will it detail the specific immunological defenses arrayed against it. Many of the symptom experiences are due to the cytokines regulating the immune response rather than to the pathogens alone. Cytokines affect the central nervous system, causing the fever, trembling, and fatigue that motivate a retreat to one's bed or den. The conscious self needs to be aware of the general status of the body to perform behaviors needed for survival. Thus, feelings of illness are sensitive to disease but nonspecific. For this reason, a variety of rules or heuristics are used to evaluate somatic changes, to identify and elaborate the nature of the systemic change, and to generate procedures and action plans to restore normal function. The body provides the basic neurophysiological machinery for detecting changes, and heuristics serve in the interpretation and elaboration of the meaning of these changes based upon a lifetime of experiences with normal functioning, prior deviations from normal, and information from direct observations, discussions with others, and public media. By assigning meaning to a somatic experience, heuristics elaborate the present and future implications of a change for physical, functional, psychological, and social self identities. These meanings create motivation for self-management.

## Heuristics Create Common-Sense Meanings for Somatic Changes

There is much that we do and much that we do not know about heuristics. It seems likely that some heuristics can be conceived of as common-sense rules for determining the meaning of a somatic change, whereas others seem more useful for deciding on a course of action. The meaning assigned to a somatic change may be less important in motivating care seeking when symptoms such as pain are extremely severe. Data exist for a half-dozen of the 13 or more heuristics that have been identified (see Table 17.1), and many of those not examined empirically are so readily recognized that it may seem superfluous to validate their existence in empirical study. Mr. X used many of these heuristics in evaluating his symptoms and in making his treatment decisions. The following sections review data for eight mental rules of thumb that seem to function intrapersonally, followed by examples of heuristics involving social comparisons.

## Identity—What Do We Call It?: Symmetry, Location, and Pattern

The "symmetry rule" is a bidirectional process that appears to be fundamental to mental functioning (Baumann, Cameron, Zimmerman, & Leventhal, 1989). It involves the search for labels to attach to somatic changes, and the search for somatic events once a person has a label (i.e., a diagnosis). An early study by Meyer, Leventhal, and Gutmann (1985) illustrated the operation of symmetry among people with elevated blood pressure. When patients in treatment for hypertension were asked, "Do you agree that *people* can't tell when their blood pressure is elevated?", 85% agreed, "People cannot tell." However, when asked later in the interview, "Can you tell when your blood pressure is up?", 90% said "Yes." This percentage (90%) was considerably higher than that of a control group of nonhypertensive patients, fewer than half of whom said they could tell when their blood pressure was elevated.

TABLE 17.1. Rules of Thumb (Heuristics) for Evaluating Somatic Change

| Heuristics | Common-sense question and answer |
|---|---|
| Heuristics reflecting basic mental operation and human anatomy | |
| Symmetry | Symptoms need labels and labels need symptoms. |
| Pattern | Pain in chest, radiation over left side of body = heart. Gastrointestinal distress, bloating, moves about, etc.—it will clear up. |
| Location | Breathless—lung, not heart. Soreness in lower left abdomen = appendicitis. |
| Rate of change | Getting worse so fast—better get help before it is unbearable! |
| Learned heuristics based upon universal somatic experience | |
| Responded to care | Took home remedy—hurt less; not serious. |
| Novelty | Unusual (sweating with chest pain)—check it out. |
| Duration | It's lasted too long—better check it out. |
| Stress–illness | It's stress—nothing medicine can do and it will go away. |
| Age–illness | If it's age, accept it. |
| Gender | Chest pain in mother—stress; in dad—heart. |
| Heuristics based upon social comparisons | |
| Similar exposures | We ate the same thing; it was food, not serious. |
| Similar vulnerabilities | Temperament same as sister and she had cancer—symptom is serious. |
| Prevalence | Everyone has it—not serious. |

Results of other laboratory experiments lend further support to the bidirectional nature of symmetry rule. Baumann and Leventhal (1985) randomly assigned students to conditions where they received either an elevated or a normal blood pressure reading prior to filling out a series of questionnaires. Students given the elevated readings were more likely than those given normal readings to report experiencing symptoms, and the symptoms they reported were the same as those reported by patients with hypertension; they did not report increases in nonhypertensive symptoms. When given labels (or readings), people search for symptoms, and as we all well know, when we have symptoms we seek explanations (i.e., labels).

The *location* and *pattern* of somatic changes are critical in establishing plausible labels and establishing the *identity* of a condition. The importance of location is clear from everyday expressions such as "I have an earache," "I have a toothache," and so on. In addition to identifying a location, these expressions usually imply that the condition is limited as to its consequence and duration, and they suggest actions for control (use eardrops, see a dentist, go to the emergency room; Bunde & Martin, 2006). The location rule provides somewhat less clear evidence with respect to the causes of a problem and little immediate evidence with respect to longer term consequences. Consequences are likely inferred from similarity with previous symptoms and their resolution. When symptoms fail to resolve spontaneously, consequences are often spelled out following a visit to a health practitioner. Location also plays a critical role in common-sense interpretations of pain. For example, the initial meaning of pain is likely to reflect where it is felt; for example, back pain can be perceived as muscular, though the pain may be referred from an internal organ, and chest pain activates fear of heart attack (Bunde & Martin, 2006).

Symptom pattern has been shown to be a factor in care-seeking following coronary attacks (Bunde & Martin, 2006; Cameron et al., 1995; Finnegan et al., 2000) and in seeking early diagnosis of potentially life-threatening cancers. Studies show that patients seek treatment sooner when the symptom pattern fits preconceived notions of a heart attack, including sharp pains in the chest, pain radiating down the arm, abrupt, partial loss of strength, and difficulty breathing. Deviation of symptoms from expected patterns and locations can create serious problems with understanding and managing cardiac conditions. For example, patients with congestive heart failure, a disease that is typically fatal within 5 years of its diagnosis, live with chronic symptoms of fatigue and breathlessness in the absence of the acute, tell-tale signs (e.g., chest pain) that are the essential signals in their minds for cardiac disease (Horowitz, Rein, & Leventhal, 2004). Unsurprisingly, many of these patients fail to seek care prior to the onset of episodes of severe cardiac decompensation, and many report that their condition "doesn't make sense," lacking clear signs signaling the need for action. Mass media messages on the "early warning signs" of breast and colon cancer and heart disease (Leventhal, Cameron, Leventhal, & Ozakinci, 2005; Martin & Leventhal, 2004) help to create the use of pattern and location in common-sense, somatic self-appraisals.

### Novelty, Duration, and Rate of Change

In contrast to pattern and location, which help to establish the identity or meaning of a symptom, the *duration* and *novelty* of symptoms have powerful effects on motivation to seek help but are ambiguous as to meaning. The *novelty* of symptoms, their lack of fit to a familiar pattern, had a very strong effect in motivating care seeking among elderly respondents who reported experiencing an acute condition, or an onset or flare-up of a chronic condition (Mora et al., 2002). Longer *duration* of these reported episodes also increased likelihood of care seeking for both acute and chronic episodes. It is likely that duration and novelty interact in complex ways, and that duration perhaps has a greater effect when symptoms are unfamiliar; this was true for Mr. X. When symptoms fit a specific pattern (e.g., heart attack, common cold, etc.), motivation for care seeking is a product of symptoms' identity or meaning; the effects of duration vary as a function of expectations with respect to the risk associated with delay. We have no empirical data on *rate of change* of somatic events, but it seems reasonable to expect that rapid increases in the intensity or extent of physical symptoms, signs, and function, will affect motivation and ring alarm bells!

Duration and novelty affected Mr. X. His self-reports included a history of difficulty falling asleep and waking up with a novel, odd feeling. Because it happened multiple times with no sign of stopping, Mr. finally sought advice.

### Causal Rules: Is It Illness, Stress, or Age?

Two other heuristics, the stress–illness and age–illness rules of thumb, contribute to the evaluation of a somatic change as a signal of illness or a sign of an alternative, nonillness event. We suspect that these heuristics function both automatically, without focused attention, and deliberatively, drawing upon conscious attention and deliberative decision making. The stress–illness "rule" questions whether a somatic change should be attributed to stress or to physical illness. The specific attribution depends on both the circumstances and the features of the stimulus. Ambiguous signals, such as fatigue, tension, and headaches, are more readily attributed to stress, whereas clear symptomatic indicators of specific conditions, such as sore throats and coughs with sputum, are attributed to illness (Cameron et al., 1995). For example, in a study of older, community-dwelling adults, symptoms that were unmistakable signs of illness were unlikely to be attributed to stress, and seeking health care for these symptoms was little affected by life stresses. On the other hand, ambiguous symptoms were attributed to stress if they were experienced in the context of an ongoing life stressor. The heuristic is simple: Distinctive symptoms, on the one hand, are not direct consequences of stress and need health care depending upon their duration and severity. Ambiguous symptoms, on the other hand, when experienced in the context of an ongoing life stressor, are seen as likely signs of stress rather than signs of illness. But ambiguous symptoms led to care seeking only when the life stressor was of long duration, suggesting that older persons perceived longer term stress as a possible cause of illness.

The age–illness heuristic, like the stress–illness heuristic, can lead people to discount the significance of symptoms as they relate to illness. Attributing symptoms to age is common among the elderly (Kart, 1981; Prohaska, Keller, Leventhal, & Leventhal, 1987) and is considered a barrier to care seeking for symptoms and dysfunctions that are often readily treated (Ryan & Zerwic, 2003). Rate of change is likely linked to the age–illness heuristic. Rapidly appearing physical symptoms are more likely to encourage care seeking (Berkanovic, Telesky, & Reeder, 1981) than symptoms, signs (e.g., spinal curvature), and functions that take place over years rather than hours, days, or weeks. Symptoms that are very slow to change are more likely to be regarded as signs of aging. It is likely that age becomes a focus for somatic appraisal in younger people during major life transitions, such as the move from school to time-demanding desk jobs, which involve major reductions in time for physical activity. There may be critical differences, however, in the way older and younger persons use this heuristic. For example, Mr. X began to suspect that his back pains might be chronic, whereas a young person might be more likely to see such changes as temporary and remediable with conditioning exercises.

### Social Comparisons: Common Exposure, Prevalence, and Common Genes

Festinger (1954) posited that people compare themselves with similar others to form and confirm beliefs that they cannot validate by objective evidence. With respect to emotions, the hypothesis was translated as saying that people could understand and validate their emotional states by choosing to be with people who were in the same situation (Schachter & Singer, 1979). The translation was based on the assumption that emotional states comprise (1) a physiological response that is inherently ambiguous, with different emotions resting on a common or indistinguishably different autonomic response pattern; and (2) a cognitive "label" created by the observation of other people's emotional behavior. When translated yet another step to the health domain, the hypothesis suggested that patients about to undergo cardiac surgery would better understand their emotional states and feel less distressed if they were in hospital rooms with patients also waiting to be wheeled into surgery; being with similar others would allow them to share their feelings and reduce uncertainty about their emotions. This expectation was inconsistent, however, with Kulik and Mahler's (1987) findings; their data showed higher levels of emotional distress among patients randomly assigned to room with similar others who were also waiting to be taken to surgery than among patients rooming with others who had completed and were recovering from surgery. The reason for this difference was simple: Waiting with postsurgical, recovering patients was reassuring. Patients anticipating surgery could see people laughing and smiling after undergoing what they could imagine to be a painful and life-threatening assault from the surgeon's knife. In short, patients waiting for surgery feel a bit fearful; they know how they feel and are receptive to evidence that their fears may be unfounded. Time and place affect the meaning of the information obtained from a social comparison and, in this case, rooming with different others provides reassuring information.

The surgical study is but one example of many in which individuals look to the social setting to evaluate the magnitude and relevance of an environmentally caused health threat. It is clear that unpleasant symptoms lead to social comparisons, and studies are needed to examine how specific symptoms shape the causal search, how the search proceeds, and other aspects of the comparative process. Social comparisons are also used to evaluate vulnerabilities seen as part of one's internal physical/physiological structure. Using a tightly controlled laboratory paradigm, Jemmot, Ditto, and Croyle (1986) showed how social consensus affects the perceived severity of a presumed pancreatic disorder (see also Croyle & Jemmot, 1991). Participants received bogus positive or negative results on a test for vulnerability to this presumed pancreatic disorder. In some cases, the student participant getting risk results was the only one of five persons tested who was found to be at risk; in other cases, students were among three of five persons who were at risk. The participants who had company in the risk category were less distressed by the finding; high prevalence reduced feelings of threat. The perception of lower threat with high prevalence makes sense in a context in which the participants have never heard of the risk and have no reason to believe that the pancreatic disorder causes widespread hospitalization or disability. Prevalence might increase threat, however, if the test disclosed vulnerability to a serious, rapidly advancing infectious disease, such as it did during the recent outbreaks of severe acute respiratory syndrome (SARS) and avian flu.

Comparison of the self to others leads not only to emotional distress or reassurance but also to the development of imagery and prototype formation. The images that develop contribute to an individual's self-system. Self-images can serve as an important factor to guide behavior (Markus & Nurius, 1986). A new physical symptom, such as wheezing perceived as chronic asthma, can convert the view of a healthy somatic self to that of a severely compromised self (Leventhal, Hudson, & Robitaille, 1997). Familiarity with active, high-functioning asthmatic individuals, however, will likely decrease the likelihood of so massive a revision in self-image. For example, believing that one's behavior caused an illness can lead to images of a destructive, irresponsible self. Conversely, a stable self-image can influence the development of a new illness representation (i.e., "I am in good shape, so my behavior could not have caused this illness" or "I am responsible and health-conscious, and will therefore always take my medication").

As in the responsible-self example, self-images can affect how people treat their illnesses. This result might be especially true later in life, because health-relevant possible selves are prevalent images of self among older adults (Hooker & Kaus, 1994). Placing more value on health-related self-images tends to lead to better health behaviors, because stronger images will be more consciously enforced. Developing positive health-related imagery with regard to the self thus increases the likelihood of carrying out relevant treatment behaviors, and different positive images contribute to different behaviors; seeing the self as responsible and health-conscious leads to regular doctor visits and medication adherence. However, it should be noted that in some cases, negative self-images might promote health behaviors as well, if these images are future-oriented. Markus and Nurius (1986) discuss negative possible selves and their reactive ability to motivate good behaviors. A patient who holds images of the future self as frail and sick, in some cases, will carry out health behaviors as a response to fear of these images.

## CONSTRUCTION OF REPRESENTATIONS, HEALTH DECISIONS, AND HEALTH BEHAVIORS

How do the accumulated data on self-appraisal heuristics reviewed earlier relate to our two major objectives as health psychologists—the development of psychological theory and contribution to practice for improving health outcomes? We believe these objectives are intimately connected; theory can best develop when it serves the needs of practice, and practice can best be improved when it serves the need for the development of theory. The studies we have reviewed illustrate how clinical practice can provide multiple clues for the conceptualization and formulation of empirical studies describing the operation of the heuristics involved in the interpretation of somatic experience that lead to care seeking. Clinical experience and basic laboratory work have also identified the substance or common-sense meanings and representations that arise from these interpretive processes. The following sections describe the substance of representations, then briefly address how contextual factors of the self, the need for efficient optimization of function with age (Baltes & Baltes, 1990), and the social context of the medical care system affect the formation of common-sense representations of both disease and treatment.

### Building Common-Sense Representations

Internal somatic stimuli, functional changes, and external social and media messages can be starting points for constructing representations of illnesses and procedures for treatment and prevention of disease. And as our example of Mr. X has shown, the individual's prior illness and treatment history affect how representations are generated by a stimulus at a specific point in time; chest pain in a middle-aged male evokes different illness representations if he has a family history of coronary disease or a personal history of gastroesophageal reflux. The "same" or highly similar somatic stimuli have very different meaning in different life contexts.

## The Five Domains of Illness and Treatment Representations

Studies have identified five content domains for the representation of illnesses, which are generated with the ongoing processing of information that uses the heuristics previously discussed.

1. *Identity* refers to the the category, name or label, and the experience of symptoms, changes in function, and visible signs. The combination of abstract and concrete experiential features "defines" or identifies the disease.
2. *Control* refers to the the expectation that a specific disease can be cured or controlled by the body's own defenses and/or in conjunction with expert intervention, and the actual experience of the effects of these interventions on specific features (symptoms and/or test results) of disease.
3. *Time line* is the expected and/or perceived duration with respect to the onset and duration of an illness, both with and without effective treatment.
4. *Cause* reflects the perception of the single or complex set of events perceived to be responsible for disease onset.
5. *Consequences* are the set of expected and perceived physical/functional, personal, and social and economic factors impacted by the illness.

The Illness Perception Questionnaire, developed by Weinman and Horne (1996), provides a basic framework for the assessment of these content factors. Factors are represented at experiential and abstract levels. The bilevel content of the variables in each of these domains defines the "anatomy" of illness representations (Leventhal, Diefenbach, & Leventhal, 1992; Martin, Lemos, & Leventhal, 2001; see Figure 17.1). Although the bilevel feature of the domains is most clear for illness identity (label and symptoms), it applies to each domain. Thus, time lines are represented abstractly as clock and calendar time, and concretely as experienced or felt time; and consequences, as verbalized expectations of effects and as concrete images of disease impact. The bilevel feature of illness and treatment representations leads to separate, sometimes conflicting goals and discrepant criteria for self-evaluations of the effectiveness of self-management procedures, and it provides two routes for the initiation of the constructive process. Disjunctions between the abstract and experiential levels of representations are likely common, though this conclusion is based upon limited data. Studies of patients with hypertension show they treat it symptomatically and stop medication when symptoms disappear, even though symptoms are uncorrelated with blood pressure (Meyer et al., 1985). Examples of nonadherence to antidepressive medication provide a dramatic example of the

**Parallel Processing and the Cognitive Factors in the common-sense model**

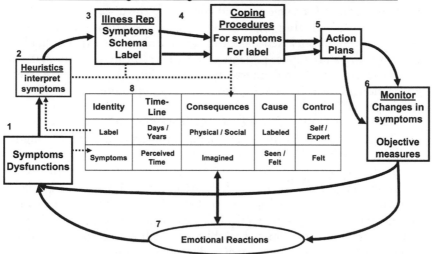

**FIGURE 17.1.** Symptoms, functional changes, and information from external sources (1) are interpreted and given meaning by heuristics (2) or rules for asking and answering simple questions. Operating automatically or consciously, heuristics activate schemas that give rise to representations (3 and 8) of a current or potential illness. Procedures (4) for management and plans (5) for implementing procedures come into play, and the outcomes are appraised (6) against expected changes. Representations of illness (3 and 8) and treatment (4) are both experiential (8: experience of symptoms; experience of time; experience of causes; imagined consequences; felt effects of treatment; etc.) and abstract (label for disease; abstract temporal expectations; conceptual label for treatment). The components comprise a bilevel control system. Actions taken for control of symptoms may differ from and be compatible or incompatible with the actions needed for control of illness. Emotional reactions (7: fear, depression, anger, etc.) are elicited by the representation of the threat and the experienced and objective effects of the procedures for avoiding and controlling the illness.

role of experiential factors in the perception of treatment time line. Although patients are told that several weeks of treatment are needed to improve mood, non-mood-related side effects of antidepressants, such as dry mouth, are felt soon after the initiation of treatment; experience contradicts the assertion that it takes weeks for the drugs to work. The experiential message is that the drugs are working and not producing the desired outcomes.

Representations are evoked through the concrete or experiential route and through the abstract or categorical route. When representations come about as a result of pains, rashes, headaches, lumps, injuries, or functional changes, they are "disturbances" that bring into play the interpretive, heuristic processes discussed earlier (Martin et al., 2001). The representations activate procedures for exploring and controlling the disturbance, and generate criteria for evaluating these actions (Carver & Scheier, 1982; Scheier & Carver, 2003). Because self-diagnostic appraisals at the experiential level are intrinsically ambiguous, patients test a variety of hypotheses that may be counterfactual to feared interpretations, asking, "Is this severe, seemingly unending headache due to a stroke or a brain tumor, or is it simply a stress response?"

Failure to generate a working representation of an illness and its treatment can arise when there is difficulty in interpreting and linking somatic symptoms to a label. Connecting the experiential and abstract levels adds depth to the representation. For example, symptoms of breathlessness and fatigue with congestive heart failure (CHF). The absence of depth can prevent the development of *breadth,* the construction of more complete representations of CHF, its cause (fluid intake is causing the symptoms of CHF), time lines (breathlessness will worsen over time), and consequences (life-threatening cardiac decompensation). When depth and breadth are lacking, there is likely no connection between the illness representation and the representation of treatment. It makes little sense to control fluid intake and use diuretics to avoid the consequences of CHF in the absence of a model of CHF that links the low-level symptoms of fatigue, edema, and mild breathlessness to the label (absence of depth), and the lack of perceived time line for worsening of symptoms with excessive fluid intake and failure to use diuretics (absence of breadth; Horowitz et al., 2004). By connecting these always present symptoms to the label, patients perceive their condition as chronic and their symptoms as cues that allow them to monitor their condition and act to avoid life-threatening episodes of cardiac decompensation. The abstract level, a time line for CHF, provides the temporal integration of otherwise discrete, concrete experiences.

We believe that the construction of illness representations will differ if the process is initiated at the abstract level by diagnostic labeling. For example, unexpected receipt of a cancer diagnosis has been described as equivalent to "a blow on the head" (Brody & Kleban, 1983), suggesting a more powerful emotional reaction than is likely when the diagnosis is preceded by days or weeks of self-appraisal in response to suspicious symptoms. It also is likely that diagnostic labeling will evoke more complete representations when individuals have a wealth of personal knowledge from either direct experience and observations of others, or media exposure, and that richly informed models may be more resistant to information from medical practitioners. We can generate hypotheses with respect to how contextual factors, specifically, the individual's sense of self and his or her medical contacts, affect how information is processed, and how representations of illnesses and treatments are generated.

## Aging Self and Social Context as Moderators of Health Decisions and Actions

All self-regulation models postulate that behavior is affected by factors at both the individual level and the social context. Some models posit additive relationships among these factors, indicating that contextual factors, such as social norms, have independent effects on behavior, in addition to the effects of individual beliefs (Ajzen & Fishbein, 1980). Self-regulation models, both the common-sense model of self-regulation and social learning models, also propose specific pathways to behavior, in which contextual factors exert their influence through representations of illness and treatment, and procedures for self-management. The common-sense model specifies pathways in which images of the self, contacts with medical practitioners, and familial and cultural beliefs shape, and are shaped by, disease and treatment representation, and management (Leventhal, Idler, & Leventhal, 1999). This bidirectional perspective is not fully captured when contextual variables are conceptualized as stable factors, with influence flowing from the social context to the individual or from the individual to disease- and treatment-specific beliefs (Christensen, Ehlers, Raichle, Bertolatus, & Lawton, 2000). A bidirectional view of the self-regulation process does not assume that the extent or rate of influence is similar in each direction; the effect of context on individual beliefs may be more extensive and occur more rapidly than influences from the individual to the context.

There are times when contextual- and individual-level factors appear to have separate, additive impacts on behavior, and times when the two sets of factors act in concert. For example, one of the older CHF patients interviewed by Horowitz et al. (2004) was both severely cognitively impaired and adherent to treatment. She was adherent because her cardiologist son-in-law called daily and reminded her to take her medication. By contrast Mr. X's appointment to seek care for his severe back and neck pains was triggered by his wife, urging him to make an appointment with an orthopedic specialist. One might interpret Mrs. X's action as a form of social influence independent of Mrs. X's representation of his condition. But in addition to giving "permission" to seek care (Zola, 1973), Mrs. X's urging confirmed an underlying feature of Mr. X's representation: that the condition posed potentially serious medical consequences. Thus, the social trigger was concordant with Mr. and Mrs. X's representation of the symptoms.

## Self as Context

Personality psychologists have expressed puzzlement over the finding that overall, measures of personality have at best very weak relationships to health outcomes in studies of participants age 65 years and older (Scheier & Bridges, 1995). These effects should not be overly surprising given the multitude of ways in which personality and self-concepts are conceptualized and measured, and given that individuals fill multiple roles and have different views of themselves depending on the situation and the time of life. Finding relationships between personality measures and health behaviors or outcomes requires conceptual clarity in the selection and assessment of views of the self that that are related to perceptions of age, and to health and illness threats (Leventhal, Patrick-Miller, Leventhal, & Burns, 1998). The *age–illness* heuristic serves as evidence that such factors exist and remain to be conceptualized.

The basic proposition underlying self-regulation theories—that biological and social factors affect how individuals experience and evaluate their physical status—suggests that experiential changes would affect self-perceptions, and that these self-perceptions would influence perceptions of vulnerability to specific health threats, shaping behavioral strategies for maintaining health. These perceptions and strategies should change over the lifespan. For example, in contrast to teenage perceptions of invulnerability (Hirschman, Leventhal, & Glynn, 1984), older individuals are likely to experience somatic changes as signs of health risk. These changes, including reductions in energy to engage in vigorous activities, the slowing of recovery from acute illnesses, and changes in physical appearance, create an awareness of a self that is living on increasingly limited resources. A question that arises is whether these changes in the perception of self at health risk alter the strategies used to maintain health and reduce risk?

Thousands of study participants have been asked the following simple question: "Would you say your health is excellent, very good, good, fair or poor?" These simple self-assessments of health (SAHs) have an impressive record in predicting future mortality and morbidity, even after controlling for respondents' age, gender, and known medical conditions. The predictions hold over relatively short time frames in samples of severely ill persons, and over years and decades in representative community samples (Idler & Benyamini, 1997). It is clear that people are sensitive to and able to make accurate judgments of their health status. Given the objective increase in chronic illness over the lifespan, one might expect to see reductions in SAHs and increased perceptions of disease risk with advancing age. However, data show relatively little change in average SAH ratings from year to year among individuals in the 8th and 9th decades of life, suggesting that SAHs are relatively insensitive to objective, age-related reductions in biological function and increases in chronic conditions; the deaths of individuals with poor ratings and shifts in the standards for judgment based on survivors within an age cohort may account for this stability. However, SAH ratings do decline over the years for some individuals among the older population. SAHs are also associated with care seeking and symptom reporting for chronic illness (Mora et al., 2002), which suggests that they can affect illness representation, likely in the severity domain. Not only SAHs but also perceived vulnerability to illness often do not increase with age (Wilcox & Stefanick, 1999).

In summary, there is relatively little evidence that aging is related to declining self-assessments of health or increasing perception of vulnerability or risk of illness. In addition, there is limited evidence showing that self-assessments are related to how individuals represent health or disease and the procedures that they engage in to stay healthy and cope with specific disease threats. These somewhat surprising conclusions reflect current data, most of which have assessed self-related perceptions and beliefs at an abstract level, examining how most reasonably healthy, aging, older persons in the United States and Western Europe think, talk, and report about themselves.

## Self-Efficacy and Self-Regulation Strategies

There is abundant evidence that older adults are highly attentive to bodily symptoms and function (Brody & Kleban, 1983), and that health maintenance and illness management are integral to the ongoing life experience of older persons. Moreover, health and its promotion, illness prevention and treatment, symptom management and encounters with the health care system are major topics of conversation for older adults, reducing perhaps the degree to which personality factors affect health behaviors. Personal characteristics relate to the processes regulating health behaviors if they influence common-sense problem solving and the exchange of health relevant information in social contexts. The concept of self-efficacy seems to meet these criteria; it can be assessed with regard to both health behaviors and social exchanges regarding these behaviors. Assessed as confidence in one's ability to perform specific behaviors, such as measuring blood sugar or using a peak flow meter, response-specific self-efficacy (Bandura, 1991) has proven to be an effective predictor of behavioral management, and sometimes health outcomes, in patients with diabetes (Krichbaum, Aarestad, & Buethe, 2003). Investigators have also interpreted and assessed self-efficacy beliefs as patients' confidence for achieving a specific outcome, such as "Can you do what you need to do to avoid emergency care for your congestive heart condition?" Assessed in this way, self-efficacy is conceptualized as belief in one's ability to reach a goal rather than to take a specific action. When defined in terms of goal attainment, self-efficacy is most likely a measure of the coherence of the individual's problem-solving skills rather than his or her confidence in ability to perform any particular act. The more broadly it is assessed, the more difficult it is to identify the specific factors responsible for high or low levels of self-efficacy, reducing the utility of the measure for developing interventions to enhance treatment adherence.

Although self-efficacy typically has a positive relationship to health outcomes, the relationship can also be negative. On the one hand, an older patient with adult-onset diabetes who is high in self-efficacy is likely to acquire skills to monitor blood sugar levels, adjust diet and use insulin, and maintain good blood sugar regulation over long periods of time (Piette, Weinberger, & McPhee, 2000). On the other hand, among patients who perceive diabetes as chronic and misunderstand its causes, such as its link to excessive weight (Jayne & Rankin, 2001), individuals high in self-efficacy may engage in behaviors that are ineffective or harmful for disease management. Similarly, patients with CHF may be confident that they can weigh themselves daily, yet not do so because they fail to see a connection between CHF and their experience of fatigue and breathlessness. Because they do not link the symptoms to the abstract label, CHF, they do not perceive that both the gain in weight and breathlessness are caused by the retention of fluid in the lungs and legs, due to the weakened pumping action of the heart (Horowitz et al., 2002). Thus, they neither weigh themselves nor take the diuretics to rid themselves of excess fluid.

Another approach to the assessment of individual differences has focused on age-related strategies for controlling one's environment. Baltes and Baltes (1990) hypothesized that strategies to conserve and to compensate for reduction of resources, and to appropriately deploy available resources are critical for successful aging. These strategies appear to motivate the use of health care (Leventhal & Crouch, 1997). For example, older adults seek medical care more swiftly and are less likely to delay than middle-aged study participants when experiencing symptoms interpreted as possible indicators of cancer or cardiac disease (Leventhal, Easterling, Leventhal, & Cameron, 1995). By reacting rapidly and giving responsibility for diagnosis and treatment to a medical practitioner, older adults *avert risk* while *conserving* mental and physical energy that would otherwise be spent ruminating about potential health catastrophes. The desire to conserve resources also reduces behavioral efforts to replace activities lost in response to a severe health episode. Giving up vigorous activities in the face of a severe illness episode is often primarily due to the severity of the illness. In contrast, finding replacements for abandoned activities, such as walking instead of jogging, is strongly and positively related to social-psychological factors such as optimism and social pressures, but negatively related to the perceived need to *conserve* resources (Duke, Brownlee, Leventhal, & Leventhal, 2002). Strategies of *conservation* and disengagement (Scheier & Carver, 2003) are common in the later years of life (Baltes & Baltes, 1990), but so too is their opposite, the belief that failure to use a skill ensures its deterioration (i.e., "Use it or lose it"). Either of these strategies can become a lifestyle, and excesses in either direction can be dangerous to health. Finding a balance between conservation and use is likely critical for sustaining physical vigor and cognitive competence.

With but one exception, the individual differences in self-perception and action discussed earlier do not appear to be related to specific personality traits, such as those assessed in the "Big Five"; the exception appears to be the factor of conscientiousness (Digman, 1989; Friedman & Martin, Chapter 9, this volume), which is a predictor of a "hard" health outcome, longevity (Roberts, Walton, & Bogg, 2005). A meta-analysis of the components comprising this factor found that the factor with the strongest influence on health was "conventionality," defined as self-reported adherence to social norms (Roberts, Chernyshenko, Stark, & Goldberg, 2005). The role of conscientiousness and conventionality in promoting conformity to medical recommendations for a healthy lifestyle may be more important in older adults, because conscientiousness increases with age (Dudek & Hall, 1991). This factor may have played a role in Mr. X's behavior; he listened to medical experts, family members who supported them, and adhered to his prescribed physical therapy. A conscientious person might be more willing to listen and to invest the effort needed to understand his medical condition better and, therefore, do a better job in using, implementing, and monitoring the efficacy of medically recommended procedures.

## Social and Cultural Context

Improvements in socioeconomic conditions, such as increased national wealth, and improved environmental hygiene and nutrition, were responsible for major improvements in population health well before the invention and widespread use of vaccination and antibiotic treatments. These societal improvements changed the top 10 causes of mortality from infectious diseases to chronic illnesses (McKinlay & McKinlay, 1986). There was a clear social class gradient for mortality both before and after this change; those who are most well off had, and still have, the best health and longest life expectancy (Hertzman, Power, Matthews, & Manor, 2001). We do not know the extent to which cultural, environmental, and socioeconomic factors altered self-management practices, including interpretation of symptoms and strategies for health maintenance and disease prevention, nor do we know whether self-management practices contributed both to the differences across nations and the social class gradient within nations, or whether these differences can be attributed exclusively to limitations in resources for creating healthy environments.

### Common-Sense Models: A Determinant of National and Class Differences?

The anthropological literature contains numerous examples of cultural and social influences on self-management processes that may account for some portion of social class differences in health. The examples cover the detection and labeling of symptoms, decisions to seek medical care, the use of traditional versus Western trained practitioners, and decisions to make lifestyle changes for illness management. The impact of cultural factors is most clearly articulated in anthropological studies of "folk illnesses"—explanatory illness models that differ from biomedical models of the same diseases (Chrisman & Kleinman, 1983). For example, *empacho*, a potentially life-threatening, gastrointestinal disorder *identified* by symptoms of stomachache, bloated stomach, cramps, and lack of appetite, is perceived by individuals in some Hispanic communities to be caused by food getting stuck in the stomach or intestines (Weller, Pachter, Trotter, & Baer, 1993, p. 121). The *location* heuristic combined with a mechanical, causal model encourages treatments to dislodge the obstruction, such as herbal teas, massage, rolling an egg on the stomach. Common-sense models define *empacho* by its surface qualities and not by its underlying bacterial or viral cause.

People appear to use medical and folk treatments in parallel, which is not problematic as long as the two have no serious interactions. Parallel use is widespread in industrialized, Western culture, where it was labeled initially as alternative or complementary medicine. The use of complementary medicine is common among well-educated individuals managing life-threatening chronic conditions (e.g., metastatic cancer; Cassileth, Lusk, Strouse, & Bodenheimer, 1984). The majority of studies on the use of complementary medicine in Western countries report on prevalence of use in patients with different chronic illnesses and do not examine the mental models driving complementary use. In many cases, however, even dissimilar cultures appear to have similar folk models and alternative treatments. Folk models are important not only because these practices can encourage practices that are ineffective for improving health but they also can create barriers to communication between physicians and patients, making it increasingly difficult for practitioners who do not understand these common-sense models to explain and justify their medical recommendations.

### Can Practitioner Behavior Shape Invalid Common-Sense Models?

Anecdotal observation suggests that many practitioners inadvertently do and say things that encourage the development of biologically incorrect common-sense models. For example, recording blood pressure is typically one of the first procedures in medical encounters. It is not unusual for these readings to be elevated, in which case the practitioner will likely suggest a second reading and observe somewhat lower numbers. This action is consistent with the commonly held view that stress is the main cause of hypertension. If practitioners reinforce this causal view in patients whose resting pressures are in fact elevated, these patients may believe it entirely correct to stop their antihypertensive medication when they are on holiday and truly unstressed. Intensive interviews revealing differences between patients' and practitioners' representation of health threats and treatments are often conducted with ethnic minorities, likely creating the false impression that education is responsible for these differences. Similar differences occur, however, for highly educated patients, as seen in Mr. X's experience with his neck and back pains.

The severity of Mr. X's back and neck pains led him to seek an orthopedic consultation. During the discussion following the physical examination, the orthopedist indicated that arthritic changes in the vertebral column and narrowing of the openings were causing irritation of the nerves. While viewing the X-rays of the afflicted area, he commented, "You have to be careful and take it easy." "Be careful and take it easy," in the framework of the uneven accumulation of bone, narrowed openings, and irritated nerves was read by "common-sense" as a grim warning that excessive motion could cut nerves, leading to crippling, and not just increased irritation and pain.

## CONCLUSION: IMPLICATIONS FOR MEDICAL TREATMENT AND FURTHER RESEARCH

Our review of the construction of common-sense representations of illness and treatment has focused on the heuristics used for interpreting somatic changes, the content domains of common-sense models, how they are structured, and how the process of construction is affected by self-perceptions and social influence. We have not discussed how elevations in threat-related fear, depression, and generalized emotional distress are affected by, and in turn affect, common-sense representations, views of the self, and perceptions of personal vulnerability to harm. Emotions play a significant role in care seeking and other aspects of self-management (DiMatteo, Lepper, & Chroghan, 2000). Consistent with our approach to cognitive heuristics, and illness and treatment representations, we propose that understanding the pathways from emotional reactions to self-management require the detailed differentiation of emotion concepts beyond trait anxiety, or trait negative affect, to affect states. Along with Gruenewald and Kemeny (Chapter 6, this volume), we propose that specific combinations or assemblies of emotion and cognition must be conceptualized to understand and describe when and how emotion and cognition interact to affect health actions. For example, the pathway from generalized affective traits to emotional and behavioral responses to illness episodes is mediated by combinations of emotion and health-specific cognitions, such as health anxiety (Maher, Mora, Leventhal, in press), and by individual history. Parallel processing of affect and cognition (Leventhal, 1970) is also clearly visible in health behaviors. Bunde and Martin (2006) found the effects of cognitive appraisals and depression on seeking care after myocardial infarction were independent of one another.

Finally, we propose that the processes involved in the common-sense construction of illnesses and treatments, and the relationships among cognitive and emotional reactions will lead to revisions in how behavioral treatments are conducted within medical settings. For example, depression and less severe forms of emotional distress are currently viewed as comorbid conditions when experienced by patients managing chronic illness, and patients receive relatively little explanation as to the interconnectedness of the "disorders." The common-sense perspective suggests that patients are likely to perceive their emotional distress as a direct product of their physical ailments rather than seeing themselves as having a second disorder. Under these conditions, referrals for psychological treatment are likely to be perceived as problematic and unnecessary, and some recommended psychological treatments, such as behavioral activation, may appear incompatible. Patients need to perceive medical and behavioral treatments as an integrated package, and to be reassured that both medical and behavioral practitioners will keep them abreast of their progress.

The integration of treatment for managing chronic illness and emotional distress requires that physicians have at least a rudimentary understanding of patients' common-sense interpretations of disease and treatment. Patients with asthma have little reason to use inhaled corticosteroids to control asthma if they perceive and believe they have asthma only when having attacks, and if they perceive that these medications are equivalent to the steroids endangering the lives of athletes. Viewing the patient's model is in many cases a less complex task than making accurate diagnoses and prescribing standard of care treatment. Addressing specific misperception, such as those we just mentioned, and dealing with broader examples, such as the tendency to view chronic conditions as unmanageable, are integral parts of clinical practice. Modern hygiene, diet, medicine, and physical therapies have provided the tools to manage the many chronic conditions that accompany the gift of a longer life.

## REFERENCES

Ajzen, I., & Fishbein, M. (1980). *Understanding attitudes and predicting social behavior.* Englewood Cliffs, NJ: Prentice-Hall.

Baltes, P. B., & Baltes, M. M. (1990). Psychological perspectives on successful aging: The model of selective optimization with compensation. In P. B. Baltes & M. M. Baltes (Eds.), *Successful aging: Perspectives from the behavioral sciences* (pp. 1–34). New York: Cambridge University Press.

Bandura, A. (1991). Self-efficacy mechanism in physiological activation and health-promoting behavior. In J. Madden, IV (Ed.), *Neurobiology of learning, emotion and affect* (pp. 229–270). New York: Raven.

Baumann, L., & Leventhal, H. (1985). I can tell when my blood pressure is up, can't I? *Health Psychology, 4,* 203–218.

Baumann, L. J., Cameron, L. D., Zimmerman, R. S., & Leventhal, H. (1989). Illness representations and matching labels with symptoms. *Health Psychology, 8*, 449–469.

Berkanovic, E., Telesky, C., & Reeder, S. (1981). Structural and social psychological factors in the decision to seek medical care for symptoms. *Medical Care, 19*, 693–709.

Bickell, N., Rojas, M., Anderson, R., & Leventhal, H. (2004). Why does it seem to take so long for patients to get to needed care? *Journal of General Internal Medicine, 19*(Supple. 1), 239.

Brody, E. M., & Kleban, M. H. (1983). Day-to-day mental and physical health symptoms of older people: A report on health logs. *Gerontologist, 23*, 75–85.

Bunde, J., & Martin, R. (2006). Depression and pre-hospital delay in the context of myocardial infarction. *Psychosomatic Medicine, 68*, 51–57.

Cameron, L., Leventhal, E. A., & Leventhal, H. (1995). Seeking medical care in response to symptoms and life stress. *Psychosomatic Medicine, 57*, 37–47.

Carver, C. S., & Scheier, M. F. (1982). Outcome expectancy, locus of attribution for expectancy, and self-directed attention as determinants of evaluations and performance. *Journal of Experimental Social Psychology, 18*, 184–200.

Cassileth, B. R., Lusk, E. J., Strouse, T. B., & Bodenheimer, B. J. (1984). Contemporary unorthodox treatments in cancer medicine. *Annals of Internal Medicine, 101*, 105–112.

Chrisman, N. J., & Kleinman, A. (1983). Popular health care, social networks, and cultural meanings: The orientation of medical anthoropology. In D. Mechanic (Ed.), *Handbook of health, health care, and the health professions* (pp. 569–590). NY: Free Press.

Christensen, A. J., Ehlers, S. L., Raichle, K. A., Bertolatus, J. A., & Lawton, W. J. (2000). Predicting change in depression following renal transplantation: Effect of patient coping preferences. *Health Psychology, 19*, 348–353.

Croyle, R. T., & Jemmott, J. B. (2001). Psychological reactions to risk factor testing. In J. A. Skelton & R. T. Croyle (Eds.), *Mental representations in health and illness* (pp. 85–107). New York: Springer-Verlag.

Damasio, A. (1999). *The feeling of what happens: Body and emotion in the making of consciousness.* New York: Harcourt Brace.

Digman, J. M. (1989). Five robust trait dimensions: Development, stability, and utility. *Journal of Personality, 57*(2), 195–214.

DiMatteo, M. R., Lepper, H. S., & Chroghan, T. W. (2000). Depression is a risk factor for noncompliance with medical treatment: Meta-analysis of the effects of anxiety and depression on patient adherence. *Archives of Internal Medicine, 160*, 2101–2107.

Dudek, S. Z., & Hall, W. B. (1991). Personality consistency: Eminent architects 25 years later. *Creativity Research Journal, 4*(3), 213–231.

Duke, J., Brownlee, S., Leventhal, E. A., & Leventhal, H. (2002). Giving up and replacing activities in response to illness. *Journals of Gerontology: Psychological Sciences and Social Sciences, Series B, 57*, 367–376.

Evangelista, L. S., Dracup, K., & Doering, L. V. (2000). Treatment-seeking delays in heart failure patients. *Journal of Heart and Lung Transplantation, 19*(10), 932–938.

Festinger, L. (1954). A theory of social comparison processes. *Human Relations, 7*, 183–201.

Finnegan, J. R., Jr., Meischke, H., Zapka, J. G., Leviton, L., Meshack, A., Benjamin-Garner, R., et al. (2000). Patient delay in seeking care for heart attack symptoms: Findings from focus groups conducted in five U.S. regions. *Preventive Medicine, 31*(3), 205–213.

Hertzman, C., Power, C., Matthews, S., & Manor, O. (2001). Using an interactive framework of society and lifecourse to explain self-rated health in early adulthood. *Social Science and Medicine, 53*, 1575–1585.

Hirschman, R., Leventhal, H., & Glynn, K. (1984). The development of smoking behavior: Conceptualization and supportive cross-sectional survey data. *Journal of Applied Social Psychology, 14*, 184–206.

Hooker, K., & Kaus, C. R. (1994). Health-related possible selves in young and middle adulthood. *Psychology and Aging, 9*, 126–133.

Horowitz, C., Rein, S., & Leventhal, H. (2004). Challenges to effective self-management of heart-failure: A grounded theory approach. *Social Science and Medicine, 58*, 631–643.

Horowitz, M., O'Donovan, D., Jones, K. L., Feinle, C., Rayner, C. K., & Sarnsom, M. (2002). Gastric emptying in diabetes: Clinical significance and treatment. *Diabetic Medicine, 19*, 177–194.

Idler, E. L., & Benyamini, Y. (1997). Self-rated health and mortality: A review of twenty-seven community studies. *Journal of Health and Social Behavior, 38*, 21–37.

Institute of Medicine. (1999). *To err is human: Building a safer health system.* Washington, DC: National Academies Press.

Jayne, R. L., & Rankin, S. H. (2001). Application of Leventhal's self-regulation model to Chinese immigrants with Type 2 diabetes. *Journal of Nursing Scholarship, 33*, 53–59.

Jemmott, J. B., Ditto, P. H., & Croyle, R. T. (1986). Judging health status: Effects of perceived prevalence an dpersonal relevance. *Journal of Personality and Social Psychology, 50*(5), 899–905.

Kart, C. (1981). Experiencing symptoms: Attribution and misattribution of illness among the aged. In M. Haug & M. P. Lawton (Eds.), *Elderly patients and their doctors* (pp. 70–78). New York: Springer.

Krichbaum, K., Aarestad, V., & Buethe, M. (2003). Exploring the connection between self-efficacy and effective diabetes self-management. *Diabetes Educator, 29*(4), 653–662.

Kulik, J. A., & Mahler, H. I. (1987). Effects of preoperative roommate assignment on preoperative anxiety and recovery from coronary-bypass surgery. *Health Psychology, 6*(6), 525–543.

Leventhal, E. A., & Crouch, M. (1997). Are there differences in perceptions of illness across the lifespan? In K. J. Petrie & J. A. Weinman (Eds.), *Perceptions of health and illness: Current research and applications* (pp. 77–102). Amsterdam, the Netherlands: Harwood Academic.

Leventhal, E. A., Easterling, D., Leventhal, H., & Cameron, L. (1995). Conservation of energy, uncertainty reduction and swift utilization of medical care among the elderly: Study II. *Medical Care, 33*, 988–1000.

Leventhal, H. (1970). Findings and theory in the study of fear communications. *Advances in Experimental Social Psychology, 5*, 119–186.

Leventhal, H., Cameron, L., Leventhal, E. A., & Ozakinci, G. (2005). Do messages from your body, your friends, your doctor, or the media shape your health behavior? In T. C. Brock & M. C. Green (Eds.), *Persuasion: Psychological insights and perspectives* (2nd ed., pp. 195–223). Thousand Oaks, CA: Sage.

Leventhal, H., Diefenbach, M., & Leventhal, E. A. (1992). Illness cognition: Using common sense to understand treatment adherence and affect cognition interactions. *Cognitive Therapy and Research, 16*(2), 143–163.

Leventhal, H., Hudson, S., & Robitaille, C. (1997). Social comparison and health: A process model. In B. P. Buunk & F. X. Gibbons (Eds.), *Health, coping, and well-being: Perspectives from social comparison theory* (pp. 411–432). Mahwah, NJ: Erlbaum.

Leventhal, H., Idler, E. L., & Leventhal, E. A. (1999). The impact of chronic illness on the self system. In R. J. Contrada & R. D. Ashmore (Eds.), *Self, social identity, and physical health: Interdisciplinary explorations rutgers series on self and social identity* (Vol 2, pp. 185–208). London: Oxford University Press.

Leventhal, H., Patrick-Miller, L., Leventhal, E. A., & Burns, E. A. (1998). Does stress–emotion cause illness in elderly people? In L. Shaie (Ed.), *Annual review of gerontology and geriatrics: Focus on emotion and adult development* (Vol. 17, pp. 138–184). New York: Springer.

Maher, M. J., Mora, P. A., & Leventhal, H. (in press). Depression as a predictor of perceived social support and demand: A componential approach using a prospective sample of older adults. *Emotion.*

Markus, H., & Nurius, P. (1986). Possible selves. *American Psychologist, 41*(9), 954–969.

Martin, R., Lemos, K., & Leventhal, H. (2001). The psychology of physical symptoms and illness behavior. In J. G. Asmundson, S. Taylor, & B. J. Cox (Eds.), *Health anxiety* (pp. 22–45). New York: Wiley.

Martin, R., & Leventhal, H. (2004). Symptom perception and health care-seeking behavior. In J. M. Raczynski & L. C. Leviton (Eds.), *Handbook of clinical health psychology: Vol. 2. Disorders of behavior and health* (pp. 299–328). Washington, DC: American Psychological Association.

McKinlay, J. B., & McKinlay, S. M. (1986). Medical measures and the decline of mortality. In P. Conrad & R. Kern (Eds.), *The sociology of health and illness: Critical perspectives* (pp. 10–23). New York: St. Martin's Press.

Meyer, D., Leventhal, H., & Gutmann, M. (1985). Common-sense models of illness: The example of hypertension. *Health Psychology, 4*, 115–135.

Mora, P., Robitaille, C., Leventhal, H., Swigar, M., & Leventhal, E. A. (2002). Trait negative affect relates to prior weak symptoms, but not to reports of illness episodes, illness symptoms and care seeking. *Psychosomatic Medicine, 64*, 436–449.

Phillips, L. S., Branch, W. T., Cook, C. B., Doyle, J. P., El-Kebbi, I. M., Gallina, D. L., et al. (2001). Clinical inertia. *Annals of Internal Medicine, 135*(9), 825–834.

Piette, J. D., Weinberger, M., & McPhee, S. J. (2000). The effect of automated calls with telephone nurse follow-up on patient-centered outcomes of diabetes care: A randomized, controlled trial. *Medical Care, 38*, 218–230.

Prohaska, T., Keller, M. L., Leventhal, E. A., & Leventhal, H. (1987). Impact of symptoms and aging attribution on emotions and coping. *Health Psychology, 6*, 495–514.

Roberts, B. W., Chernyshenko, O. S., Stark, S., & Goldberg, L. R. (2005). The structure of conscientiousness: An empirical investigation based on seven major personality questionnaires. *Personnel Psychology, 58*(1), 103–139.

Roberts, B. W., Walton, K. E., & Bogg, T. (2005). Conscientiousness and health across the life course. *Review of General Psychology, 9*(2), 156–168.

Ryan, C. J., & Zerwic, J. J. (2003). Perceptions of symptoms of myocardial infarction related to health care seeking behaviors in the elderly. *Journal of Cardiovascular Nursing, 18*(3), 184–196.

Safer, M. A., Tharps, Q. J., Jackson, T. C., & Leventhal, H. (1979). Determinants of three stages of delay in seeking care at a medical clinic. *Medical Care, 17,* 11–29.

Schachter, S., & Singer, J. (1979). Comments on the Maslach and Marshall-Zimbardo experiments. *Journal of Personality and Social Psychology, 37*(6), 989–995.

Scheier, M. F., & Bridges, M. (1995). Person variables and health: Personality predispositions and acute psychological states as shared determinants for disease. *Psychosomatic Medicine, 57,* 255–268.

Scheier, M. F., & Carver, C. S. (2003). Goals and confidence as self-regulatory elements underlying health and illness behavior. In L. D. C. H. Leventhal & L. D. Cameron (Eds.), *The self-regulation of health and illness behaviour* (pp. 17–41). London: Routledge/Taylor & Francis.

Wang, Z., Wu, Y., Zhao, L., Li, Y., Yang, J., Zhou, B., et al. (2004). Trends in prevalence, awareness, treatment and control of hypertension in the middle-aged population of China, 1992–1998. *Hypertension Research, 27*(10), 703–709.

Weinman, J., & Horne, R. (1996). The Illness Perception Questionnaire: A new method for assessing the cognitive representation of illness. *Psychology and Health, 11,* 431–445.

Weller, S. C., Pachter, L. M., Trotter, R. T., & Baer, R. D. (1993). *Empacho* in four Latino groups: A study of intra- and inter-cultural variation in beliefs. *Medical Anthropology, 15*(2), 109–136.

Wilcox, S., & Stefanick, M. L. (1999). Knowledge and perceived risk of major diseases in middle-aged and older women. *Health Psychology, 18*(4), 346–353.

Zola, I. K. (1973). Pathways to the doctor: From person to patient. *Social Science and Medicine, 7,* 677–689.

# CHAPTER 18

# The Role of Clinical Health Geropsychology in the Health Care of Older Adults

SARA HONN QUALLS *and* CHARLES C. BENIGHT

The role for psychologists to help chronically ill patients maximize their well-being is expanding, with mounting empirical evidence for effective interventions and growing opportunities for reimbursement. Clinicians can now implement effective interventions based on available empirical data from health psychology, behavioral medicine, and the broader field of clinical psychology. Although controversies surround the implementation of evidence based practice (Chambless & Ollendick, 2001; Persons & Silberschatz, 1998), psychological interventions designed to improve health have received growing attention in the American Psychological Association Health Psychology Division (38), the Society for Behavioral Medicine, and the American Psychosomatic Society, as is evident even from their websites. To date, no formal recommendations have been published to provide practitioners with guidelines for evidence-based practice in this area, although efforts to produce guidelines are currently under way.

Given the lack of formalized recommendations, we have reviewed the literature, focusing on the common chronic illnesses that practitioners are most likely to face with older adults, and on the mental and family challenges commonly encountered in health care settings. We have also attempted to gather empirical investigations that focus directly on older adults and chronic illness management. Although our review is not exhaustive, it does provide a base in which practitioners can anchor their work with older adults suffering from chronic illness. In this review, we present an overview of the types of interventions utilized for different groups of chronically ill patients (e.g., general chronic illness interventions, treatments for diabetes), followed by empirical evidence for these different interventions in general and in older adults specifically. We then discuss the impact of the new Medicare Health and Behavior Codes on chronic illness psychological interventions. Finally, we summarize literature on the treatment of mental disorders in chronic illness populations, and on interventions that target family members of patients in health care settings.

Intervention research on chronic illnesses has taken two primary approaches: (1) a broad-based focus on overall self-management of chronic illness across disease types, or (2) specific interventions targeted toward different disease groups. The more general intervention approaches are reviewed first, followed by a select review of the different disease groups. Specific intervention studies that have targeted older adults' adjustment and management of a chronic disease are offered when available.

## CHARACTERISTICS OF INTERVENTION RESEARCH TARGETING CHRONIC ILLNESS

Any chronic illness can challenge management of the disease progression, critical physical limitations and losses, and fear of death, as well as profoundly affect quality of life. Patients must gain important behavioral and emotional self-regulatory skills to optimize their level of functioning and quality of life. Most interventions for chronic disease management have utilized psychoeducational approaches combined with cognitive-behavioral strategies (Lorig, 1995). These programs attempt to assist patients in gaining greater knowledge about their disease process, as well as skills to improve communication with health providers, pain management, positive health behaviors, and ability to reduce negative health habits.

## GENERAL CHRONIC DISEASE INTERVENTIONS

Research on self-management training for people with chronic disease has shown promise for assisting patients in general (Lorig et al., 1999; Lorig, Ritter, et al., 2001; Lorig, Sobel, Ritter, Laurent, & Hobbs, 2001) and chronically ill older adults specifically (Ersek, Turner, McCurry, Gibbons, & Kraybill, 2003; Leveille et al., 1998; Rybarczyk, DeMarco, De La Cruz, Lapidos, & Fortner, 2001). The topics typically covered in these individual or group programs include disease education, general self-management principles, problem solving, exercise, pain management, psychological adjustment, nutrition, family and health provider communication, and goal setting. The interventions take place in a variety of settings (e.g., in the home, senior centers, community clinics) and are provided by various providers, including nurse practitioners, lay tutors, psychologists, and intervention teams including a physician, a nurse, and a pharmacist.

Randomized controlled trials show positive findings, with intervention groups demonstrating improvements in psychological and physical functioning maintained over extended follow-up periods (Ersek et al., 2003; Lorig et al., 1999; Lorig, Ritter, et al., 2001; Rybarczyk et al., 2001).

## INTERVENTIONS FOR COMMON CHRONIC DISEASE GROUPS

Interventions to assist patients with disease management and adjustment have also been tested for specific disease groups (e.g., diabetes, cancer, cardiovascular disease). For an excellent review of psychosocial and biobehavioral management of specific chronic illnesses, see Schneiderman, Antoni, Saab, and Ironson (2001). The most common diseases among older adults are reviewed next.

### Diabetes

The incidence of diabetes mellitus worldwide is exploding. The number of individuals with diabetes across the world is estimated to be 221 million by 2010, up from only 124 million in 1997 (Björk, 2001). Diabetes is a leading cause of disability among adults, with complications including blindness, kidney disease, coronary heart disease, stroke, peripheral neuropathy, amputation, and sexual dysfunction (Feifer & Tansman, 1999). Diabetes is typically divided into Type I and Type II diabetes. Type I, which accounts for a small percentage (approximately 10%) of cases, is the result of the inability of the pancreas to produce insulin and is typically diagnosed in childhood or young adulthood. Type II (approximately 90% of cases), which is usually diagnosed in adulthood, results from inability of the cells to utilize effectively the available insulin (i.e., insulin resistance), thereby increasing the glucose levels in circulation. Type II diabetes is often characterized as a disease of negative health lifestyle, including a poor diet (high in fat and carbohydrates) and lack of exercise, both leading to excessive weight. As such, most intervention programs for Type II diabetics target dietary intake, physical activity, or both.

#### Psychosocial Interventions

Psychosocial interventions to assist diabetics range from educational interventions that focus on increasing patients' knowledge about diabetes to more tailored behavioral modification interventions that attempt to change poor health habits and improve psychosocial functioning (Clark & Hampson,

2001; Delamater et al., 2001). Typical interventions focus on diet modification, increase in regular aerobic or resistant exercise, self-monitoring instruction, stress management, and disease education (Padgett, Mumford, Hynes, & Carter, 1988). Primary physical outcome assessments focus on glycosylated hemoglobin (HbA1c), lipid profiles (low-density lipoproteins [LDL], very-low-density lipoproteins), and body mass index. Psychosocial outcomes include improved emotional states (e.g., decreased depression or anxiety), reduced stress levels, and improvement in perceived quality of life.

Interventions have been completed in-hospital and in the physician's office. Programs have been offered through one-on-one counseling in groups and computer programs followed-up by telephone contact (Karlsen, Idsoe, Dirdal, Hanestad, & Bru, 2004; Glasgow et al., 1997). As with the other chronic illnesses already discussed, these interventions are provided by a host of different professionals, including physicians, nurses, psychologists, social workers, and pharmacists. No systematic investigation into the differential effectiveness of the providers has been completed.

## Non-Age-Specific Findings

In general, research has demonstrated that psychosocial interventions have been relatively effective in improving physical outcome, knowledge levels, emotional distress, and compliance (Padgett et al., 1988). The strength of these effects over time has been questioned. For example, short-term improvements in glycemic control can be achieved with very basic educational interventions, although the effects drop off after about a year (Sarkadi & Rosenqvist, 2004).

A more detailed, personalized computer-based program has shown some promise in reducing serum cholesterol levels and calories consumed from fat. This program focuses on behavioral issues related to dietary self-management and includes a follow-up phone call and videotape intervention. The benefits, identified in cholesterol levels and reduction of calories consumed from fat, were found at a 12-month follow-up assessment (Glasgow et al., 1997).

## Older-Adult-Specific Studies

Most of the research completed to date has included age-diverse samples and has not focused specifically on older adults with diabetes. Exceptions are reviewed below.

Interventions to assist older adults with Type II diabetes have demonstrated positive findings on a number of the critical outcomes for diabetes self-care, such as glycemic control, HbA1c, weight, and caloric intake (Castaneda et al., 2002; Glasgow et al., 1992; Miller, Edwards, Kissling, & Sanville, 2002). As with the other interventions, these programs have focused on a variety of biopsychosocial aspects of diabetic self-management, including dietary intake, exercise, problem solving, and self-efficacy.

A randomized controlled trial on older adults with Type II diabetes tested the effectiveness of a theory-based nutrition education program (Miller et al., 2002). Drawing on the theory of meaningful learning, the information-processing model, and social cognitive theory, the intervention was a comprehensive, 10-week program designed to help patients adopt more healthy eating behaviors outlined by a registered dietitian. Significant differences between the intervention group and a usual care control group included improvement in glycemic control, fasting plasma glucose, HbA1c levels, and total and LDL cholesterol and triglyceride levels. Indeed, the intervention group demonstrated two times the reduction in triglyceride levels as the control group. The key components in this intervention appear to be solid educational strategies, goal setting, self-monitoring, reinforcement, and support within the group sessions. This study supports a multimodal intervention for Type II older adult (over 65 years old) diabetics to assist in dietary behavior, but it is unclear from the intervention description how the program was tailored specifically for older adults.

Castaneda et al. (2002) conducted a 16-week, randomized, controled trial with a sample of Latino older adults with Type II diabetes. The intervention group received progressive resistance training (i.e., weight lifting) three times per week for 16 weeks. Significant reductions were found for the intervention group for HbA1c levels, in dose of prescribed diabetes medication, and in muscle glycogen stores. The control group demonstrated opposite results.

Glasgow et al. (1992) compared a 10-week self-management program that targeted self-efficacy and problem-solving skills in older adults with Type II diabetes. In this randomized wait-list control group study, the group intervention resulted in reductions in caloric intake, weight, and percent of calories from fat, and produced increases in frequency of glucose testing compared to the delayed-treatment group. The immediate-treatment group also showed significant reductions in weight, and reported greater problem-solving ability and a greater number of problem-solving strategies utilized at a 6-month follow-up assessment.

Recent guidelines in the treatment of diabetes mellitus in geriatric populations have stressed the importance of targeting not only the standard factors associated with diabetes, such as glycemic control and cardiovascular risk factors, but also those geriatric syndromes that are more common in older adults with this disorder (e.g., depression, cognitive impairment, urinary incontinence, falls, pain, and polypharmacy; Olson & Norris, 2004). To date, the completed psychosocial intervention studies have been limited to the management of specific aspects of diabetes (e.g., glycemic control, weight management) and have not attempted to intervene in a broader, multifaceted approach for older adults.

In summary, research with older adult patients with Type II diabetes has demonstrated that direct interventions to assist patients in dietary behaviors, problem solving, and exercise can influence important diabetes mediating factors and outcomes. Future research is needed to determine specific intervention components that are most influential for different outcomes (e.g., behavioral strategies, educational components, cognitive strategies, etc.) in older adults, along with guidance about the extent to which interventions need to be tailored distinctively for older, as opposed to younger or middle-aged, adults.

## Cardiovascular Disease

The prevalence of heart disease in older adults is remarkable. A conservative estimate indicates that more than half of all older adults have significant cardiovascular disease. People over the age of 65 account for over 80% of the deaths associated with heart disease (Fair, 2003). Surprisingly, modifiable risk factors are the same whether the focus is on older or younger adults. The primary biopsychosocial risk factors for cardiovascular disease include cigarette smoking, elevated cholesterol levels, obesity, insulin resistance, advanced age, sedentary lifestyle, family history of coronary heart disease (CHD), low perceived emotional support, isolation, depression, hostility, Type A behavior, anxiety, and work-related stress (Schneiderman et al., 2001). Furthermore, recent research suggests that risk factor modification reduces CHD risk in older adults (over 65 years of age) as effectively as it does in younger patients (Levine & Kannel, 2003).

### Psychosocial Interventions

As with the more general chronic disease management interventions, the psychoeducational interventions for reducing the plethora of negative CHD risk factors are commonly conducted in variety of settings: hospital-based (e.g., acute cardiac rehabilitation), outpatient, private practice, and home-based. As with the more general programs, these interventions are also provided by a variety of practitioners, including nurses, physicians, psychologists, and social workers. The programs are offered individually or in groups.

### Non-Age-Specific Findings

In general, research has demonstrated positive findings for biological and psychological outcomes. Improvements have been demonstrated in cholesterol levels, exercise, weight, smoking, systolic blood pressure, anxiety, depression, and Type A behavior, as well as in morbidity and mortality levels (Bracke & Thoresen, 1996; Dusseldorp, van Elderen, Maes, Meulman, &

Kraaij, 1999; Linden, Stossel, & Maurice, 1996; Mendes de Leon, Powell, & Kaplan, 1991; O'Connor et al., 1989; Oldridge Guyatt, Fischer, & Rimm, 1988; Rejeski et al., 2003).

The most impressive strategy for reducing morbidity and mortality in patients with CHD has been with aerobic exercise (O'Connor et al., 1989; Oldridge et al., 1988). These meta-analyses show that submaximal aerobic exercise in patients with CHD decreases reinfarction and demonstrates a 25% reduction in mortality due to cardiovascular or other causes of mortality compared to usual care. Psychosocial interventions have also shown beneficial effects.

The Recurrent-Coronary-Prone Prevention Project (Friedman et al., 1986; Mendes de Leon et al., 1991) was a randomized controlled trial to reduce the risk of another infarction in individuals who had already had one heart attack. The group-based program provided education on the pathophysiology of Type A behavior and CHD; diagnostic signs of Type A; the emotional, attitudinal, and cognitive belief structures of Type A; the role of self-esteem and self-worth in Type A; and the importance of reducing impatience, competitiveness, and hostility (Bracke & Thoresen, 1996). Results from this investigation demonstrated a significant reduction in Type A behavior and a 44% reduction of reinfarction (Mendes de Leon et al., 1991).

Ornish et al. (1990, 1998) completed a randomized, controlled trial utilizing a multimodal, nonmedical intervention that included stress management; strict, low-fat vegetarian diet; aerobic exercise; yoga; and group support. This investigation demonstrated that a comprehensive nonmedical psychosocial intervention was able to produce actual reversal of CHD that was maintained for 5 years. However, this intervention should not be seen as a panacea, because not all patients comply with such a strict intervention.

Thus, evidence supports the effectiveness of psychosocial interventions that focus on the biological, psychological, and social risk factors in reducing CHD risk factors, disease morbidity, and mortality. However, this research has not utilized diverse study populations or sophisticated research designs, which limits confidence in both the authority of the supportive evidence and the generalizability to different potential study populations (e.g., women, ethnic minorities, older adults). Most crucial to this discussion is whether these psychosocial interventions are more or less effective dependent on age. In general, this remains an empirical question that awaits future research.

## Older-Adult-Specific Studies

Although most of the programs reviewed have included older adults due to the age of most individuals with CHD, to our knowledge, the literature that focus specifically on older adults and biopsychosocial interventions for risk factor reduction is extremely limited. A randomized controlled study with older adults (ages 50–80) at risk for, or with documented CHD demonstrated that a cognitive-behavioral exercise offered in a group context was successful in increasing physical fitness activity levels, fitness, and self-efficacy perceptions compared to usual care cardiac rehabilitation (Focht, Brawley, Rejeski, & Ambrosius, 2004; Rejeski et al., 2003). Interestingly, gender and baseline levels (of the outcome variables) moderated the effects, with men and lower functioning individuals making the greatest improvements. Although the description for this intervention was quite detailed, no information was provided on how the program was specifically designed for older adults.

Inpatient smoking cessation counseling with older adults (over age 65) following an acute myocardial infarction demonstrated improved survival rates even after adjusting for myriad other health and demographic variables (Brown et al., 2004). In this retrospective chart review study, patients were considered counseled on smoking cessation if they had documentation of viewing a smoking cessation video or having received brochures or handouts on stopping smoking. Clearly, these "counseling" interventions were not tailored in any way to older adults, and the lack of experimental control over the intervention impacted the findings.

Although not an empirical study, Sheahan's (2002) study does address the specific needs of older adults relative to smoking cessation. This article, which provides useful clinical information relative to how older adult smokers may differ, might be useful for future development and research on interventions tailored for older adults.

In summary, the general research on interventions for CHD consistently finds that biopsychosocial interventions reduce risk factors, and improve morbidity and mortality rates. Specifically designed interventions for older adults to reduce risk factors for CHD await future research.

## Cancer

Age is considered the single greatest risk factor for cancer, with dramatic increases in incidence rates of cancer in populations over the age of 65 (Calabresi & Freeman, 1997; Yancik, 1997). Interestingly, although older adults incur an increased prevalence of cancer diagnosis, age is negatively associated with emotional distress (Andersen, 1992). Studies of patients with advanced cancer have typically included older adults (age 55), yet age has not been examined as a factor to investigate differential responses to interventions. Future research is critical to uncover possible age-related interactions with therapy components to enhance therapy effectiveness for older adults living with cancer.

## Psychosocial Interventions

Coping with cancer is a multistage process that begins with prevention and evolves through diagnosis and adaptation to different aspects of cancer treatment. Antoni (2002) suggests six stages: (1) prevention, (2) diagnosis, (3) treatment, (4) recurrence, (5) recurrence and dying, and (6) bereavement of family members. Consistent with the focus of this volume on management of chronic illness, we focus on *adjustment* to cancer. Readers may also want to note the significant research on psychosocial factors that influence preventive behaviors (Schneiderman et al., 2001).

Clinical intervention to assist in the management of cancer typically involves methods to improve quality of life, while dealing with the demands of the medical treatments. Elevated distress in patients with cancer can impede treatment decision making, increase unnecessary health care visits, interfere with curative or palliative treatment, and compound caregiver burden (Schneiderman et al., 2001).

Intervention programs have utilized cognitive-behavioral strategies or existential/experiential methods to assist cancer patients. The cognitive-behavioral programs typically are conducted in a supportive group format, with a focus on teaching self-management skills (e.g., relaxation strategies), cognitive restructuring, coping skills training (e.g., interpersonal relationship skills), anger management, and assertiveness training. The goal for these interventions is to reduce psychological distress; increase effective coping; foster emotional expression; improve pain management, illness knowledge, and self-image; increase sense of hope; manage specific noxious aspects of medical intervention; and gain relaxation skills (Antoni, 2002).

## General Empirical Findings

Intervention studies have varied in their methodological rigor, yet have been relatively consistent in demonstrating positive outcomes (for excellent reviews, see Andersen, 1992; Schneiderman et al., 2001). Important improvements have been shown in pain management, nausea control, emotional distress, physical symptom management, alteration of immune and neuroendocrine parameters, positive and negative health behaviors, and general quality of life. Improvements do seem to covary with severity of the illness, with more positive findings in persons with moderate or advanced cancer (Andersen, 1992; Antoni, 2002; Oldervoll, Kaasa, Hjermstad, Lund, & Loge, 2004).

One well-researched program, the B-SMART (Breast Cancer Stress Management and Relaxation Training; Antoni, 2002) intervention, has demonstrated efficacy for decreasing depression, reducing stress and reproductive hormones, and improving general optimism and immune cell proliferation response.

The existential/experiential group approach has focused primarily on providing a supportive group environment for patients to confront death-related concerns and to have an outlet for negative emotions (Schneiderman et al., 2001). These studies have demonstrated mixed results, with some reporting benefits for survival rates (Spiegel, Bloom, Kraemer, & Gottheil, 1989), but not others (Goodwin et al., 2001). Methodological differences, as well as changes in medical treatment for cancer, are likely suspects for the disparate findings. Most interventions utilizing this format have found improvements in quality of life and decreases in emotional distress.

### Older-Adult-Specific Studies

Over 25% of cancer survivors, the vast majority of whom are older adults, report clinical levels of depression (Deimling, Kahana, Bowman, & Schaefer, 2002). No outcome studies of interventions that targeted aging patients with cancer were identified in our review of the literature, however. Obviously, future intervention research that focuses specifically on the elderly is critically needed.

## Summary

The empirical research has provided a strong foundation for the efficacy of psychosocial interventions, with more global chronic illness interventions, as well as more focused, disease-specific treatments. The data for how these interventions work, or do not work, in older adults remains largely unexplored. Moreover, interventions specifically tailored to help older adults with chronic illness are virtually nonexistent. The next step in linking science with practice is to make it feasible for practicing health psychologists to utilize these types of interventions and to receive reimbursement.

## MEDICARE HEALTH AND BEHAVIOR CODES

In January 2002, psychologists for the first time were allowed to bill Medicare for services provided to help older adults manage chronic illnesses. These codes were not included under mental health services, but were instead included in the accepted medical treatment for chronic illnesses. This was truly a breakthrough for health psychology and a validation of the role behavioral factors play in the primary chronic illnesses facing older adults. The inclusion of these codes into Medicare reimbursement was accomplished through the combined efforts of the American Psychological Association's Practice Directorate (2004) and the cooperation of many APA divisions, including Divisions 12, 17, 22, 38, 40, and 54 (i.e., the Interdivisional Healthcare Committee). These codes cover a variety of health interventions, assisting patients with (1) adherence to medical treatment, (2) symptom management, (3) reduction of negative health behaviors, (4) increasing positive health behaviors, and (5) adjustment to their disease. These codes are not for primary prevention efforts; patients need to have a chronic illness diagnosed by a physician to be eligible for intervention under these codes. Specific information about the codes and their use are available on websites for the American Psychological Association Practice Directorate, as well as the Centers for Medicare and Medicaid Services.

The impact of these codes on the role of psychology in health care reflects one of the largest expansions of the scope of psychological practice since psychologists became eligible for direct Medicare reimbursement. No study of the impact of these codes on training, research, and practice patterns has yet been conducted, but the broadening of psychology's role in health care appears likely to increase the importance of research such as that summarized in this volume.

## MENTAL DISORDERS IN PRIMARY CARE SETTINGS

Epidemiological data on mental disorders in older adults show that approximately 20% of persons over age 65 have mental disorders (Gatz & Smyer, 2001), with higher rates presented in acute and chronic care settings (Blazer, 1999). Depression rates in primary care clinics are estimated at 9.5%–14% for diagnosable conditions, with an additional 10–20% for minor depression (Lyness, Caine, King, Cox, & Yoediono, 1999; Oxman, Barrett, Barrett, & Gerber, 1990). Other disorders, such as anxiety, insomnia, and substance abuse, are even more prevalent than depression in older adults in community samples that rely on outpatient care (Lyness et al., 1999). Advanced age is an added risk factor for subsyndromal depression and cognitive impairment.

Several factors likely contribute to the high rate of presentation of mental disorders in medical settings. Chronic medical illnesses generally have high rates of comorbidity with psychological disorders (Montano, 1999). Furthermore, serious illnesses and psychological disorders have mutually deleterious effects, often generating a downward spiral that results in loss of function, excessive disability, and premature mortality (Beekman, Deeg, Braam, Smit, & Tilburg, 1997; Katon & Ciechanowski, 2002). Finally, mental disorders can generate conditions that foster chronic illness (Verbrugge & Jette, 1994).

### Challenges of Detecting Mental Disorders

Within primary care, rates of missed detection of mental disorders are extraordinary for adults of all ages: 30–70% of depressive disorders are missed by primary care physicians (Perez-Stable, Miranda, Munoz, & Ying, 1990). In their defense, researchers argue that these may be the depressions that produce little functional impairment or that remit more spontaneously (Coyne, Schwenck, & Fechner-Bates, 1995; Coyne, Thompson, Klinkman, & Nease, 2002). For complex reasons, few diagnosed older adults receive appropriate treatments (e.g., because of diagnostic complexity, lack of acceptance of psychiatric nosology by primary care providers, patient and provider variables) for disorders that are not simple to resolve (Coyne et al., 2002; Unützer, 2002; Unützer et al., 1999).

Left untreated, mental disorders are very costly (Rost et al., 1998; Katon, Lin, Russo, & Unützer, 2003). The impact on cost of health services is substantial because of the high rates of medical care utilization, especially among those with depression and chronic illnesses for whom health costs are approximately 50% higher than for nondepressed individuals (Katon, et al., 2003). Even subclinical levels of mental disorders generate disability, reduced well-being, and greater health care utilization (Beekman et al., 1997). Finally, the most catastrophic cost for the individual is mortality from illness or suicide (Montano, 1999). Among older patients age 75 or older who commit suicide, 60–75% have diagnosable depression (Conwell, 1993).

## Interventions for Mental Disorders in Primary Care

Mental disorders respond to treatment in primary care settings, and those benefits extend beyond mental well-being to physical improvements in chronic illnesses such as arthritis (e.g., Lin et al., 2003). Unfortunately, across the mental disorders, rates of treatment access are low. Older adults are less likely than other age groups to seek help from mental health professionals, relying exclusively on their primary care providers for mental health treatment (Unützer et al., 1999).

Primary care settings have been the target of a variety of efforts to improve both rates of detection of mental disorders and interventions (Coyne et al., 2002; Kroenke, Taylor-Vaisey, Dietrich, & Oxman, 2000; Stanley et al., 2003). The strongest research base exists for improving rates of detection and treatment of depression. Several studies report efficacy rates for various quality improvement strategies, similar to those found with other medical interventions with positive outcomes, including reduced burden, medical cost offset, and increased number of days at work (Rost, Nutting, Smith, & Werner, 2000; Schoenbaum et al., 2001; Simon et al., 2001; Tutty, Simon, & Ludman, 2000; Unützer et al., 2001). Specific intervention strategies include educating clinicians and patients, screening routinely, engaging care managers for medication follow-up, making psychotherapy accessible on site, and telephone contact, (Schoenbaum et al., 2001; Sherbourne et al., 2001).

Despite these successes, serious challenges must still be overcome. Significant work must be done to address the full range of mental disorders seen in primary care. Research is needed to clarify whether the types of disorders seen in primary care have the same characteristics, treatment outcomes, and course as those seen in outpatient mental health settings (Coyne et al., 2002). We must also learn about patient characteristics that influence help seeking, openness to various types of intervention, and predictors of relapse into debilitating disorders from lower intensity conditions (Coyne et al., 2002). The level and mechanisms of systemic intervention needed to sustain change in health providers' patterns of detection, referral, or treatment must be identified (Kroenke et al., 2000). Cost–benefit analyses of effective interventions are needed to persuade payors to fund delivery models not currently supported by Medicare (e.g., telephone contact or case management; Coyne et al., 2002; Katon et al., 2003). The role of families and significant others in the improvement of physical and mental well-being represents another key area for future research.

## FAMILIES OF AGING PATIENTS IN HEALTH CARE SETTINGS

A critical focus for health care providers concerned with promoting physical and emotional well-being in older adults is the family. Families are key components of the health care delivery system for older adults. Frail elders receive 80% of their needed daily assistance from family members (National Center for Health Statistics, 1999), including help with basic activities of daily living (e.g., bathing, dressing, feeding), as well as activities necessary for independence, referred to as "instrumental activities of daily living" (e.g., medication monitoring, managing doctors appointments). Although the type of involvement varies according to geographic distance between caregiver and care recipient, the rate of involvement is very high. Even following placement into an institutional environment, family members remain intensively involved in decisions about health and daily care (High & Rowles, 1995).

The strong positive relationship between family support, both instrumental and emotional, and health and well-being in older adults is well documented (Antonucci & Akiyama, 1995; George, 1996). Furthermore, the absence of family support is associated with poorer response to treatment for illness, as well as greater risk of mental disorders (Oxman & Hull, 2001). Of course, increased rates of family contact do not equate simplistically with improved support, because not all contact is supportive (Antonucci,

Akiyama, & Lansford, 1998), and negative family contact adversely influences well-being (e.g., Druley, Stephens, Martire, Ennis, & Wojno, 2003). Furthermore, family health habits can impede positive components of health care by compromising medication compliance, undermining recommendations for diet or exercise, or increasing stress (Ewart, 1990).

## Family Roles in Health Care

Families are not always visible to health care providers for reasons that relate to the family's process of engaging in the caregiving role, as well as structures in the health care delivery system (Frank & McDaniel, 2004). Families usually become involved in the health and well-being of older adults rather gradually over the course of the aging process (Aneshensel, Pearlin, Mullin, Zarit, & Whitlatch, 1995; Fortinsky Tennen, Frank, & Affleck, Chapter 12, this volume). Unless the health care settings structure care to engage families purposively, family members' role in health care may not be visible to the health care system until quite late in the caregiving process, when a patient's physical functioning deteriorates so much that long term care services are needed. Delaying explicit engagement risks losing coordination with a major partner in health care, as well as compounding risks to families and patients from unrecognized stress and burden on caregivers (Rusin & Lawson, 2001).

Health psychologists need to understand the paths by which families become involved in older adults' health care. Family involvement with patients with dementia has been mapped onto a continuum (Qualls, 1997) that ranges from one extreme, in which the aged person and family share the type of interest that mutually autonomous adults show in each other, to the other, in which the family maintains full legal and ethical responsibility for care. The roles shift as family members gradually become involved in the lives of older adults, long before anyone is defined as a "caregiver" (Qualls, 1999). The role changes are gradual, shifting from simply showing interest to observing purposefully for signs of health or problems, to active monitoring of well-being and risks. Informal observations suggest that families move along that continuum unconsciously, responding to subtle cues that lack universal identity or clear mandates for role change, and with considerable uncertainty (Qualls, 1997). Furthermore, the process of moving from one end of that continuum to the other has no clear signposts that mark the role transitions.

The career conceptualization of caregiving for patients with dementia emphasizes the caregiver's process of engaging in the necessary roles over time, as marked by distinct periods of role induction, role enactment, and role disengagement (Aneshensel et al., 1995). Relatively little is known about when and how family members decide to take on particular roles related to the health of older persons, particularly in the early role changes, prior to establishment of the caregiver role. However, characteristics of family structure and decision-making style influence the content and timing of key decisions such as institutional placement (Lieberman & Fisher, 1999). Furthermore, the challenge of getting the entire family to agree on either the principles or outcomes of a particular decision is substantial (Roberto, 1999).

Regardless of decision-making style, families make decisions with, or on behalf of, the patient as a key component of family responsibility for persons with chronic illness (Corcoran, 1994; Wackerbarth, 1999b). Health systems often emphasize individual autonomy in decision making, a contrast to the interdependence in which families function (Haley et al., 2002). Ethicists have cautioned that the recent emphasis on individual autonomy may actually constrain health systems from engaging intimate others in making health decisions in ways that preserve the integrity of the individual's identity and autonomy (Jecker, 1990).

As the patterns by which patients and families make decisions together becomes clearer, the ethical principles and intervention processes by which health providers can guide the decision-makers in a family to balance the well-being and autonomy of individuals and families must be clarified (Bata & Power, 1995; Moody, 1988). For example, a useful distinction can be made between family members who plan ahead in anticipation of transitions and those who make decisions almost exclusively in the context of crises (Wackerbarth, 1999a). Furthermore, family decision making can be conceptualized as invoking a sequence of steps, such as considering, discussing, planning, and deciding (Bromley & Blieszner, 1997). Health care providers potentially play a key role in stimulating appropriate planning, although relatively little is known about how families and health care delivery systems interact to shift those roles on behalf of older patients.

Older adults almost universally want families involved in their health decisions, leading adults without family into a dilemma about whom to appoint in surrogate decision-making roles (High, 1988, 1991; Hopp, 2000). Indeed, having families involved in decisions is more important than the principles used for making the decisions (e.g., the choice between ethical principles of substituted judgment or best interests'). Decisions for long term care strategies on behalf of older patients with seriously debilitating chronic illnesses are far more likely to involve family than to involve the patients themselves (McAuley & Travis, 1997). End-of-life decisions are influenced by factors as diverse as the cognitive impairment status of the patient, cultural contexts of the family (Allen-Burge & Haley, 1997), and generational position within the family (Karel & Gatz, 1996).

## Strategies for Engaging Families in Primary Care

A quick perusal of the environment in which health care is delivered produces the immediate observation that routine health delivery practices discourage or even impede an integrated team approach that involves multiple providers, the patients, and their families (Haley, 1996). Families are not routinely engaged as informants about functioning, health practices, or other aspects of well-being. Indeed, health privacy laws raise concerns about mechanisms and appropriateness of family involvement and pragmatically constrain communication. Thus, families caring for a mildly cognitively impaired older adult living independently cannot receive information about the results of medical evaluations or treatment recommendations without the patient initiating the involvement of family. Outpatient offices often lack space for family members; hospital operators may not provide information about the presence or absence of family members; and rehabilitation settings often lack space and staff time to coach families into roles as therapy assistants.

Current practice innovations to improve family engagement include gathering regular screening data from family informants (Jorm, 2003) and adding collateral interviews to enhance knowledge about daily functioning (Blazer & Siegler, 1984). Family members can be included in assessment feedback and treatment decisions, with patient consent, or under conditions in which patient capacity to make use of the information is compromised. Proactive efforts to identify caregiver distress within the primary care context can prevent crisis decision making for the target patient, as well as prevent deterioration in the caregiver's health (see Fortinsky et al., Chapter 12, this volume).

## CONCLUSION

The practice of psychology has shifted dramatically as opportunities to apply knowledge from health psychology, behavioral medicine, and clinical psychology in health care settings have expanded (Frank & McDaniel, 2004). Respect for the fundamental interplay among physical health, health behavior, and psychosocial well-being secures a key role for psychologists in health care settings as diverse as primary care, rehabilitation hospitals, acute medical care, and long term care settings. This volume illustrates the rapidly growing knowledge base for practicing clinical health psychology. The content and skills of health psychology almost certainly will play a larger part in training curricula at the predoctoral and internship levels (Anderson & Lovejoy, 2000; Zeiss, 2000). The future of health care depends on psychologists continuing at an aggressive pace in research, education, and practice expansion of health care issues and settings.

## REFERENCES

Allen-Burge, R., & Haley, W. E. (1997). Individual differences and surrogate medical decisions: Differing preferences for life-sustaining treatments. *Aging and Mental Health, 1,* 121–131.

Andersen B. L. (1992). Psychological interventions for cancer patients to enhance the quality of life. *Journal of Consulting and Clinical Psychology, 60,* 552–568.

Anderson, G. L., & Lovejoy, D. W. (2000). Predoctoral training in collaborative primary care: An exam room built for two. *Professional Psychology: Research and Practice, 31,* 692–697.

Aneshensel, C. S., Pearlin, L. I., Mullan, J. T., Zarit, S. H., & Whitlatch, C. J. (1995). *Profiles in caregiving: The unexpected career.* San Diego: Academic Press.

Antoni, M. (2002). *Stress management intervention for women with breast cancer.* Washington, DC: American Psychological Association.

Antonucci, T. C., & Akiyama, H. (1995). Convoys of social relations: Family and friendships within a life span context. In R. Blieszner & V. H. Bedford (Eds.), *Handbook of aging and the family* (pp. 355–371). Westport, CT: Greenwood Press.

Antonucci, T. C., Akiyama, H., & Lansford, J. E. (1998). Negative aspects of close social relations. *Family Relations, 47,* 379–384.

Bata, E. J., & Power, P. W. (1995). Facilitating health care decisions within aging families. In G. C. Smith, S. S. Tobin, E. A. Robertson Tchabo, & P. W. Power (Eds.), *Strengthening aging families: Diversity in practice and policy* (pp. 143–157). Thousand Oaks, CA: Sage.

Beekman, A. T. F., Deeg, D. J. H., Braam, A. W., Smit, J. H., & Tilburg, W. V. (1997). Consequences of major and minor depression in later life: A study of disability, well-being and service utilization. *Psychological Medicine, 27,* 1397–1409.

Björk, S. (2001). The cost of diabetes and diabetes care. *Diabetes Research and Clinical Practice, 54* (Suppl. 1), S13–S18.

Blazer, D. G. (1999). Epidemiology of late-life depression. In W. R. Hazzard, J. P. Blass, W. H. Ettinger, Jr., D. B. Halter, & J. G. Ouslander (Eds.), *Principles of geriatric medicine and gerontology* (4th ed., pp. 1331–1339). New York: McGraw-Hill.

Blazer, D. G., & Siegler, I. C. (1984). *A family oriented approach to health care of the elderly.* Menlo Park, CA: Addison-Wesley.

Bracke, P. E., & Thoresen, C. E. (1996). Reducing Type A behavior patterns: A structured-group approach. In R. Allen & S. Scheidt (Eds.), *Heart and mind: The practice of cardiac psychology* (pp. 255–290). Washington, DC: American Psychological Association.

Bromley, M. C., & Blieszner, R. (1997). Planning for long-term care: Filial behavior and relationship quality of adult children with independent parents. *Family Relations, 46,* 155–162.

Brown, D. W., Croft, J. B., Schenck, A. P., Malarcher, A. M., Giles, W. H., & Simpson, R. J., Jr. (2004). Inpatient smoking-cessation and all-cause mortality among the elderly. *American Journal of Preventive Medicine, 26,* 112–118.

Calabresi, P., & Freeman, H. (1997). Cancers of special populations: Cancer and the aging population. *Cancer, 80,* 1258–1260.

Casteneda, C., Layne, J. E., Munoz-Orians, L., Gordon, P. L., Walsmith, J., Foldvari, M., et al. (2002). A randomized controlled trial of resistance exercise training to improve glycemic control in older adults with Type 2 diabetes. *Diabetes Care, 25,* 2335–2341.

Chambless, D., & Ollendick, T. H. (2001). Empirically supported psychological interventions: Controversies and evidence. *Annual Review of Psychology, 52,* 685–716.

Clark, M., & Hampson, S. E. (2001). Implementing a psychological intervention to improve lifestyle self-management in patients with Type 2 diabetes. *Patient Education and Counseling, 42,* 247–256.

Conwell, Y. (1993). Suicide in elderly patients. In L. S. Schneider, C. F. Reynolds, & B. D. Lebowitz (Eds.), *Diagnosis and treatment of depression in later life* (pp. 397–418). Washington, DC: American Psychiatric Press.

Corcoran, M. A. (1994). Management decisions made by caregiver spouses of persons with Alzheimer's disease. *American Journal of Occupational Therapy, 48,* 38–45.

Coyne, J. C., Schwenck, T. L., & Fechner-Bates, S. (1995). Nondetection of depression by primary care physicians reconsidered. *General Hospital Psychiatry, 17,* 3–12.

Coyne, J. C., Thompson, R., Klinkman, M. S., & Nease, D. E. (2002). Emotional disorders in primary care. *Journal of Consulting and Clinical Psychology, 70,* 798–809.

Deimling, G. T., Kahana, B., Bowman, K. F., & Schaefer, M. L. (2002). Cancer survivorship and psychological distress in later life. *Psychooncology, 11,* 479–494.

Delamater, A. M., Jacobson, A. M., Anderson, B., Cox, D., Fisher, L., Lustman, P., et al. (2001). Psychosocial therapies in diabetes: Report of the psychosocial therapies working group. *Diabetes Care, 24,* 1286–1292.

Druley, J. A., Stephens, M. A. P., Martire, L. M., Ennis, N., & Wojno, W. C. (2003). Emotional congruence in older couples coping with wives' osteoarthritis: Exacerbating effects of pain behavior. *Psychology and Aging, 18,* 406–418.

Dusseldorp, E., van Elderen, T., Maes, S., Meulman, J., & Kraaij, V. (1999). A meta-analysis of psychoeducational programs for coronary heart disease patients. *Health Psychology, 18,* 506–519.

Ersek, M., Turner, J. A., McCurry, S. M., Gibbons, L., & Kraybill, B. M. (2003). Efficacy of a self-management group intervention for elderly persons with chronic pain. *Clinical Journal of Pain, 19,* 156–167.

Ewart, C. K. (1990). A social problem-solving approach to behavior change in coronary heart disease. In S. A. Shumaker, E. B. Schron, & J. K. Ockene (Eds.), *The handbook of health behavior change* (pp. 153–190). New York: Springer.

Fair, J. M. (2003). Cardiovascular risk factor modification: Is it effective in older adults? *Journal of Cardiovascular Nursing, 18,* 161–168.

Feifer, C., & Tansman, M. (1999). Promoting psychology in diabetes primary care. *Professional Psychology: Research and Practice, 30,* 14–21.

Focht, B. C., Brawley, L. R., Rejeski, W. J., & Ambrosius, W. T. (2004). Group-mediated activity counseling and traditional exercise therapy programs: Effects on health-related quality of life among older adults in cardiac rehabilitation. *Annals of Behavioral Medicine, 28,* 52–61.

Frank, R. G., & McDaniel, S. H. (2004). *Primary care psychology.* Washington, DC: American Psychological Association.

Friedman, M., Thoresen, C. E., Gill, J. J., Ulmer, D., Powell, L. H., Price, V. A., et al. (1986). Alteration of Type A behavior and its effect on cardiac recurrences in post myocardial infarction patients: Summary results of the Recurrent Coronary Prevention Project. *American Heart Journal, 112,* 653–665.

Gatz, M., & Smyer, M. A. (2001). Mental health and aging at the outset of the twenty-first century. In J. Birren (Ed.), *Handbook of the psychology of aging* (5th ed., pp. 523–544). San Diego: Academic Press.

George, L. K. (1996). Social factors and illness. In R. H. Binstock & L. K. George (Eds.), *Handbook of aging and the social sciences* (pp. 229–252). San Diego: Academic Press.

Glasgow, R. E., La Chance, P., Toobert, D. J., Brown, J., Hampson, S. E., & Riddle, M. C. (1997). Long term effects and costs of brief behavioral dietary intervention for patients with diabetes delivered from the medical office. *Patient Education Counseling, 32,* 175–184.

Glasgow, R. E., Toobert, D. J., Hampson, S. E., Brown, J. E., Lewinsohn, P. M., & Donnelly, J. (1992). Improving self-care among older patients with Type II diabetes: The "Sixty Something . . . " study. *Patient Education Counseling, 19,* 61–74.

Goodwin, P. J., Leszcz, M., Ennis, M., Koopmans, J., Vincent, L., Guther, H., et al. (2001). The effect of group psychological support on survival in metastatic breast cancer. *New England Journal of Medicine, 345,* 1719–1726.

Haley, W. E. (1996). The medical context of psychotherapy with the elderly. In S. H. Zarit & B. G. Knight (Eds.), *A guide to psychotherapy and aging* (pp. 221–240). Washington, DC: American Psychological Association.

Haley, W. E., Allen, R. S., Reynolds, S., Chen, H., Burton, A., & Gallagher-Thompson, D. (2002). Family issues in end-of-life decision making and end-of-life care. *American Behavioral Scientist, 46,* 284–298.

High, D. M. (1988). All in the family: Extended autonomy and expectations in surrogate health care decision-making. *Gerontologist, 28* (Suppl.), 46–51.

High, D. M. (1991). A new myth about families of older people? *Gerontologist, 31,* 611–618.

High, D. M., & Rowles, J. (1995). Nursing home residents, families, and decision-making: Toward an understanding of progressive surrogacy. *Journal of Aging Studies, 9,* 101–117.

Hopp, F. P. (2000). Preferences for surrogate decision makers, informal communication, and advance directives among community-dwelling elders: Results from a national study. *Gerontologist, 40,* 449–457.

Jecker, N. S. (1990). The role of intimate others in medical decision making. *Gerontologist, 30,* 65–71.

Jorm, A. F. (2003). The value of informant reports for assessment and prediction of dementia. *Journal of the American Geriatrics Society, 51,* 881–882.

Karel, M. J., & Gatz, M. (1996). Factors influencing life-sustaining treatment decisions in a community sample of families. *Psychology and Aging, 11,* 226–234.

Karlsen, B., Idsoe, T., Dirdal, I., Hanestad, B. R., & Bru, E. (2004). Effects of a group-based counseling programme on diabetes-related stress, coping, psychological well-being and metabolic control in adults with Type 1 or Type 2 diabetes. *Patient and Education Counseling, 53*(3), 299–308.

Katon, W., & Ciechanowski, P. (2002). Impact of major depression on chronic medical illness. *Journal of Psychosomatic Research, 53,* 859–863.

Katon, W. J., Lin, E., Russo, J., & Unützer, J. (2003). Increased medical costs of a population-based sample of depressed elderly patients. *Archives of General Psychiatry, 60,* 897–903.

Kroenke, K., Taylor-Vaisey, A., Dietrich, A. J., & Oxman, T. E. (2000). Interventions to improve provider diagnosis and treatment of mental disorders in primary care: A critical review of the literature. *Psychosomatics, 41,* 39–52.

Leveille, S. G., Wagner, E. H., Davis, C., Grothaus, L., Wallace, J., LoGerfo, M., et al. (1998). Preventing disability and managing chronic illness in frail older adults: a randomized trial of a community-based partnership with primary care. *Journal of the American Geriatrics Society, 46,* 1191–1198.

Levine, B. S., & Kannel, W. B. (2003). Coronary heart disease risk in people 65 years of age and older. *Progressive Cardiovascular Nursing, 18,* 135–140.

Lieberman, M. A., & Fisher, L. (1999). The effects of family conflict resolution and decision making on the provision of help for an elder with Alzheimer's disease. *Gerontologist, 39,* 159–166.

Lin, E. H. B., Katon, W., Von Korff, M., Tang, L., Williams, J. W., Kroenke, K., et al. (2003). Effect of improving depression care on pain and functional outcomes among older adults with arthritis. *Journal of the American Medical Association, 290*(18), 2428–2434.

Linden, M. W., Stossel, C., & Maurice, J. (1996). Psychosocial interventions for patients with coronary artery disease. *Archives of Internal Medicine, 156,* 745–752.

Lorig, K. (1995). Patient education: Treatment or nice extra [Editorial]. *British Journal of Rheumatology, 34,* 703–706.

Lorig, K., Ritter, P., Stewart, A., Sobel, D., Brown, B., Bandura, A., et al. (2001). Chronic disease self-management program: 2-year health status and health care utilization outcomes. *Medical Care, 39,* 1217–1223.

Lorig, K., Sobel, D., Ritter, P., Laurent, D., & Hobbs, (2001). Effectiveness of a self-management program on patients with chronic disease. *Effective Clinical Practice, 4,* 256–262.

Lorig, K., Sobel, D., Stewart, A., Brown, B., Bandura, A., Ritter, P., et al. (1999). Evidence suggesting that a chronic disease self-management program can improve health status while reducing hospitalization: A randomized trial. *Medical Care, 37,* 5–14.

Lyness, J. M., Caine, E. D., King, D. A., Cox, C., & Yoediono, Z. (1999). Psychiatric disorders in older primary care patients. *Journal of General Internal Medicine, 14,* 249–254.

McAuley, W. J., & Travis, S. S. (1997). Positions of influence in the nursing home decision. *Research on Aging, 19,* 26–46.

Mendes de Leon, C. F., Powell, L. H., & Kaplan B. H. (1991). Change in coronary-prone behaviors in the recurrent coronary prevention project. *Psychosomatic Medicine, 53,* 407–419.

Miller, C. K., Edwards, L., Kissling, G., & Sanville, L. (2002). Nutrition education improves metabolic outcomes among older adults with diabetes mellitus: Results from a randomized controlled trial. *Preventive Medicine, 34,* 252–259.

Montano, C. B. (1999). Primary care issues related to the treatment of depression in elderly patients. *Journal of Clinical Psychiatry, 60*(Suppl. 20), 45–51.

Moody, H. R. (1988). From informed consent to negotiated consent. *Gerontologist,* 28(Suppl.), 64–70.

National Center for Health Statistics. (1999). *Health, United States, 1999, With health and aging chartbook* [Online]. Retrieved July 12, 2006 from www.cdc.gov/nchs/data/hus/hus99.pdf.

O'Connor, G. T., Buring, J. E., Yusuf, S., Goldhaber, S. Z., Olmstead, E. M., & Paffenbarger, R. S. (1989). An overview of randomized trials of rehabilitation with exercise after myocardial infarction. *Circulation, 80,* 234–244.

Oldervoll, L. M., Kaasa, S., Hjermstad, J. J., Lund, J. A., & Loge, J. H. (2004). Physical exercise results in improved subjective well-being of a few or is effective rehabilitation for all cancer patients? *European Journal of Cancer, 40,* 951–962.

Oldridge, N. B., Guyatt, G. H., Fischer, M. E., & Rimm, A. A. (1988). Cardiac rehabilitation after myocardiac infarction: Combined experience of randomized clinical trials. *Journal of the American Medical Association, 260,* 945–950.

Olson, D. E., & Norris, S. L. (2004). Overview of AGS guidelines for the treatment of diabetes mellitus in geriatric populations. *Geriatrics, 59,* 18–25.

Ornish, D., Brown, S. E., Scherwitz, L. W., Billings, J. H., Armstrong, W. T., Ports, T. A., et al., (1990). Can lifestyle changes reverse coronary heart disease? *Lancet, 336,* 129–133.

Ornish, D., Scherwitz, L. W., Billings, J. H., Gould, L., Merritt, T. A., & Sparler, S. (1998). Intensive lifestyle changes for reversal of coronary heart disease. *Journal of the American Medical Association, 280,* 2001–2007.

Oxman, T. E., Barrett, J. E., Barrett, J., & Gerber, P. (1990). Symptomatology of late life minor depression among primary-care patients. *Psychosomatics, 31,* 174–180.

Oxman, T. E., & Hull, J. G. (2001). Social support and treatment response in older depressed primary care patients. *Journals of Gerontology: Psychological Sciences and Social Sciences, Series B, 56,* P35–P45.

Padgett, D., Mumford, E., Hynes, M., & Carter, R. (1988). Meta-analysis of the effects of educational and psychosocial interventions on management of diabetes mellitus, *Journal of Clinical Epidemiology, 41,* 1007–1030.

Perez-Stable, E. J., Miranda, J., Munoz, R. F., & Ying, Y. W. (1990). Depression in medical outpatients: Underrecognition and misdiagnosis. *Archives of Internal Medicine, 150,* 1083–1088.

Persons, J. B., & Silberschatz, G. (1998). Are results of randomized controlled trials useful to psychotherapists. *Journal of Consulting and Clinical Psychology, 66,* 126–135.

Qualls, S. H. (1997). Transitions in autonomy: The essential caregiving challenge. *Family Relations, 46,* 41–45.

Qualls, S. H. (1999). Realizing power in intergenerational family hierarchies: Family reorganization when older adults decline. In M. Duffy (Ed.), *Handbook of counseling and psychotherapy with older adults* (pp. 228–241). New York: Wiley.

Rejeski, W. J., Brawley, L. R., Ambrosius, W. T., Brubaker, P. H., Focht, B. S., Foy, C. G., et al. (2003). Older adults with chronic disease: Benefits of group-mediated counseling in the promotion of physically active lifestyles. *Health Psychology, 22,* 414–423.

Roberto, K. A. (1999). Making critical health care decisions for older adults: Consensus among family members. *Family Relations, 48,* 167–175.

Rost, K., Nutting, P. A., Smith, J., & Werner, J. J. (2000). Designing and implementing a primary care intervention trial to improve the quality and outcome of care for major depression. *General Hospital Psychiatry, 22,* 66–77.

Rost, K., Zhang, M., Fortney, J., Smith, J., Coyne, J., & Smith, G. R. (1998). Persistently poor outcomes of undetected major depression in primary care. *General Hospital Psychiatry, 20,* 12–20.

Rusin, M. J., & Lawson, K. J. (2001). Behavioral interventions and families: A medical rehabilitation perspective. *Journal of Clinical Geropsychology, 7,* 255–269.

Rybarczyk, B., DeMarco, G., De La Cruz, M., Lapidos, S., & Fortner, B. (2001). A classroom mind/body wellness intervention for older adults with chronic illness: Comparing immediate and 1-year benefits. *Behavioral Medicine, 27,* 15–27.

Sarkadi, A., & Rosenqvist, U. (2004). Experience-based group education in Type 2 diabetes: A randomized controlled trial. *Patient Education and Counseling, 53,* 291–298.

Schneiderman, N., Antoni, M., Saab, P., & Ironson, G. (2001). Health psychology: Psychosocial and biobehavioral aspects of chronic disease management. *Annual Review of Psychology, 52,* 555–580.

Schoenbaum, M., Unützer, J., Sherbourne, C., Duan, N., Rubenstein, L. V., Miranda, J., et al. (2001). Cost-effectiveness of practice-initiated quality improvement for depression. *Journal of the American Medical Association, 286,* 1325–1330.

Sheahan, S. L. (2002, December). How to help older adults quit smoking. *Nurse Practitioner,* pp. 27–33.

Sherbourne, C. D., Well, K. B., Duan, N., Miranda, J., Unützer, J., Jaycox, L., et al. (2001). Long-term effectiveness of disseminating quality improvement for depression in primary care. *Archives of General Psychiatry, 58,* 696–703.

Simon, G. E., Katon, W. J., Von Korff, M., Unützer, J., Lin, E. H. B., Walker, E. A., et al. (2001). Cost-effectiveness of a collaborative care program for primary care patients with persistent depression. *American Journal of Psychiatry, 158,* 1638–1644.

Spiegel, D., Bloom, J. R., Kraemer, H. C., & Gottheil, E. (1989). Effect of psychosocial treatment on survival of patients with metastatic breast cancer. *Lancet, 2,* 888–891.

Stanley, M. A., Hopko, D. R., Diefenbach, G. J., Bourland, S. L., Rodriguez, H. L., & Wagener, P. (2003). Treatment of generalized anxiety disorder in primary care: Treatment development and initial outcomes. *American Journal of Geriatric Psychiatry, 11,* 92–96.

Tutty, S., Simon, G., & Ludman, E. (2000). Telephone counseling as an adjunct to antidepressant treatment in the primary care system: A pilot study. *Effective Clinical Practice, 4,* 170–178.

Unützer, J. (2002). Diagnosis and treatment of older adults with depression in primary care. *Biological Psychiatry, 52,* 285–292.

Unützer, J., Katon, W., Russo, J., Simon, G., Bush, T., Walker, E., et al. (1999). Patterns of care for depressed older adults in a large-staff model HMO. *American Journal of Geriatric Psychiatry, 7,* 235–243.

Unützer, J., Rubenstein, L., Katon, W. J., Tang, L., Duan, N., Lagomasino, I. T., et al. (2001). Two-year effects of quality improvement programs on medication management for depression. *Archives of General Psychiatry, 58,* 935–942.

Verbrugge, L. M., & Jette, A. M. (1994). The disablement process. *Social Science in Medicine, 38,* 1–14.

Wackerbarth, S. (1999a). Modeling a dynamic decision process: Supporting the decisions of caregivers of family members with dementia. *Qualitative Health Research, 9,* 294–314.

Wackerbarth, S. (1999b). What decisions are made by family caregivers? *American Journal of Alzheimer's Disease, 14,* 111–119.

Yancik, R. (1997). Cancer burden in the aged: An epidemic and demographic overview. *Cancer, 80,* 1273–1283.

Zeiss, A. M. (2000). Reenvisioning internship training in clinical and counseling psychology: Developments in the Department of Veterans Affairs system. *Professional Psychology: Research and Practice, 31,* 310–314.

# CHAPTER 19

# Effects of Changes in Diagnostic Thresholds on Health Care for Older Adults

## ROBERT M. KAPLAN

Older adults comprise the largest health care consumer group. One of the most challenging problems in contemporary America is the solvency of the Medicare system. When the system was founded, approximately eight people paid into the system for each person who received benefits. By 2050 only two workers will support each recipient. Decisions in Medicare policy can affect older people in at least two ways. First, policy can dictate what services adults will receive. Second, some policies may place a financial burden on the system. When Medicare becomes financially troubled, some services may need to be cut back. This chapter explores the unintended consequences of well-intentioned proposals for changes in treatment guidelines.

In 1992 Geoffrey Rose published *The Strategy of Preventive Medicine*. Many consider the book to be one of the most important statements about epidemiology and public health produced in the 20th century. Rose noted that there is systematic relationship between risk factors for coronary heart disease and poor health outcomes. For example, the current threshold for high systolic blood pressure (SBP) is 140 mm Hg. However, the relationship between SBP and deaths from both heart disease and stroke moves systematically upward with SBP above 110 mm Hg (Goldstein et al., 2001; Howard & Howard, 2001). Similarly, the British Heart Protection Study demonstrated that lowering low-density lipoprotein (LDL) cholesterol using simvastatin (Zocor) reduces the development of vascular disease independent of the initial levels of serum cholesterol ("MRC/BHF Heart Protection Study," 2002).

Rose argued that only a small portion of cardiovascular events occur in persons with risk factor scores above levels now believed to be thresholds for treatment. For example, in comparison to persons with a SBP less than 120 mm Hg, only about 24% of the excess deaths from stroke accrue to those with SBP higher than 160 mm Hg (Marmot & Poulter, 1992). The great majority of cases of coronary heart disease (CHD) and stroke occur in those with risk factor scores below the therapeutic threshold. Too much attention, according to Rose, has been devoted to case identification and treatment, and not enough attention has been paid to shifting the entire curve of blood pressure and cholesterol downward (Rose & Day, 1990). This argument is summarized in Figure 19.1. A population-based intervention that shifts the distribution of blood pressure toward the left will have greater impact on population health than will targeted screening (Marmot & Poulter, 1992). Rose did not suggest changing the thresholds for treatment. Instead, he argued that everyone in the population should be exposed to healthy lifestyle interventions. This argument formed the basis for population-based preventive medicine.

Rose argued that population-based preventive measures must meet several criteria. First, they must be low cost. Second, interventions must be minimally invasive. Any intervention applied to an entire population must produce as little pain and discomfort as possible. Rose did not argue for changing the diagnostic threshold for treating disease, nor did he advocate for the use of high-cost pharmaceutical products (Rose, 1992). Nevertheless, Rose's arguments have been used to justify more aggressive treatment

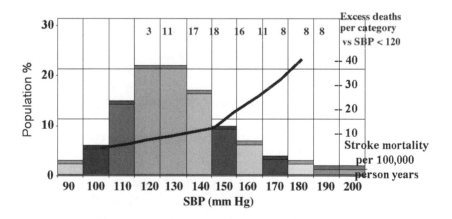

**FIGURE 19.1.** Population blood pressure and excess stroke mortality: the Whitehall study (Marmot & Poulter, 1992). Men 40–64 years old at entry; 18-year follow-up.

of CHD risk factors using expensive pharmaceutical interventions ("Summary of the Second Report," 1993).

Over the course of the last decade, there have been several changes in the thresholds for intervention on CHD risk factors (Schwartz & Woloshin, 1999). These thresholds are the points along the continuum where therapeutic intervention is recommended. The purpose of this chapter is to examine the rationale for these changes and to estimate the impact of changing diagnostic thresholds upon population health. Change in disease or risk factor identification may have at least three effects. First, it affects the number of people diagnosed and treated for risk factors. Second, it may have an effect on population health status. Third, changes in diagnostic thresholds may have a significant impact on health care costs. Rising health care costs have other effects, including an increase in the number of people who have no health insurance (Gilmer & Kronick, 2001).

## DEFINITION OF HEALTH OUTCOME

The purpose of health care is to improve health. We have argued that health outcomes should be defined in terms in both quantity and quality of life; a successful treatment is one that makes people live longer and/or improves quality of life (Kaplan, 1994; Kaplan & Wingard, 2000). If a treatment neither extends life expectancy nor improves life quality, we must challenge whether it has benefit. Similarly, the definition of disease must separate true disease from pseudodisease (Black & Welch, 1997). A true disease is one that impacts life expectancy or life quality. Prostate cancer that causes early death or causes symptoms prior to death is an example of true disease. On the other hand, prostate cancer discovered at autopsy, which was unknown to the patient or treating physician, might be considered pseudodisease. Diagnostic maneuvers that identify pathology that would never affect life course might lead to increased identification of pseudodisease, without the potential to improve population health (Welch & Black, 1997).

## THE DISEASE RESERVOIR HYPOTHESIS

Modern diagnostic technology has revealed that disease is common, particularly among older adults. If we look hard for disease, then we are likely to find it. Yet much of identified disease is pseudodisease (Welch & Black, 1997). If left alone, these conditions would have little effect. Organizations such as the American Cancer Society, the American Heart Association, the American Diabetes Association, and others have all advocated for the greater use of screening. They suggest that observed disease in the community is only the tip of the iceberg, and that population screening programs would identify a vast number of new cases. However, among these cases, although some will be true disease, the majority are likely to be pseudo-disease. As a result of this problem, considerable controversy has developed around the screening for common cancers, such as breast, prostate, and colorectal cancer (Black & Welch, 1997).

In each of the cancer examples, clinicians are faced with the presence of a tumor that can be identified by a pathologist. The controversy concerns whether the observed pathology has clinical significance—whether it is true disease or pseudodisease. In addition to problems identifying pathology, a new set of problems has recently emmerged. In some cases, the identification of a disease depends on the threshold defined by a peer committee. Based upon evidence-based reviews, consensus is used to pick a point along a continuum to define the threshold for disease. Schwartz and Woloshin (1999) discussed four changes in diagnostic thresholds for common health conditions. The Expert Committee on the Diagnosis and Classification of Diabetes Mellitus ("Report of the Expert Committee," 1997) recommended that the threshold for diabetes be changed from a fasting blood glucose level of 140 mg/dL to 126 mg/dL. More recently, the Expert Committee on the Diagnosis and Classification of Diabetes Mellitus recommended that the lower limit for impaired fasting glucose (IFG) be reduced from 110 mg/dL to 100 mg/dL (or down to 5.6 mmol/L; Genuth et al., 2003).

The Joint National Committee on Detection, Evaluation, and Treatment of High Blood Pressure recommended that the threshold for initiation of treatment of high blood pressure be moved from SBP of 160 mm Hg to 140 mm Hg. They also recommended the threshold for diagnosis of elevated diastolic pressure (DBP) be moved from 100 mm Hg down to 90 mm Hg. The most recent committee goes a step further by defining a new condition known as prehypertension. Individuals in this category have an SBP of 120–139 mm Hg or a DBP of 80–89 mm Hg (Chobanian et al., 2003). Following the Air Force/Texas Coronary Athroscorosis Prevention Study, an expert committee recommended that the threshold for hypercholesterolemia be reduced from 240 mg/dL down to 200 mg/dL. In terms of LDL cholesterol, early guidelines were concerned only with LDL levels above 200 mg/dL. Later, this threshold was moved to 160, then to 130; in 2004 it was lowered to 100 (Grundy et al., 2004).

Finally, the National Heart, Lung, and Blood Institute and the World Health Organization suggested that the threshold for being overweight be reduced from 27 kg/m$^2$ to 25 kg/m$^2$. Using data from the National Health and Nutrition Examination Survey (NHANES; "Plan and Operation," 1994), Schwartz and Woloshin (1999) estimated the number of new cases of diabetes, hypertension, hypercholesterolemia, and overweight created by changes in diagnostic thresholds. With a simple change in disease definition, diabetes increased 14%, hypertension increased 35%, overweight in-

creased 42%, and hypercholesterolemia increased 86%! Furthermore, few
people in the NHANES data set were ineligible for a chronic disease diagnosis. Considering just these four conditions, three out of four American
adults qualified for a treatable chronic condition. We recently reanalyzed
the NHANES data with these latest thresholds in mind. Figure 19.2 shows
the percentage of the age 60+ population eligible for a diagnosis under the
early guidelines, under the guidelines cited by Schwartz and Woloshin
(1999), and under the most recent proposals. For blood glucose, the threshold for concern increased from about 14% of the older adult population to
28%, and now to 88%. For SBP, the threshold increased from 35% to 55%
to 82%.

How will the changes in disease definition affect the number of individuals diagnosed, the health status of the population, and medical care
costs? In the following sections I explore these effects for three conditions:
hypertension, hypercholesterolemia, and overweight. Hypertension was
chosen as an example because it may represent the case with the best justifi-
cation for lowering diagnostic thresholds. Overweight is the case for which
evidence is weakest, and hypercholesterolemia is the intermediate case.

## HYPERTENSION

According to a variety of data sets, about 24% of the adult population
have prevalent hypertension (Burt et al., 1995). Using population surveys,
the proportion of the population with "hypertension," defined as SBP

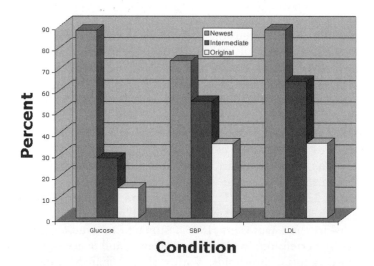

**FIGURE 19.2.** Percent of U.S. population age 60+ qualifying for diagnosis under different thresholds (based on analysis of NHANES).

greater than 140 mm Hg or DBP greater than 90 mm Hg, has remained stable over the last 40 years. However, the proportion of the population diagnosed by physicians and treated for hypertension has systematically increased (Vallbona & Pavlik, 1992). Changing the diagnostic threshold for hypertension from 160/95 to 140/90 approximately doubled the number of cases (Vallbona & Pavlik, 1992). Between 1970 and 2000, there were systematic increases in the proportion of people who were aware that they had hypertension, those treated for high blood pressure, and those whose blood pressure was controlled (Whelton et al., 2002).

It appears that more aggressive management of hypertension and the change in diagnostic threshold has produced results. For example, MacMahon (1990) pooled the results from seven observational studies with stroke outcomes and nine observational studies on CHD outcomes. The relative risk of stroke began to increase systematically with DBP exceeding 91mm Hg. Persons with DBPs at 105 mm Hg were nearly 3.5 times more likely to experience stroke than those with DBPs at 90 mm Hg or lower. Similarly, the risks for CHD doubled for those with a DBP of 105 mm Hg or higher (MacMahon, 1990). The Joint National Commission on High Blood Pressure noted that between 1960 and 1990, aggressive treatment of high blood pressure coincided with significant declines in stroke ("The Fifth Report," 1993). However, some questions have been raised. For example, the decrease in strokes exceeds what would be expected given studies on the effect of blood pressure control. In one analysis that pooled results from nine clinical trials, a 5.6 mm Hg decrease in DBP was associated with 38% decrease in stroke. Between 1970 and 1980, there was about a 1 mm Hg decline in DBP, which should have resulted in about an 18% decrease in stroke. However, the actual observed decline was 43%. The Minnesota Heart Study showed significant annual declines in stroke over the course of time, but the decline in stroke was uncorrelated with hypertension in that population (Luepker et al., 1988). Factors other than medical care may account for this decline.

In summary, changes in the diagnostic threshold have led to the identification of 13 million new cases of high blood pressure. The consequences of high blood pressure, including stroke and CHD, have systematically declined, and it appears that the change in diagnostic threshold has resulted in better population health. However, the observed decline in stroke and CHD has been much more rapid than would be expected from changes in blood pressure. Nevertheless, aggressive control of blood pressure seems most justified among the three examples we considered.

## LOWERING CHOLESTEROL

Following the Coronary Primary Prevention Trial ("The Lipid Research Clinics: I," 1984; "The Lipid Research Clinics: II," 1984), the National

Cholesterol Education Program has argued for the aggressive management of elevated serum cholesterol. Multiple arguments favor population-based lowering of cholesterol. Perhaps the two most persuasive arguments come from the Multiple Risk Factor Intervention Trial (MRFIT; Stamler et al., 2000) and the British Medical Research Council/British Heart Foundation Heart Protection Study ("MRC/BHF Heart Protection Study," 2002). The MRFIT study demonstrated that the relationship between total cholesterol and death from CHD over a 16- to 34-year interval was systematic and independent of the original level. Reducing total cholesterol from 300 to 280, for example, provided the same percentage reduction in death from CHD as would be afforded someone who reduced their total cholesterol from 220 to 200 (Stamler et al., 2000). Ironically, the MRFIT study was an intervention trial that failed to demonstrate a change for intervening on risk factors. (Multiple Risk Factor Intervention Trial Research Group, 1982).

The Coronary Primary Prevention Trial (CPPT) used cholestyramine to reduce elevated serum cholesterol for men at risk for CHD. Over the next decade, there was significant controversy about the benefits of lowering cholesterol. Meta-analyses consistently showed benefits for reduction in deaths from heart disease, but no benefit for total mortality (Muldoon, Manuck, & Matthews, 1991; Muldoon et al., 2001). Furthermore, there was concern that reductions in deaths from heart disease were compensated for by increases in deaths from other causes (Golomb, 1998).

The introduction of the statin medications helped to silence this controversy. Studies involving statins tended to show reductions in both deaths from heart disease and total mortality (Caro et al., 1997; Downs et al., 1998). Nevertheless, some controversy remained. The MRC/BHF Heart Protection Study was particularly important because it was large ($n = 20{,}536$) and randomized ("MRC/BHF Heart Protection Study," 2002). Perhaps the most interesting finding was that simvastatin was given to a wide range of individuals at risk for CHD. There was a benefit in terms of CHD mortality, irrespective of the initial cholesterol concentrations. Consumption of 40 mg of simvastatin daily was associated with reductions in myocardial infarction, stroke, and the number of the revascularization procedures. The study has been interpreted as suggesting the need for greater use of statin drugs in the population ("MRC/BHF Heart Protection Study," 2002). Despite widespread advocacy for the use of statins, controversy remains. For example, meta-analyses show no benefits of statin therapy for lowering total mortality in women (Walsh & Pignone, 2004).

Changing the diagnostic threshold for hypercholesterolemia may have profound effects on the number of people eligible for treatment. Figure 19.3, based on our recent analysis of the NHANES, shows that eligibility based on total cholesterol is approximately normally distributed in the population. Under the old diagnostic threshold of 240 mg/dL, about 35% of the population over age 60 is eligible for a diagnosis. With the first revision of the guidelines the number of eligible persons doubled to 70%, and under

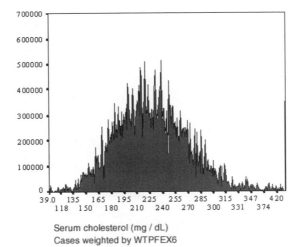

Serum cholesterol (mg / dL)
Cases weighted by WTPFEX6

**FIGURE 19.3.** Distribution of total cholesterol in the United States for adults age 60+. Data from NHANES 3 (analysis original).

the most recent proposal, nearly 95% of older adults are eligible for a diagnosis. From the NHANES weights, we estimated that about 40,101,197 Americans are age 60 or over. The change in diagnostic threshold takes the treatable population from about 14 million older adults to about 38 million— an increase of 166%.

It is clear that many more people will become eligible for treatment. How will this change in diagnostic threshold affect health outcome and cost?

To address this issue, we attempted to estimate the rate of cholesterol screening, the rate at which cholesterol-lowering agents will be prescribed, and the rate of compliance to cholesterol-lowering drugs. Using data reported by Nelson, Norris and Mangione (2002), we estimated that about 60% of the population would be screened for cholesterol and about 20% would receive a prescription for a lipid-lowering drug. Rates of compliance to drug therapy were estimated to be 70% in the Nelson et al. analysis, and were comparable for men and women. Simulation was used to estimate the expected benefit of lowering cholesterol for hypothetical cases. Figure 19.4 provides one example. Using Framingham equations available through the National Heart, Lung, and Blood Institute (NHLBI) and the Adult Treatment Panel (ATP-III) website, we estimated the absolute risk reduction for treatment of three persons. The first was a 55-year-old nonsmoker with an HDL of 50 and untreated SBP of 120. The second was a 60-year-old nonsmoker with an HDL of 30 and untreated systolic blood pressure of 140. The third case was a 65 year old smoker with an HDL of 30 and SBP treated to 130 mm Hg. The X-axis in the figure shows hypothetical baseline total cholesterol and assumes that treatment normalizes total choles-

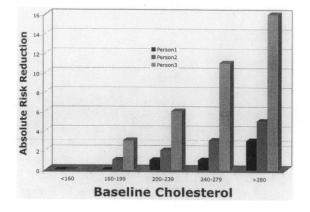

**FIGURE 19.4.** Change in absolute risk reduction for three hypothetical women. Adapted from Khaleghi and Kaplan (unpublished).

terol. Absolute risk reduction for persons 1 and 2 is relatively modest and increases linearly but slightly with increasing initial total cholesterol. Absolute risk reduction increases steeply for person 3, with multiple risk factors.

Figure 19.5 shows the number needed to treat to prevent one death given that the initial total cholesterol level was 240, 280, or 280. This analysis uses data from the MRFIT (Stamler et al., 2000) and assumes that treatment reducing total cholesterol to less than 200 mg/dL can be achieved, and that lowering cholesterol reduces risk to what has been observed for individuals with similar, low cholesterol levels in observational studies. We described this as the best case. The figure also shows the "best

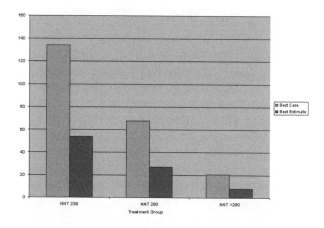
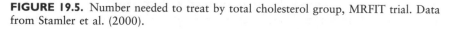

**FIGURE 19.5.** Number needed to treat by total cholesterol group, MRFIT trial. Data from Stamler et al. (2000).

estimate," which takes into consideration estimated rates of diagnosis, treatment, and compliance as reported by Nelson et al. (2002). Numbers needed to treat decreased dramatically as initial risk increases. However, cost remains relatively stable with increasing risk.

In collaboration with M. Khaleghi, I have been building models of the cost-effectiveness of interventions for heart disease prevention. Figures 19.6a and 19.6b show the cost-effectiveness of various diagnostic thresholds for men and women. The analysis focuses on dollars to reduce the absolute risk by one percentage point. As the figure shows, cost per unit reduction in absolute risk is a function of other risk factors and initial cholesterol level. In particular, the cost per unit reduction for low-risk men and women is very high, unless total cholesterol exceeds 240 mg/dL. These results are consistent with other reports in the literature. For example, Prosser et al. (2000) considered cost per quality adjusted life year (QALY) for treating elevated LDL cholesterol with pravastatin. Cost-effectiveness varied as a function of age and initial risk factors. The least efficient use of resources involved using medicine to treat elevated LDL in younger adults with no other risk factors.

In summary, statin medications have been remarkably successful in managing elevated serum cholesterol. However, the wisdom of using these medications for those with mildly elevated cholesterol values remains a matter of controversy. Although some benefit may be derived from treating those with total cholesterol values between 200 and 240, the costs will be substantial. About 30% of the adult population has total cholesterol values between 200 and 240 mg/dL. Risk of cardiovascular events is modified only slightly for these individuals, whereas cost of medication is similar to that for those at higher risk. The findings from the Heart Protection Study suggest that the benefits of lowering total cholesterol by 10 mg/dL are equivalent, independent of the initial total cholesterol level ("MRC/BHF Heart Protection Study," 2002). Similar conclusions were suggested by observational studies such as MRFIT (Stamler et al., 2000). The fallacy in these arguments, however, is that the goal of therapy is to reduce total cholesterol by 10 mg/dL. For individuals with initial values at 300 mg/dL, effective treatment is designed to reduce to total cholesterol by 100 mg/dL, whereas for the individual with initial values of 210 mg/dL, the goal of therapy may be a reduction of 10 mg/dL. Thus, the expected absolute risk reduction for the high-risk patient is considerably greater than what it would be for the low-risk patient.

## OVERWEIGHT

The body mass index (BMI) is calculated as weight in kilograms divided by height in meters squared. In 1998 the National Institute of Health (NIH)

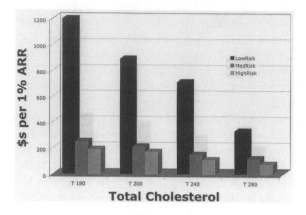

**FIGURE 19.6a.** Cost per 1% reduction in absolute risk for men.

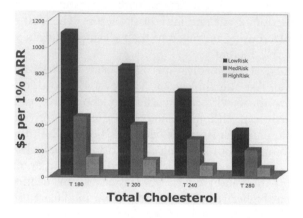

**FIGURE 19.6b.** Cost per 1% reduction in absolute risk for women.

and the World Health Organization (WHO) redefined standards for overweight and obesity based on BMI. Under the WHO classification, underweight is defined is a BMI less than 18.5, and normal weight is defined as a BMI between 18.5 and 24.9. The most controversial aspect of the new classification system was the change in threshold for overweight, from a BMI of 27 down to a BMI of 25. Obesity was defined as a BMI 30. There is legitimate concern about obesity in America. For example, NHANES showed that the rate of obesity in the United States increased from 23% in 1994 to over 30% in 2000 (Schwartz & Woloshin, 1999).

Concerns about the new definitions of overweight began to emerge when seemingly fit individuals were labeled as overweight. For example, a 5'9" man weighing 170 pounds is overweight. Extremely fit professional athletes, with very little body fat, qualify for obesity. For example, professional baseball player Barry Bonds has a BMI of approximately 30, which defines him as obese.

The rationale for overweight was based on epidemiological studies summarized by the NHLBI Joint National Commission on High Blood Pressure ("The Fifth Report," 1993). Considering the range of BMI between 25 and 30, there is a systematic, graded relationship between BMI and the percent of the population with elevated blood pressure for both men and women (see Figure 19.7), and a similar but weaker relationship was shown between BMI and the percentage of the population with elevated serum cholesterol (see Figure 19.8).

However, considering the BMI range of 25–27, there appears to be little or no relationship with health status outcomes. For example, we reviewed data reported by Allison, Fontaine, Manson, Stevens, and VanItallie (1999) summarizing major population studies from Alameda County; Framingham; Massachusetts; Tecumseh, Michigan; American Cancer Society Cancer Prevention Study; Nurses Health Study; and the NHANES. Relationships between BMI and mortality for each of these studies are summarized in Figure 19.9. Aggregated across studies, there is a U-shaped relationship, with BMI less than 23 associated with a slightly elevated risk and the risk of mortality beginning to increase with BMI's above 28. The range 25–27 appears flat.

Using data from the Rancho Bernardo cohort, we examined the relationship between BMI and health-related quality of life using the Quality of Well-Being Scale (Kaplan et al., 1998). Obese participants (BMI > 30) have significantly reduced quality-of-life scores. However, those with BMI scores between 25.0 and 29.9 do not differ significantly from persons of normal weight (Groessl, Kaplan, Barrett-Conner, & Ganiats, 2004). Similarly, we

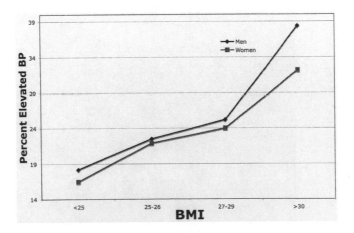

**FIGURE 19.7.** Relationship between BMI and high blood pressure. Data from NHLBI.

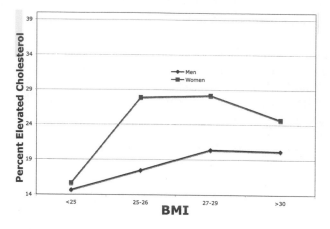

**FIGURE 19.8.** Relationship between BMI and high cholesterol. Data from NHLBI.

examined the relationship between BMI measured 15–20 years ago and current quality of life. Again, persons in the overweight category do not differ significantly from those with normal weight. There is a significant decline in quality of life for persons who are obese (BMI > 30) and an even more severe decrements for those who are severely obese (BMI > 35).

In summary, the reduction of the threshold for overweight from 27 to 25 created nearly 30 million new cases in the United States. In fact, nearly

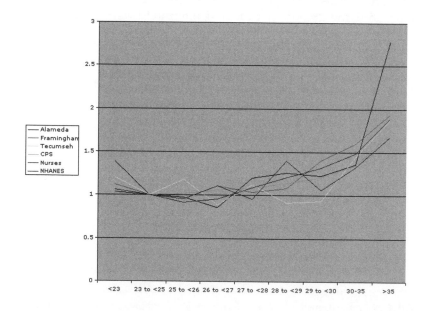

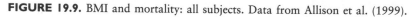

**FIGURE 19.9.** BMI and mortality: all subjects. Data from Allison et al. (1999).

65% of the American population now qualifies as being overweight or obese. Although being overweight may be related to risk factors, we find no evidence that individuals with BMI levels between 25 and 27 are at increased risk for mortality or for reduced-health related quality of life. Thus, aggressive treatment programs for individuals in this range will not produce population health benefits.

## THE COST PROBLEM

Geoffrey Rose promoted population-based medicine, because he felt it would be a better use of health care resources. He strongly advocated for behaviorally based population intervention programs. Clearly, he did not advocate for more aggressive population screening and for methods that would identify, in some cases, half of the population as having a "disease." One of the consequences of changes in diagnostic thresholds is that health care in the United States has become considerably more expensive. Change in the diagnostic thresholds for hypercholesterolemia, for example, created the potential for 45–55 million new cases to be treated.

Pharmaceutical costs are the most rapidly growing component of the health care system. The number of prescriptions in the United States went from 2 billion in 1992 to nearly 3 billion in 2002, an increase of 50% in just one decade. Low-income patients without prescription drug coverage may be forced to choose between food, rent, and expensive medications for chronic conditions such as hypercholesterolemia and hypertension.

A "back of the envelope" calculation estimates the impact of changing thresholds for hypercholesterolemia from 240 mg/dL to 200 mg/dL. We assume that patients would use Lipitor (atorvastatin) 40-mg tablets. The retail cost (from Epocrates) is $94.99 for 30 tablets, or just over $3 per pill. Zocor (simvastatin) costs $123.99 for 20-, 30-, or 40-mg tablets ($4.13 per tablet). Furthermore, we estimate that the compliance rate would be only 50%, but that the average patient would use the prescription for 20 years. We assume that only about one-third of the patients eligible for a diagnosis would actually get a prescription. Using these assumptions, we estimated that the lifetime cost per patient would be nearly $5,000 and that the market size would be as high as 30 million. Thus, the total cost of the change in diagnostic threshold would be $150,000,000,000. Of course, we must factor in the reduced cost to the health care system if heart attacks are prevented. Furthermore, significant savings might be gained from bulk purchase of the mediations or the use of generic equivalents (Russell & Wolff, 2002).

It is notable, however, that several of the top-selling pharmaceutical products are those for which mass markets have been opened up by changing diagnostic thresholds (Rosenthal, Berndt, Donohue, Frank, & Epstein, 2002). Lipid-lowering agents and antidepressants each have market sales greater than $6 billion per year.

## HOW DOES THIS AFFECT OLDER ADULTS?

Most older patients think about diagnoses and treatments in binary terms. A disease is either present or absent and the treatment is either effective or not effective. In the preceding sections I have argued that most biological processes are continua. Peer groups identify points along these continua as thresholds for diagnosis, but there is often debate about the selection of these points. Furthermore, many treatments offer benefit to only a small portion of those treated. The remainder pay the costs of the treatments and become exposed to the side effects without benefit.

In an ideal world, a patient could approach a physician with a list of symptoms and problems. The physician would identify the problem and administer a remedy. The service should be inexpensive and painless. However, this scenario is not common. For most medical decisions, judgments about disease are not perfectly reliable, and even when an early diagnosis is available, it is not always clear what treatment is the best option (Lenert & Kaplan, 2000). Choices about what treatments should be offered have typically been left to the physician. For a variety of reasons, however, patients are becoming activated in the decision process. These include changes in the standard of informed consent in making and implementing treatment decisions, increased access to information among patient through the Internet, and a growing recognition of the importance of patient preferences in making clinical decisions (Frosch & Kaplan, 1999).

Shared decision making is the process by which the patient and physician join in partnership to decide whether the patient should undergo diagnostic testing or which, if any, therapy to receive. Often, shared decision making involves formal decision aids that provide patients with detailed information about their options. The information is usually presented through interactive video disks, decision boards, descriptive consultations, or through the Internet (Frosch & Kaplan, 1999; Lenert & Cher, 1999). Using these decision aids, patients complete exercises to inform them of the risks and benefits of treatment options, then evaluate these with their physician relative to patient preferences for outcomes (Frosch & Kaplan, 1999).

Decision aids are valuable for both patients and physicians. One of the challenges of contemporary primary care medicine is that patient visits are short. Typically, the entire visit is limited to 15 minutes. During this time, the physician must greet the patient, do routine evaluations such as taking blood pressure, review medical history, determine the presenting complaint, perform a physical examination, make a diagnosis, write a prescription, discuss treatment plans, write notes in the patient's chart, and be on to the next patient. If at the end of this interaction, the patient asks a difficult question (e.g., "Should I be on hormone replacement therapy?"; "Should I get a PSA [prostate-specific antigen]; test?" or "Do I need a mammogram?"), the physician knows that there is not enough time to discuss the issue properly. For each of these issues, the literature is complex and conflicting. Instead of dealing with the complexity, it is much easier to simply say that the test or treatment is recommended. However, each of these decisions may have important consequences for the patient.

The decision to get a PSA test, for example, may lead to a significant chance of having a false-positive result, creating unnecessary anxiety, or heading down a pathway toward further evaluation. Not getting the test might mean that a cancer goes undetected. The decision whether to get the test is fiercely debated among scientists and physicians, and there is significant uncertainty as to whether the test is of value. Shared decision making allows patients to gain a better understanding of this uncertainty and to make an informed choice.

Shared decision making is not patient decision making. In other words, there are technical aspects of medical decisions for which patients are not be well equipped (Deber, Kraetschmer, & Irvine, 1996). For example, patients are not expected to know what approach to surgery is best, or the advantages or disadvantages of particular medications. On the other hand, patients have a perspective that only they fully understand. For instance, surgical treatment of prostate cancer may make a man impotent. For some men, this is a major concern, even at older ages. Other men may not be sexually active, and impotence may not be a concern. The patient provides the perspective that is typically unknown to the physician. Use of decision aids allows these preferences to be expressed. The patient's personal issues can be merged with the physician's technical concerns and dispassionate evaluation of risks and benefits.

Because time in medical encounters is so limited, shared decision making often involves a referral to a decision laboratory. The physician may advise the patient to use a decision aid, often under the supervision of another health care professional. Once the patient has interacted with the decision aid, physician and patient can efficiently address the key issues that are most relevant.

Although shared decision making is a relatively new field, several decision aids have now been evaluated (Weinstein, 2000). Further research is necessary to determine how to best present data on risks and benefits of different treatment options to the health care consumer (Edwards, Elwyn, Smith, Williams, & Thornton, 2001), but studies completed to date have shown that use of decision aids is associated with increases in patient knowledge about the problem in question, a greater subjective sense of feeling informed, more conservative treatment choices, and a greater desire to participate in medical decision making (O'Connor et al., 1999).

One specific example considered a decision aid to help men decide whether they should be screened for prostate cancer with the PSA test (Frosch, Kaplan, & Felitti, 2001). The men were all enrolled in a clinic that provides a wide variety of medical screening tests. In an experiment, the men were randomly assigned to one of four groups in a two-by-two factorial design. One factor was use of a decision video. Men either watched or did not watch a video that systematically reviewed the risks and benefits of PSA screening. The video featured a debate between a urologist who favored PSA screening and an internist who opposed PSA screening. Furthermore, the video systematically reviewed the probabilities of false positives, false negatives, and the risks of prostate cancer. It also systematically reviewed the evidence for the benefits of treatment for prostate cancer. The other factor in the experimental design was whether men had the opportunity to discuss the decision with others. The design resulted in four groups: usual care, discussion alone, video alone, and video plus discussion. All the men were asked whether they wanted the PSA test, and Frosch et al. obtained medical records to determine whether the test was completed.

The study showed that there was a systematic effect of the video and discussion groups. In the usual care control group, virtually all men (97%) got the PSA test. In other words, with no new information, men typically take the test. In the other groups, having more information led to a conservative bias. In contrast to the usual care control, men in the other groups were more sensitive to the risks of the test in relation to its benefits. Among those participating in the discussion group, 82% got the PSA test. For those watching the video, 63% completed the test. Those men watching the video and participating in those discussions had only a 50% PSA completion rate (see Figure 19.10). The study demonstrates that as patients become better informed, they are less likely to take the PSA test. The study also obtained information on patient knowledge. As knowledge increased, the likelihood of getting the PSA test deceased, stressing that better informed patients make more conservative decisions.

## CONCLUSION

It has been more than a decade since the publication of Geoffrey Rose's (1992) epic monograph, *The Strategy of Preventive Medicine*. Rose argued that we must be more aggressive in bringing prevention to the masses. Changes in the population distribution for risk factors can have substantial effects on population health. Rose's arguments have been used to stimulate more aggressive intervention for individuals previously thought not to need treatment. However, Rose's arguments may have been misused. He favored aggressive intervention using low-cost behavioral and public health methods. Instead, we have seen greater use of aggressive screening and interventions with high-cost pharmaceutical products.

One of the most interesting trends in current medicine is advocacy for the most expensive pharmaceutical interventions. For instance, evidence suggests that reserpine is an effective intervention for adults with high blood pressure. It is well tolerated and well proven in randomized clinical trials. However, reserpine is almost never used in current medicine. The cost of a 1-year supply of reserpine is less than the cost of a 1-week supply

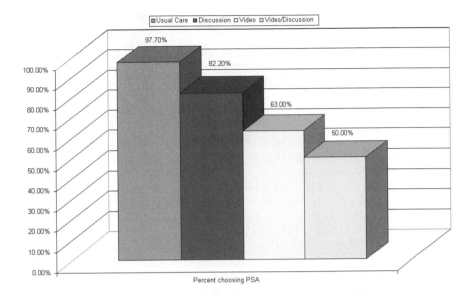

**FIGURE 19.10.** Men choosing PSA test by intervention group. Data from Frosch et al. (2001).

of currently advocated treatment (Lederle, Applegate, & Grimm, 1993). Cost has been ignored as a component of the decision process.

Choices to pursue the most expensive options create opportunity cost problems. Aggressive management of risk factors with expensive interventions uses resources that might have been put to better use elsewhere. For example, there appear to be only very modest benefits from treating low-spectrum disease. However, because of the need to comply with guidelines, many managed care plans use the lowered thresholds for treating common risk factors. Because their budgets are limited, they must give up funding other services. Smoking cessation programs, know to produce large health benefits, are common targets for elimination.

In summary, there have been significant reductions in diagnostic thresholds for many diseases or risk factors. These policy changes have had a significant impact on the number of individuals diagnosed and the number treated for various conditions. The impact on population health has been less clearly evaluated. In the case of hypertension, population health has probably benefited. It is also possible that population health benefits will result from the change in the definition of hypercholesterolemia. The population health benefit for changing the definition of overweight remains to be demonstrated. Changes in diagnostic thresholds have had an enormous impact on health care costs, particularly through the use of high-cost prescription medications. As a result, we may be losing the opportunity to invest precious health care resources in interventions where they will do more good.

# REFERENCES

Allison, D. B., Fontaine, K. R., Manson, J. E., Stevens, J., & VanItallie, T. B. (1999). Annual deaths attributable to obesity in the United States. *Journal of the American Medical Association, 282*(16), 1530–1538.

Black, W. C., & Welch, H. G. (1997). Screening for disease. *American Journal of Roentgenology, 168*(1), 3–11.

Burt, V. L., Whelton, P., Roccella, E. J., Brown, C., Cutler, J. A., Higgins, M., et al. (1995). Prevalence of hypertension in the us adult population: Results from the third National Health and Nutrition Examination Survey, 1988–1991. *Hypertension, 25*(3), 305–313.

Caro, J., Klittich, W., McGuire, A., Ford, I., Norrie, J., Pettitt, D., et al. (1997). The West of Scotland Coronary Prevention Study: Economic benefit analysis of primary prevention with pravastatin [see comments]. *British Medical Journal (Clinical Research Ed.), 315*(7122), 1577–1582.

Chobanian, A. V., Bakris, G. L., Black, H. R., Cushman, W. C., Green, L. A., Izzo, J. L., Jr., et al. (2003). The seventh report of the Joint National Committee on Prevention, Detection, Evaluation, and Treatment of High Blood Pressure: The JNC 7 report. *Journal of the American Medical Association, 289*(19), 2560–2572.

Deber, R. B., Kraetschmer, N., & Irvine, J. (1996). What role do patients wish to play in treatment decision making? *Archives of Internal Medicine, 156*(13), 1414–1420.

Downs, J. R., Clearfield, M., Weis, S., Whitney, E., Shapiro, D. R., Beere, P. A., et al. (1998). Primary prevention of acute coronary events with lovastatin in men and women with average cholesterol levels: Results of AFCAPS/TEXCAPS: Air Force/Texas Coronary Atherosclerosis Prevention Study [see comments]. *Journal of the American Medical Association, 279*(20), 1615–1622.

Edwards, A., Elwyn, G., Smith, C., Williams, S., & Thornton, H. (2001). Consumers' views of quality in the consultation and their relevance to "shared decision-making" approaches. *Health Expectations, 4*(3), 151–161.

The fifth report of the Joint National Committee on Detection, Evaluation, and Treatment of High Blood Pressure (JNC V). (1993). *Archives of Internal Medicine, 153*(2), 154–183.

Frosch, D. L., & Kaplan, R. M. (1999). Shared decision making in clinical medicine: Past research and future directions. *American Journal of Preventive Medicine, 17*(4), 285–294.

Frosch, D. L., Kaplan, R. M., & Felitti, V. (2001). The evaluation of two methods to facilitate shared decision making for men considering the prostate-specific antigen test. *Journal of General Internal Medicine, 16*(6), 391–398.

Genuth, S., Alberti, K. G., Bennett, P., Buse, J., Defronzo, R., Kahn, R., et al. (2003). Follow-up report on the diagnosis of diabetes mellitus. *Diabetes Care, 26*(11), 3160–3167.

Gilmer, T., & Kronick, R. (2001). Calm before the storm: Expected increase in the number of uninsured Americans. *Health Affairs (Project Hope), 20*(6), 207–210.

Goldstein, L. B., Adams, R., Becker, K., Furberg, C. D., Gorelick, P. B., Hademenos, G., et al. (2001). Primary prevention of ischemic stroke: A statement for healthcare professionals from the Stroke Council of the American Heart Association. *Stroke, 32*(1), 280–299.

Golomb, B. A. (1998). Cholesterol and violence: Is there a connection? *Annals of Internal Medicine, 128*(6), 478–487.

Groessl, E. J., Kaplan, R. M., Barrett-Connor, E., & Ganiats, T. G. (2004). Body mass index and quality of well-being in a community of older adults. *American Journal of Preventive Medicine, 26*(2), 126–129.

Grundy, S. M., Cleeman, J. I., Merz, C. N., Brewer, H. B., Jr., Clark, L. T., Hunninghake, D. B., et al. (2004). Implications of recent clinical trials for the National Cholesterol Education Program Adult Treatment Panel III guidelines. *Circulation, 110*(2), 227–239.

Howard, G., & Howard, V. J. (2001). Ethnic disparities in stroke: The scope of the problem. *Ethnicity and Disease, 11*(4), 761–768.

Kaplan, R. M. (1994). The ziggy theorem: Toward an outcomes-focused health psychology. *Health Psychology, 13*(6), 451–460.

Kaplan, R. M., Ganiats, T. G., Sieber, W. J., & Anderson, J. P. (1998). The Quality of Well-Being Scale: Critical similarities and differences with SF-36 [see comments]. *International Journal for Quality in Health Care, 10*(6), 509–520.

Kaplan, R. M., & Wingard, D. L. (2000). Trends in breast cancer incidence, survival, and mortality. *Lancet, 356*(9229), 592–593.

Khaleghi, M., & Kaplan, R. M. (2006). *Effects of changing illness thresholds on healthcare costs and health outcomes.* University of California, San Diego, unpublished manuscript.

Lederle, F. A., Applegate, W. B., & Grimm, R. H., Jr. (1993). Reserpine and the medical marketplace. *Archives of Internal Medicine, 153*(6), 705–706.

Lenert, L., & Kaplan, R. M. (2000). Validity and interpretation of preference-based measures of health-related quality of life. *Medical Care, 38*(Suppl. 9), II138–II150.

Lenert, L. A., & Cher, D. J. (1999). Use of meta-analytic results to facilitate shared decision making. *Journal of the American Medical Informatics Association, 6*(5), 412–419.

The Lipid Research Clinics Coronary Primary Prevention Trial results: I. Reduction in incidence of coronary heart disease. (1984). *Journal of the American Medical Association, 251*(3), 351–364.

The Lipid Research Clinics Coronary Primary Prevention Trial results: II. The relationship of reduction in incidence of coronary heart disease to cholesterol lowering. (1984). *Journal of the American Medical Association, 251*(3), 365–374.

Luepker, R. V., Jacobs, D. R., Jr., Folsom, A. R., Gillum, R. F., Frantz, I. D., Jr., Gomez, O., et al. (1988). Cardiovascular risk factor change—1973–74 to 1980–82: The Minnesota Heart Survey. *Journal of Clinical Epidemiology, 41*(9), 825–833.

MacMahon, S. (1990). Antihypertensive drug treatment: The potential, expected and observed effects on vascular disease. *Journal of Hypertension: Supplement, 8*(7), S239–S244.

Marmot, M. G., & Poulter, N. R. (1992). Primary prevention of stroke. *Lancet, 339*(8789), 344–347.

MRC/BHF Heart Protection Study of cholesterol lowering with simvastatin in 20,536 high-risk individuals: A randomised placebo-controlled trial. (2002). *Lancet, 360*(9326), 7–22.

Muldoon, M. F., Manuck, S. B., & Matthews, K. A. (1991). Does cholesterol lowering increase non-illness-related mortality? *Archives of Internal Medicine, 151*(7), 1453–1454.

Muldoon, M. F., Manuck, S. B., Mendelsohn, A. B., Kaplan, J. R., & Belle, S. H. (2001). Cholesterol reduction and non-illness mortality: Meta-analysis of randomised clinical trials. *British Medical Journal, 322*(7277), 11–15.

Multiple Risk Factor Intervention Trial Research Group. (1982). Multiple risk factor intervention trial: Risk factor changes and mortality results. *Journal of the American Medical Association, 248*(12), 1465–1477.

Nelson, K., Norris, K., & Mangione, C. M. (2002). Disparities in the diagnosis and pharmacologic treatment of high serum cholesterol by race and ethnicity: Data from the third National Health and Nutrition Examination Survey. *Archives of Internal Medicine, 162*(8), 929–935.

O'Connor, A. M., Rostom, A., Fiset, V., Tetroe, J., Entwistle, V., Llewellyn-Thomas, H., et al. (1999). Decision aids for patients facing health treatment or screening decisions: Systematic review [comment]. *British Medical Journal, 319*(7212), 731–734.

Plan and operation of the third National Health and Nutrition Examination Survey, 1988–94: Series 1. Programs and collection procedures. (1994). *Vital Health Statistics, 1*(32), 1–407.

Prosser, L. A., Stinnett, A. A., Goldman, P. A., Williams, L. W., Hunink, M. G., Goldman, L., et al. (2000). Cost-effectiveness of cholesterol-lowering therapies according to selected patient characteristics. *Annals of Internal Medicine, 132*(10), 769–779.

Report of the Expert Committee on the Diagnosis and Classification of Diabetes Mellitus. (1997). *Diabetes Care, 20*(7), 1183–1197.

Rose, G., & Day, S. (1990). The population mean predicts the number of deviant individuals. *British Medical Journal, 301*(6759), 1031–1034.

Rose, G. A. (1992). *The strategy of preventive medicine.* Oxford, UK/New York: Oxford University Press.

Rosenthal, M. B., Berndt, E. R., Donohue, J. M., Frank, R. G., & Epstein, A. M. (2002). Promotion of prescription drugs to consumers. *New England Journal of Medicine, 346*(7), 498–505.

Russell, L. B., & Wolff, N. (2002). The impact of drug pricing policies on the health of the elderly. *American Journal of Preventive Medicine, 22*(3), 151–155.

Schwartz, L. M., & Woloshin, S. (1999). Changing disease definitions: Implications for disease prevalence: Analysis of the third National Health and Nutrition Examination Survey, 1988–1994. *Effective Clinical Practice, 2*(2), 76–85.

Stamler, J., Daviglus, M. L., Garside, D. B., Dyer, A. R., Greenland, P., & Neaton, J. D. (2000). Relationship of baseline serum cholesterol levels in 3 large cohorts of younger men to long-term coronary, cardiovascular, and all-cause mortality and to longevity. *Journal of the American Medical Association, 284*(3), 311–318.

Summary of the second report of the National Cholesterol Education Program (NCEP) Expert Panel on Detection, Evaluation, and Treatment of High Blood Cholesterol in Adults (Adult Treatment Panel II). (1993). *Journal of the American Medical Association, 269*(23), 3015–3023.

Vallbona, C., & Pavlik, V. (1992). Advances in the community control of hypertension: From epidemiology to primary care practice. *Journal of Hypertension: Supplement, 10*(7), S51–S57.

Walsh, J. M., & Pignone, M. (2004). Drug treatment of hyperlipidemia in women. *Journal of the American Medical Association, 291*(18), 2243–2252.

Weinstein, J. N. (2000). The missing piece: Embracing shared decision making to reform health care. *Spine, 25*(1), 1–4.

Welch, H. G., & Black, W. C. (1997). Using autopsy series to estimate the disease "reservoir" for ductal carcinoma *in situ* of the breast: How much more breast cancer can we find? *Annals of Internal Medicine, 127*(11), 1023–1028.

Whelton, P. K., He, J., Appel, L. J., Cutler, J. A., Havas, S., Kotchen, T. A., et al. (2002). Primary prevention of hypertension: Clinical and public health advisory from the National High Blood Pressure Education Program. *Journal of the American Medical Association, 288*(15), 1882–1888.

# CHAPTER 20

# Health Psychology and Aging

## Moving to the Next Generation of Research

CAROLYN M. ALDWIN, CRYSTAL L. PARK,
and AVRON SPIRO III

This handbook opened with the simple question: Are older adults more or less vulnerable to stressors than younger adults? We asked health psychologists to consider the role of aging in their models, and gerontologists to consider the role of health in their models. In most of the chapters, the answer was "We don't know yet." For the most part, the extant research does not provide a sufficient basis to answer the question. Comparative studies of this sort have seldom been conducted, and most of these have been cross-sectional. Thus, nearly all of the authors called for longitudinal studies to investigate how particular processes change with age. However, the various chapters contain hints as to what the answer to our question might be, and most of the authors took advantage of this wide-open situation to develop possible models. Thus, our aim in this chapter is to examine those proposed models to find common threads as a means of gaining insight into how psychosocial factors can affect the aging process.

In examining the current state of the literature, we borrow the framework of Friedman and Brownell (1995), who, in their review of obesity research, argued that the development of research fields follows a particular pattern. In the first generation of research, the main research design is comparative; that is, two groups are compared, often on a single variable, and inconsistent results are often found. Thus, in the health psychology and aging field, early studies simply asked, "Do older adults have more or less of X than do younger adults?" Examples of X could include stress, stress hormones, or immune factors. Thus, it is not surprising that there is much inconsistency in these early studies.

In the second generation of research, according to Friedman and Brownell (1995), researchers begin examining clusters of risk factors within a given population, using more sophisticated analytical designs, and begin to identify who is at risk. In the third generation, prospective designs are used, with multiple types of measures assessed at frequent intervals, and development of sophisticated analytical models leading to the identification of causes and effects.

As all good developmentalists know, there are limitations to simple stage theories. However, it is reasonably safe to conclude that health psychology and aging research is, at best, in the early stages of the second generation of research. The value of this book lies not only in the compilation and synthesis of the extant knowledge of health psychology and aging but also in the development of different models, which, we hope, will allow us to progress to the third generation of research.

## EMERGING THEMES

In Chapter 3, Berg, Smith, Henry, and Pearce argue that the roots of successful aging lie in early developmental processes. However, they argue, it is a mistake simply to have cognitive and physical functioning as outcomes of psychosocial processes. Rather, they argue for transactional models of adaptation across the lifespan, in which cognitive and physical functioning play a role in successful psychosocial adaptation to changing roles. In contrast, health psychologists Young and Vitaliano (Chapter 4) organize the emerging stress–illness–mortality model around the primary–secondary aging distinction in gerontology. They argue that normative, age-related changes in the body's reserve capacity lead to changes in the ability to adapt to stress. The combination of primary aging in stress-response systems, coupled with the emergence of chronic stress in later life, leads to an increased vulnerability to secondary aging, or disease. This argument parallels that found in the biogerontology literature—that the hallmark of aging is the decreased capacity to response to stress (see Aldwin & Gilmer, 2004, for a review). However, Young and Vitaliano emphasize that psychosocial factors such as health behavior habits may moderate the rate of primary aging and decreases in reserve capacity.

The three chapters in the biological issues section of this volume examine in depth several biological pathways that can result in increased vulnerability in later life. Gruenewald and Kemeny (Chapter 6) examine the inflammatory process, which is regulated by neuroendocrine and immune factors. Dysregulation of biological systems and heightened inflammatory processes underlie many of the chronic illnesses found in later life, especially cardiovascular disease and cognitive impairment. However, psychosocial factors, such as social support and positive mood, may moderate inflammatory processes, and may thus be especially protective in later life.

Epel, Burke, and Wolkowitz (Chapter 7) focus on the anabolic/catabolic balance in the neuroendocrine system. Whereas anabolic hormones promote tissue growth, catabolic processes promote the necessary breakdown of the tissues. Nearly all biological systems reflect this balance. The skeleton is a prime example, with bone buildup and breakdown occurring at all points in the lifespan; the relative balance between anabolic and catabolic processes determines whether the skeleton continues growing and increases in density, or becomes less dense and therefore more frail. Epel et al. argue that changes in the anabolic/catabolic balance may presage the development of overt disease in later life, including osteoporosis, atherosclerosis, cognitive impairment, and depression. Increases in basal levels of a stress-related hormone, cortisol, may antedate changes in the anabolic/catabolic balance, again placing stress squarely in the rate of aging equation. Psychosocial factors such as exercise, benefit finding, and social support may support a healthier anabolic/catabolic balance.

Cooper, Katzel, and Waldstein (Chapter 8) examine cardiovascular reactivity to stress as the underlying mechanism for all forms of cardiovascular disease. Again, the balance between sympathetic and parasympathetic tone regulates age-related changes in heart rate variability, with a low variability (responsiveness) related to cardiovascular morbidity and mortality. Psychosocial factors also contribute to the development of poor cardiovascular reactivity, with hostility, depression, chronic stress, and health behavior habits such as smoking all increasing its likelihood.

A clear pattern has emerged from these chapters. The three primary factors underlying both primary and secondary aging are inflammatory processes, anabolic/catabolic balance, and cardiovascular reactivity. In most of the instances, these processes each become more dysregulated with age and these changes both lead to and are accelerated by disease. The unifying factor in all of these dysregulating processes is stress, which affects patterns of regulation and dysregulation. However, psychosocial factors may moderate all of these processes, providing theoretical insights into how the psychosocial context may influence aging processes. Thus, the third section of the book examines key psychosocial factors and their effects on health.

From a biological point of view, the surprising thing is how many psychosocial factors moderate the aging process, including personality and mental health, sense of control, coping, social support, and religiousness. Berg et al. (Chapter 3) remind us of the untoward effect of hostility on many aspects of health, and how it can undermine positive factors such as social support. While admitting the existence of a "disease prone personality," Friedman and Martin (Chapter 9) also describe a "self-healing personality," in which a key factor may be the trait of conscientiousness. Conscientious individuals are not only more likely to avoid poor health behaviors, such as smoking and excessive drinking, but are also more likely to have successful careers and marriages—all factors leading to greater longevity.

Health psychologists have long investigated sense of control as a major factor in health, especially in later life. As Skaff (Chapter 10) points out, though, the prevailing "primary–secondary" model, with "primary" referring to control over external events and "secondary" referring to control over internal states, may be too simplistic. There are many different ways of conceptualizing control, from global senses to those that are domain-specific. Furthermore, there are cultural, societal, and cohort differences in control and what it means. For example, in some cultures, control over internal states is central to any sort of action. Thus, disentangling the relationships among age, control, and health is highly complex, although there is some evidence that a sense of control does have positive effects on health in later life.

Coping shows a similarly complex relationship with age. According to Aldwin, Yancura, and Boeninger (Chapter 11), whether coping changes with age depends upon the conceptualization of coping. Again, very few studies examine whether (and which) coping strategies are particularly efficacious for older adults. Some tantalizing hints in the literature indicate that there may be qualitative shifts in coping in later life, with older adults more likely to conserve resources and refocus on meaning. Furthermore, age-appropriate coping may be efficacious in at least maintaining positive mental health. Aldwin et al. point out that many studies of coping with chronic disease utilize older samples, but almost none have examined how these processes vary by age. The few that do suggest that coping may have greater impact on health in relatively healthy samples, but that chronic disease may overwhelm any beneficial effect of individuals' coping efforts.

All too often, chronic illness in later life is paired with caregiving. Fortinsky, Tennen, Frank, and Affleck (Chapter 12; also Young & Vitaliano, Chapter 4) review the tremendous amount of evidence that caregiving is a chronic stressor that affects many different aspects of psychological well-being and physical health, especially among those with prior health conditions. It is even associated with higher levels of mortality (Schulz & Beach, 1999). Caregiving for patients with Alzheimer's disease is particularly stressful, especially for women. However, certain types of coping strategies, including benefit-finding and cognitive-behavioral problem solving, appear to mitigate the stressfulness of caregiving and result in long-term positive outcomes. In part, finding benefits may have positive outcomes because it helps individuals to focus on positive emotions during times of stress.

Davis, Zautra, Johnson, Murray, and Okvat (Chapter 13) review evidence that positive emotions are associated with better psychological, cognitive, and physical health, including better cardiovascular and immune function, and may even predict greater longevity. Older adults are better at focusing on positive experiences and avoiding negative ones than are younger adults, and emotional complexity is thought to increase with age. Under stress, however, affective structure tends to simplify; rather than relatively independent dimensions, positive and negative affect become more closely linked. Individuals who are more adept at emotion regulation are more able to maintain complex emotional processing under stress, thus maintaining positive emotions in the face of stress.

Another way of maintaining positive affect in the face of stress, including disability, in later life is to maintain close, harmonious personal ties with others (Rook, Mavandadi, Sorkin, & Zettel, Chapter 14); social support has also been positively associated with multiple dimensions of health. However, social support can lead to worse outcomes if there is a pattern of negative interaction patterns, or if one's social support network encourages the adoption of a "sick role," which can lead to greater functional disability. Certain coping strategies, such as forgiveness or emotional self-restraint, may mitigate the harmful effects of negative social interactions, and more work is needed to understand dyadic coping strategies in later life.

Yee and Chiriboga (Chapter 15) remind us that the impact of both culture and gender on aging and health processes is highly understudied. They present the intriguing hypothesis that one reason women and members of ethnic minorities appear to be more vulnerable to the effects of stress is a problem of power differential, which may lead to impaired emotion regulation. This is particularly interesting in light of Park's (Chapter 16) observation that religion and spirituality are most likely to have positive associations with health in members of minority communities. This suggests that some of the discrepancy in the religion–health literature reflects a lack of attention to the function of religion and religious coping. Pargament, Koenig, and Perez (2000) differentiate between positive and negative religious coping. One could hypothesize that religious coping that serves to enhance emotional regulation may be associated with better health, whereas those religious coping strategies that result in negative emotional arousal may be harmful to health.

Thus, the common theme running through the psychosocial chapters is that of emotion regulation. Personality, social support, coping, gender, culture, and religiousness all play a role in the regulation of emotion, which in turn is hypothesized to assist in physiological regulation. Thus, it is not surprising that this theme also emerges in the clinical chapters. Leventhal, Forster, and Leventhal (Chapter 17) explicitly examine aging and self-regulation. In later life, chronic illnesses are the norm, requiring a great deal of self-management, which in turn is dependent on how one perceives physical symptoms. Leventhal et al. have developed a complex model identifying the lay heuristics that individuals use to recognize and categorize pain, including location, rate of change, novelty, and duration, and have shown how misidentification of the cause and importance of symptoms may lead to inadequate coping and more dysfunction. The authors call for more work with health care providers to assist older adults in self-management.

Qualls and Benight (Chapter 18) review interventions to enhance management of chronic illness in later life. Typical interventions include both psychoeducational and cognitive-behavioral aspects, but those that specifically target older adults are rare (despite the fact that older adults are highly overrepresented in the chronically ill population). The few studies that have focused specifically on older adults often find very positive outcomes of interventions on diabetes and heart disease, but it is unclear how these programs were modified to accommodate the needs of older adults. Sadly, there are no studies of age-specific interventions for cancer patients, despite the dramatic increase in incidence of cancer in later life. Depression may also be underdiagnosed in older adults, especially those who are chronically ill, and little is known about the efficacy of interventions there. Families play a key role in helping to manage chronic illnesses, and understanding how to promote their positive involvement is also important.

Kaplan (Chapter 19), however, raises serious questions about the value of medical interventions in later life. He points out the dangers inherent in medicalizing old age and presents some very sobering statistics showing that empirically substantiated medical interventions may reduce disease-specific morbidity and mortality but not have much effect on all-cause mortality. This leads to the serious question: What should be the goal of intervention? Is the aim longer life, or increased quality of life?

## TOWARD A LIFESPAN DEVELOPMENTAL THEORY OF HEALTH AND OPTIMAL AGING

Golub and Langer (Chapter 2) point out that theories are absolutely necessary for organizing knowledge, but that basic assumptions may end up doing more harm than good. In particular, they take exception to the idea that "age is associated only with biological decline, and that the major developmental task of aging is coping with loss" (p. 16). Even among those theories that include supposedly positive development, this is typically defined as compensation for age-related deficits. They argue that "these assumptions may increase vulnerability to health problems among older adults to the extent to which they are unquestioningly applied to all older persons irrespective of context" (p. 17). In other words, theories that assume that aging is synonymous with decline feed into negative stereotypes of aging, and Levy, Slade, Kunkel, and Kasl (2002) have shown that individuals who adopt these negative stereotypes are at greater risk for premature mortality. Golub and Langer (Chapter 2) argue that it is time for developmental theories to look at aging in a new light, one that focuses on what new abilities emerge in later life, instead of couching everything in terms of loss of old abilities.

Spiro (Chapter 5) has provided a broad theoretical framework for what a lifespan developmental approach to health and aging should look like. He identifies four basic tenets of a lifespan developmental approach: (1) development is lifelong; (2) it is pluralistic, requiring a multidisciplinary approach; (3) it is located within a contextual worldview; and (4) there are individual differences in developmental pathways. Using this theoretical approach, we attempt to synthesize the findings of this volume to present a preliminary theory of how vulnerability and resilience to psychosocial stress may change across the life course, using the self-regulation rubric.

## Development Is Lifelong

The development of self-regulatory processes begins quite early in life (Eisenberg & Zhou, 2000). At first, parents regulate infants' emotional reactions, but gradually young children learn to regulate themselves. This process consists of learning not only coping strategies to regulate emotions but also, more generally, strategies to regulate both the internal and external expression of emotions in culturally appropriate ways. Both processes are based on the effortful regulation of attention; that is, being able to shift and refocus attention, as well as use cognitive distraction. Self-regulation also includes strategies such as positive cognitive restructuring. Note that this also can serve to regulate social interaction, which is based upon the recognition of and response to emotional cues.

Aldwin and Levenson (2005) suggested that these self-regulatory processes also underlie the development of emotional maturity in early adulthood. They identified several components of emotional maturity, including increased emotional stability, acceptance of responsibility for one's own actions, and the ability to self-generate goals and goal-related activity, but also the ability to modify them according to environmental demands and contingencies, to accept critical feedback, and to work in group settings. Thus, emotional maturity combines a complex pattern of emotional stability, but with sufficient direction and enthusiasm to provide motivation to pursue goals, as well as autonomy combined with the ability to work cooperatively. This echoes Davis et al.'s (Chapter 13) acknowledgment of increasing emotional complexity with age, which allows both positive and negative emotions to be relatively autonomous. Furthermore, emotional complexity allows one to find benefits in stressful situations, presumably leading to stress-related growth. This suggests a parallel—that the type of complexity of self-regulation hypothesized by Aldwin and Levenson (2005) might also promote stress-related growth.

Other psychosocial protective factors may also show increased complexity with age. Rook et al. (Chapter 14) remind us that social support dynamics change, with some older individuals focusing more on close, personal relationships. Similarly, Skaff (Chapter 10) also supports the notion that control may increase in complexity with age, as simplistic, global notions of control give way to more differentiated, domain-specific control—including not only external domains but also internal ones. The idea of attention regulation and cognitive restructuring hypothesized to underlie self-regulation may also help explain Aldwin et al.'s (Chapter 1) findings that older individuals are less likely to appraise situations as being problematic. Park's (Chapter 16) assertion that older adults may derive greater health-related benefits from religiousness/spirituality also suggests that the latter may also play a role in self-regulation in later life. All of these factors may help to explain how older individuals are able to focus more on positive emotions than on negative ones (Davis et al., Chapter 13), which in turn may enable older adults to avoid the sort of negative neuroendocrine cascades associated with stress. *Thus, there are health-related trajectories that develop over the lifespan.*

## Development Requires a Multidisciplinary Approach

Changes in physiology with age underlie vulnerability to *physical* stressors, and both primary and secondary age-related changes feed into this process. Thus, *ceteris paribus*, older adults may be physiologically vulnerable to *psychosocial stressors* as well, to the extent that these trigger a cascade of physiological reactions that older adults are likely to find more difficult to regulate. However, *ceteris* are not always *paribus*—that is, all things are not equal for all people, and a variety of factors may protect older adults from this increased vulnerability. For example, there well may be survivor effects; that is, individuals who survive until late life may be those who are more resilient to the effects of stress. Thus, Williams's (2000) findings that hostility may have its greatest adverse effects in midlife, while having little effect in later life, may reflect the fact that individuals with less healthy cardiovascular systems simply do not make it to late life. Berg et al. (Chapter 3) present a cogent case for recursive processes among psychological, cognitive, and physical health throughout the lifespan, arguing for a dynamic, transactional model of development across domains in adulthood. *In short, there are interlocking trajectories of health-related factors across the lifespan.*

## Contextual Issues

Individual health does not exist independent of context. Growing evidence suggests that successive cohorts are becoming healthier, with changes in nutrition, public health, and medicine providing optimal aging opportunities to develop across the lifespan. Other contextual factors may provide adverse influences. In particular, the epidemic of obesity in this country may well lead to both increased vulnerability in later life and a shortened lifespan (Aldwin, Spiro, & Park, 2006). In addition, factors in the immediate context may also provide an opportunity for change. For example, a health scare or the birth of a child may provide prompt changes in health behavior habits.

In life-course theory, such opportunities for change are called "turning points" (Elder & Shanahan, 2006). Turning points may be related to the larger organization of the society (e.g., institutions that help adolescents transition to adulthood, such as the military or higher education), or they may be more closely linked to the individual's microcontext, (e.g., developing a relationship with a mentor, or hooking up with the "wild crowd" in high school and adopting very risky behaviors). *These turning points provide opportunities for change, whether positive or negative, that may affect the developmental course of health-related trajectories.*

## There Are Individual Differences in Development

A core tenet of a lifespan developmental approach to health psychology and aging is that there are individual differences in optimal aging. A major contribution of this volume is the suggestion that older adults can develop psychosocial resistance factors that forestall psychoneuroendocrine cascades in response to stress. In other words, there may be quantitative and qualitative changes in self-regulation with age may protect individuals from adverse consequences of psychosocial stress, thus contributing to optimal aging.

Mroczek, Spiro, Griffin, and Neupert (in press) discussed the problems of older adults who have failed to develop adequate regulatory processes. "Kindling," defined as heightened reactivity to stress, may be a function of personality traits such as neuroticism, prior exposure to trauma, or mental illness. Mroczek et al. present evidence that individuals who remain high in neuroticism in late life have far higher negative affect levels in response to daily stressors than any other age group. In contrast, older adults who are low in neuroticism report the lowest negative affect levels of any group. Older adults who are high in emotional stability may be most likely to exhibit optimal physical and mental aging (Aldwin, Levenson, Spiro, & Cupertino, 2001).

Thus, older adults who are able to self-regulate successfully in later life may focus on forestalling the stress process. Indeed, if they are physiologically more vulnerable to stress, then it makes sense that those individuals who survive to old age have developed ways to appraise situations to decrease the amount of stress they experience (Boeninger, Shiraishi, Aldwin, & Spiro, 2006), thereby avoiding stress-related neuroendocrine cascades that would disrupt their homeostasis. These strategies might focus on the positive aspects of the situation and their social support networks, be flexible in their goals to realistically reflect their abilities and environmental opportunities, focus on those aspects of the situation and their selves that they can control, and use religion and/or spirituality to help them deal with less controllable problems.

Aldwin and Gilmer (2004) argued that a wisdom, critical but neglected element of successful aging in later life, may be one of those positive abilities that Golub and Langer (Chapter 2) argue may emerge in later adulthood.

Using data from the Normative Aging Study, Jennings, Aldwin, Levenson, Spiro, and Mroczek (2006) found that stress-related growth predicted self-reported wisdom some 14 years later in a sample of middle-aged and older men. Thus, self-regulation gives rise to emotional maturity, which allows benefit finding and other aspects of stress-related growth to develop, which in turn may eventually result in wisdom. Wisdom may not be unique to older adults, and certainly not all older adults are wise, reflecting individual differences in this developmental process. Furthermore, what is considered wise may vary across cultures and cohorts, reflecting contextual contingencies. Nonetheless, wisdom may be a resource that both develops under stressful conditions and allows one better regulatory control under stress.

Figure 20.1 presents a diagram of this theoretical model. It described two different trajectories that might stem from childhood stress: kindling and resilience. Early childhood stress, in the context of childhood poverty and poor social support, may lead to impulsive behaviors. These may in turn lead to increased exposure to stressors, especially if individuals adopt negative coping behaviors, such as escapism, or external regulation of emotions through drug and alcohol use. In turn, these may lead to the early onset of chronic illnesses in midlife, such as cardiovascular disease or diabetes, creating an increased physiological vulnerability to stress in later life.

In contrast, childhood stress in the context of supportive environments may lead to the development of emotional maturity and positive coping

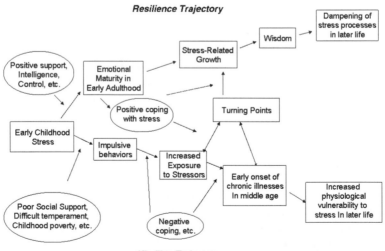

**FIGURE 20.1.** Theoretical model describing two trajectories.

strategies. In turn, this may lead to stress-related growth and wisdom in later life, which are hypothesized to lead to the ability to dampen or forstall adverse physiological reactions to stress. Note that these trajectories are not necessarily set in stone; turning points may allow vulnerable individuals to develop resilience resources, or they may create insurmountable problems that lead to kindling processes and greater vulnerability in later life. *Thus, individual differences in developmental trajectories may result in optimal or impaired aging.*

## SUMMARY

Stress is integral to the aging process, on both physiological and psychosocial levels. On a physiological level, vulnerability to stress may both contribute to and reflect both primary and secondary aging processes. To the extent that old age is characterized by difficulty in physiological regulation, older adults may also be more vulnerable to psychosocial stress. However, stress throughout the lifespan affords individuals the ability to develop better self-regulation and emotional maturity, in turn leading to the potential to engage in stress-related growth and to develop wisdom. This development of psychosocial resources under stress may help older adults in forstalling excessive physiologically reactions to stressors in later life, to the extent that they can modulate their appraisal processes to define situations either as less problematic or as less stressful than do younger adults in similar situations. However, depending on the context and psychosocial resources available, stress may also lead to kindling effects, rendering individuals more vulnerable and reactive to stressors in later life.

This synthesis is at best preliminary, and much more empirical work is needed to test various aspects of this model. However, a lifespan developmental approach provides a useful heuristic that may enable an integrated field of health psychology and aging to advance toward the third generation of research.

In particular, the question that was the original impetus for this volume may need to be reframed. Rather than asking, "Are older individuals more or less vulnerable to psychosocial stress?" we need to recognize the individual differences that become accentuated over the life course, and instead ask, "Which older adults have heightened vulnerability to stress in later life, and which are more resilient?" Indeed, redefining successful aging in terms of stress resilience would align psychosocial gerontological research efforts not only with the biogerontologists but also with the growing literature on the development of resilience in early life (e.g., Goldstein & Brooks, 2005). This would allow a true multidisciplinary developmental theory of stress vulnerability and resilience across the lifespan to emerge. After all, as Kurt Lewin said, there is nothing so practical as a good theory.

# REFERENCES

Aldwin, C. M., & Gilmer, D. F. (2004). *Health, illness, and optimal aging: Biological and psychosocial perspectives.* Thousand Oaks, CA: Sage.

Aldwin, C. M., & Levenson, M. R. (2005). Military service and emotional maturation: The Chelsea Pensioners. In K. W. Schaie & G. Elder, Jr. (Eds.), *Historical influences on lives and aging* (pp. 255–281). San Diego: Academic Press.

Aldwin, C. M., Spiro, A., III, Levenson, M. R., & Cupertino, A. P. (2001). Longitudinal findings from the Normative Aging Study: III. Personality, individual health trajectories, and mortality. *Psychology and Aging, 16,* 450–465.

Aldwin, C. M., Spiro, A., III, & Park, C. L. (2006). Health, behavior, and optimal aging: A lifespan developmental perspective. In J. Birren & K. W. Schaie (Eds.), *Handbook of the psychology of aging, sixth edition* (pp. 85–104). San Diego: Academic Press.

Boeninger, D. K., Shiraishi, R. W., Aldwin, C. M., & Spiro, A., III (2006). *Contributions of age, personality, and stressor type to primary stress appraisals: Findings from the Normative Aging Study.* Manuscript under review.

Eisenberg, N., & Zhou, Q. (2000). Regulation from a developmental perspective. *Psychological Inquiry, 11,* 167–171.

Elder, G. H., Jr., & Shanahan, M. J. (2006). The life course and human development. In R. M. Lerner (Ed.), *Handbook of child psychology* (Vol. 1, 6th ed., pp. 665–715). New York: Wiley.

Friedman, M. A., & Brownell, K. D. (1995). Psychological correlates of obesity: Moving on to the next research generation. *Psycholological Bulletin, 117,* 3–20.

Goldstein, S., & Brooks, R. B. (Eds.). (2005). *Handbook of resilience in children.* New York: Kluwer.

Jennings, P. A., Aldwin, C. M., Levenson, M. R., Spiro, A., III, & Mroczek, D. (2006). Combat exposure, perceived benefits of military service, and wisdom in later life: Findings from the Normative Aging Study. *Research on Aging, 28,* 115–124.

Levy, B. R., Slade, M. D., Kunkel, S. R., & Kasl, S. V. (2002). Longevity increased by positive self-perceptions of aging. *Journal of Personality and Social Psychology, 83,* 261–270.

Mroczek, D.K., Spiro, A., III, Griffin, P.W., & Neupert, S. (in press). Social influences on adult personality, self-regulation, and health. In L. Carstensen & K. W. Schaie (Eds.), *Social structure, aging and self-regulation.* New York: Springer.

Pargament, K. I., Koenig, H. G., & Perez, L. M. (2000). The many methods of religious coping: Development and initial validation of the RCOPE. *Journal of Clinical Psychology, 56,* 519–543.

Schulz, R., & Beach, S. (1999). Caregiving as a risk factor for morbidity: The Caregiver Health Effects Study. *Journal of the American Medical Association, 282,* 2215–2260.

Williams, R. B. (2000). Psychological factors, health, and disease: The impact of aging and the life cycle. In S. B. Manuck, R. Jennings, R. S. Rabin, & A. Baum (Eds.), *Behavior, health, and aging* (pp. 135–151). Mahway, NJ: Erlbaum.

# Author Index

425

# Subject Index